Approaching Global Oncology

The win-win model

IOP Series in Global Health and Radiation Oncology

Series editor

Wilfred Ngwa
Dana-Farber/Harvard Cancer Center, University of Massachusetts Lowell, Johns Hopkins University, USA

Editor biography

Wilfred Ngwa is the Director of the Global Health Catalyst, a cross-institutional collaboration initiative launched at Harvard to catalyze high impact collaborations in global health. He currently serves as Adjunct Professor at the University of Massachusetts, as Associate Professor of Radiation Oncology at Johns Hopkins University and as ICTU Distinguished Professor of Public Health. He is a chair of the Lancet Oncology Commission for Sub-Saharan Africa, has published three books on global health and serves on the editorial board of a number journals, including ASCO's *Journal of Global Oncology, Ecancermedicalsciences*, and *Frontiers in Oncology*. He has won many awards from Harvard, the USA National Institutes of Health, and International professional organizations for his innovations and leading work in global health to address disparities in the USA and globally.

Aims and scope

This series includes books in the emerging area of global radiation oncology and its applications in global health. Building on the published book by the series editor entitled *Emerging Models for Global Health in Radiation Oncology*, it will further detail the work being done globally to promote cancer research and awareness, particularly in lower-income countries.

Approaching Global Oncology

The win-win model

Edited by

Ahmed Elzawawy

Clinical Oncology and Nuclear Medicine Department, Faculty of Medicine, Suez Canal University, Ismailia, Egypt and chair of Alsoliman Clinical and Radiation Oncology Center, Port Said, Egypt

Wilfred Ngwa

Dana-Farber/Harvard Cancer Center, University of Massachusetts Lowell, and Johns Hopkins University, USA

IOP Publishing, Bristol, UK

ISBN 978-0-7503-3075-6 (ebook)
ISBN 978-0-7503-3073-2 (print)
ISBN 978-0-7503-3076-3 (myPrint)
ISBN 978-0-7503-3074-9 (mobi)

DOI 10.1088/978-0-7503-3075-6

Version: 20220601

IOP ebooks

British Library Cataloguing-in-Publication Data: A catalogue record for this book is available from the British Library.

Published by IOP Publishing, wholly owned by The Institute of Physics, London

IOP Publishing, Temple Circus, Temple Way, Bristol, BS1 6HG, UK

US Office: IOP Publishing, Inc., 190 North Independence Mall West, Suite 601, Philadelphia, PA 19106, USA

From both editors: this book is dedicated to all who are working to eliminate global cancer health disparities and increase access to cancer care.

From Ahmed Elzawawy:

To my father and my mother, who were very keen to teach me that all human beings were originally one family. To my wife Mona (Dr Mona Fahmy) and daughters Aya and Miriam who supported me; they are eager to see hand-in-hand contributions and partnerships from many in the world, as part of the win-win initiative, in order to be able to serve millions of cancer patients everywhere.

To the souls of my mentor Professor Alain Laugier (Paris, France) and his wife Yvone Werth Laugier, who guided my way in clinical oncology and taught me to find a global scope for my career for many years, from the time when I was a medical postgraduate student and a young clinical oncologist in Paris in the seventies and early eighties until the present.

—Ahmed Elzawawy

From Wilfred Ngwa:

For my dad, John Ngwa, who taught me about hard work and discipline. To my mom, Catherine Befu Ngwa, who wakes up each day thinking about how to help the poor and needy in our communities and inspired my passion for addressing healthcare disparities. To my wife Lydia, my greatest blessing and answered prayer.

—Wil Ngwa

Contents

Part V Perspectives of leading industries of equipment of radiation therapy and informatics systems and the win-win movement

Part VI Examples of initiatives and actions

Preface

To all readers, to all stakeholders in the fields of cancer care around the globe; to clinical oncologists, scientists, international and national cancer care societies and organizations, to industrialists, governments, business persons; investors and leaders in different communities and to all human beings in the world who are concerned with relieving the burden of lack of affordability of better-value cancer care in the world: this book, **'Approaching Global Oncology: The win-win model'**, is not just our book; it is mostly **yours**. We don't claim to have a magic wand, but we present a Win-Win forum based on scientific, practical, classic, and innovative approaches. The Movement and this forum are open for all to share in the same objective, which is focused on how to increase the affordability of better-value cancer care in the upcoming years, starting from now.

When Wilfred Ngwa suggested editing this book and obtained an agreement with the publisher IOP that its title would be 'Approaching global oncology: the win-win model', our idea was to present to the international community how we can contribute together and how different stakeholders in the world can collaborate to approach better access to affordable and good-value global oncology, with scientific approaches and win-win scenarios.

The Win-Win initiative was proposed by Ahmed Elzawawy in December 2007. The Win-Win initiative became a part of the Global Health Catalyst Summit at Harvard Medical School in April, 2016. In 2020, it became the Win-Win Global Health Catalyst Movement (Win-Win GHC), which includes stakeholders at Harvard Medical School, Pennsylvania University, Oxford University (UK), the University of Heidelberg (Germany), Argentina, Tanzania, Egypt, the University of Gothenburg (Sweden), and in collaboration with all organizations, societies, institutes, individuals, experts, and all stakeholders who share the same objective; to narrow the big gap in access to better-value cancer care in the world. Examples of involved organizations are the European Societies of Surgical Oncology, the African Organization for Research and Training in Cancer (AORTIC), Africa—Oxford–Harvard–Hopkins Cancer Research and Clinical Trials Consortium (AFROX-H2 Clinical Trials Network) and the Latin American and Caribbean Society of Medical Oncology (SLACOM). The challenges and the gap are so huge that there is plenty of room for everyone to do a lot.

To be clear, we are mainly focused on increasing clinical oncology care. By clinical oncology services, we mean surgical oncology and clinical oncology (medical and radiation oncology). There are many other respectable international efforts and works on other extremely important aspects of cancer control. To all readers and to all who might be interested in the world: we emphasized the concept that the Win-Win Movement belongs to all. Hence, we state here that this book is yours too! But how did we translate this meaning in editing this book?

One of the growing problems that book publication is facing is that at the moment of reading the first hard copy of a book, the reader finds that some of its parts are already outdated or that there are recently published articles or articles on the internet and in the media that convey newer data or advances!

In this book, for the first time, we will apply what Ahmed Elzawawy proposes as a model for publishing books in the third decade of the twenty-first century, namely a combination of five approaches: (1) hard copy; (2) electronic copy; and (3) in addition, we will receive the feedback, comments, ideas, new information, new achievements, scientific research, and proposals of readers. There are at least two links available that can be used to send feedback http://icedoc.net/feedback.html and http://icedoc.org/feedback.html. (4) In addition to classical references, links to videos and YouTube—such as those of some of the presentations in the win-win sessions of the GHC Summits and GHC webs—are included. (5) This is a new era for book publication, one in which readers will contribute by making progress in the forthcoming years. So, senders may receive replies via emails and via websites as well as by e.g. ecancerforall (previously ecancer4all), http://www.icedoc.org/Books.htm and http://www.icedoc.net/Books.htm. Some of the feedback in Spanish and English will appear in the new website of the Latin American and Caribbean Medical Oncology Society (SLACOM) led by Professor Eduardo Cazap in partnership with the Network of Latin American Cancer Institutes (RINC). That relates to the short-term replies and interactions between contributors. It is what Ahmed Elzawawy describes as **'a living book!'**. (6) For the longer term, the feedback will be filtered, summarized, and edited in special chapters or in the main text in a next edition or a next book.

This edition is a concise book. Most of the chapters are short.

To all readers: you will make the progress of this Movement and of the book. We—the editors—do not claim any credit or glory.

All stakeholders—particularly millions of our human beings, i.e. cancer patients everywhere—will win!

Ahmed Elzawawy
Wilfred Ngwa

Special dedication and acknowledgement

The late Dr Tabaré Vázquez, Past president of the Republic of Uruguay was deceased on 6 December 2020 after his contribution in chapter 7 'Turning impact of COVID-19 on cancer care into positive'. President Tabaré Vázquez, was a radiation and clinical oncologist, known for his great efforts in pioneering tobacco, cancer and non-communicable diseases control measures in Uruguay, the Americas and the world. He was named a Public Health Hero of the Americas by the Pan American Health Organization/World Health Organization (PAHO/WHO) on 21 September 2018 in Washington, D.C., USA[1]. According to the Constitution of the Republic of Uruguay, a president serves only one term for five years. Dr Tabaré Vázquez served as the 39th President of Uruguay from 2005 to 2010. Due to his popularity he was re-elected by his people to be the 41st President of Uruguay from 2015 to 2020.

On behalf of The editors and all contributors in this book, including his friend Professor Eduardo Cazap, Former President of the UICC, President of Latin American and Caribbean society of Medical Oncology (SLACOM) and one of the main leaders of the Global Health Catalyst Win-Win movement, we specially dedicate this work in honor and deepest appreciation of the late Dr Tabaré Vázquez. We ask all readers to continue his great work on cancer control and for the good of humanity.

[1] Video Public Health Hero of the Americas, President Tabaré Vázquez https://youtu.be/PQP2RN0xfzo.

Editor biographies

Ahmed Elzawawy

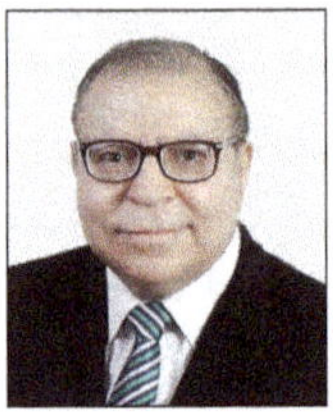

Dr Ahmed Elzawawy is a professor of clinical oncology at Suez Canal University and the chair of the Alsoliman Clinical and Radiation Oncology Center, Port Said, Egypt. His postgraduate studies and the early years of his medical career took place at the Tenon Hospital, Centre René Huguenin, and Institute Curie, Paris, France. He is the president of the International Campaign for the Establishment and Development of Oncology Centers (ICEDOC) and the chair of the Global Health Catalyst win-win scientific initiative (GHC win-win) initiated at Harvard. The latter is a scientific global initiative that aims to increase the affordability of better-value cancer treatment globally. He proposed the win-win scientific initiative in 2007; the initiative then became a main part and concept of the Global Health Catalyst (GHC) program at Harvard in November 2015 and was announced in April 2016. Dr Ahmed Elzawawy chairs the board of directors of Global Oncology University (GO-U). He is also a past president of the African Organization for Research and Training in Cancer (AORTIC) and co-president of the South and East College of Oncology (SEMCO). He contributed to the World Health Organization's (WHO) cancer strategy for the new millennium, its professional cancer education, its global strategy for radiotherapy, and the WHO list of medical device priorities for cancer management. He has contributed to scientific, educational, and consultancy missions for ICEDOC, the Programme of Action for Cancer Therapy (PACT), the International Agency for Atomic Energy (IAEA), and the American Society of Clinical Oncology (ASCO) in Africa, Asia, and East Europe. He has contributed to the ASCO's resource-stratified guidelines advisory group, the European Society of Medical Oncology's Global Policy Committee, and the International Network for Cancer Research and Treatment (INCTR). He is a reviewer for many journals and has contributed to the editorial boards of several journals, e.g. *e*cancer, Lancet Oncology, JCO Global Oncology, the World Journal of Surgical Oncology, and Cambridge Scholars Publishing, UK.

Wil Ngwa

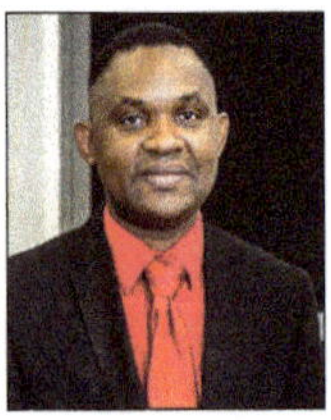

Dr Wil Ngwa is a professor in radiation oncology at Harvard Medical School, and a distinguished professor of public health. He is a founding director of the Global Health Catalyst program launched at the Harvard Radcliffe Institute in 2015, and dedicated to catalyzing high-impact collaborations to reduce global health disparities, especially involving the USA and low- and middle-income country institutions (LMICs). He is also Association Professor of Radiation Oncology at Johns Hopkins University.

He currently chairs the Africa Health and Infrastructure Committee advising the USA Government on global health. He has also been serving as a chair of the Lancet Oncology Commission for Sub-Saharan Africa. Dr Ngwa has held professorships at the University of Massachusetts and Tufts University and guest professorships at the University of Pennsylvania (USA) and the University of Heidelberg (Germany). He is a co-founder (with Prof Ahmed Elzawawy and others) of GO-U, which has an award-winning win-win collaborative educational model that offers everyone access to the same world-class education and training available from professors at the world's best institutions. Dr Ngwa has published four books and over 100 peer-reviewed articles, some of which were published in prestigious journals, such as: Nature, Science, The Lancet, the Proceedings of the National Academy of Sciences (PNAS), and the International Journal of Radiation Oncology, Biology, Physics. He currently chairs a Lancet Oncology Commission and sits on the editorial boards of different journals including ASCO's Journal of Global Oncology and Frontiers in Oncology, and he is the lead editor of the IOP Science series on global health. Dr Ngwa is widely recognized for his strong commitment as a leader in enhancing diversity and inclusion related to minorities in the USA, for building high-impact collaborations between the USA and LMICs to eliminate global oncology disparities, and for working with individuals, institutions, the diaspora, industry, and government to ensure sustainability and impact. Dr Ngwa has won numerous awards, including over 18 prestigious awards/honors in the past six years alone from Harvard, the United States National Institutes of Health, the American Association of Physicists in Medicine, and international professional societies and organizations for his leading efforts in global health and radiation oncology.

Foreword by Sir Professor Muir Gray

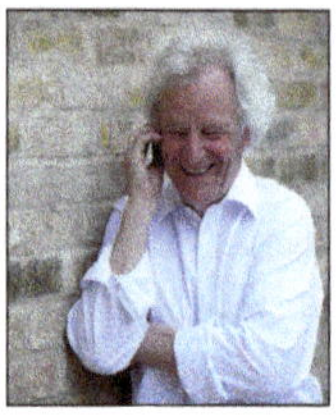

The first healthcare revolution was the public health revolution directed primarily at infectious diseases, such as tuberculosis and cholera. Its success resulted in the population ageing, which increased the incidence of cancer, as did many of the consequences of the first industrial revolution which changed the nature of society, of how we eat, how much we move, and of course, how much we smoke. The second healthcare revolution has been the high-tech revolution, which has resulted in amazing developments, such as chemotherapy and radiotherapy, which have changed cancer from being regarded as a fatal condition to being a long-term condition. However, another revolution is taking place accelerated by the COVID-19 pandemic but evidenced before that, which is the need to take into account the third industrial revolution driven by citizens, knowledge, and the internet; this will revolutionize cancer care in a third and a fourth revolution.

From the perspective of the population, there will be a growing recognition of the need for clinicians to be accountable to that population for the outcomes achieved and the use of resources. In countries committed to universal healthcare, this will include the need to be accountable for equity, namely, ensuring that members of the most deprived subgroups of the population have an outcome as good as that of people in the least deprived groups.

From the perspective of the individual, there will be a need to take into account the fact that the person called the patient now has the opportunity to access the best knowledge available, for example, from the Cochrane Collaboration, remembering that they will also find misleading and wrong information on the internet as well.

A new paradigm is emerging in the way in which knowledge is used. We need evidence—knowledge from research about effectiveness and cost effectiveness; we need information—knowledge from data collection and analysis—about the quality and efficiency of service delivery, but we also need knowledge about value.

We need to think about and discern value from the perspective of the individual. What did they think about the additional chemotherapy course? Did they feel that it added value because they were desperate to see a grandchild born, or did they, in retrospect, feel they should have been given more information about the options and more support in reaching the decision? We also need to think about value from the population perspective: are people with cancer from the most deprived subgroups of the population accessing cancer services as quickly as those from the least deprived subgroups, or is there inequity? What value does the new drug provide when it is routinely prescribed to everyone with a particular cancer and not just to the subgroups of that patient group for which there is strong evidence in the published report? More broadly, we need to ask whether the additional resources invested in treatment, while undoubtedly providing some benefit, would have provided more benefit if they had been invested in services to help people stop smoking. These are value questions for which there is no easy answer. There is no formula that can make this decision. Neither is there a single ethical principle that can be used. There just need to be good, open, and honest debates about value.

So, we need not just more evidence about new chemotherapy, radiotherapy, and surgery; we need a different perspective, and this book provides that perspective very clearly.

Sir Muir Gray, CBE, DSC, MD, FRCPSGals, FECLIP
The Oxford Centre for Triple Value Healthcare https://www.3vh.org/

List of Contributors

Nicholas A Othieno-Abinya
Professor, Medical Oncology, University of Nairobi, Kenya
Leader in win-win movement

Isaac F Adewole
Former Minister of Health, Nigeria
Department of ObGyn, College of Medicine/University College Hospital, University of Ibadan, Nigeria

Victoria Ainsworth
University of Massachusetts Lowell, USA

James Alaro
National Cancer Institute Center for Global Health, USA

Gemma Aldetron
Senior Editor, *Science*

Francisco Alves
Mercurius Health SA, Lisboa, Portugal

Lydia Asana
University of South Florida, Tampa, FL, USA
and GHC

Riccardo Audisio
Editor in Chief, *European Journal of Surgical Oncology*
Professor, Department of Surgery, Institute of Clinical Sciences, Sahlgrenska University Hospital, Göteborg, Sweden
Main leader, win-win movement

Stephen Avery
Professor, University of Pennsylvania
Main leader, win-win movement

Hasin Anupama Azhari
United International University (UIU), Dhaka, Bangladesh
and
Gono Bishwabidyalay (University), Savar Dhak, Bangladesh

I O Morhason-Bello
South Asia Centre for Medical Physics and Cancer Research (SCMPCR), Alo Bhubon Trust (Alo-BT), Dhaka, Bangladesh

Ross Berbeco
Brigham and Women's Hospital, Dana-Farber Cancer Institute
and
Harvard Medical School, Boston, MA USA

Noella Bih
Dana Farber Cancer Institute, University of Massachusetts Lowell, USA
and
win-win movement

Arben Bislimi
Oncology Clinical Center, University Clinical Center of Kosovo, Pristina, Kosovo

Danny Burke
Associate CEO, *e*cancer

Sumera Butt
Shaukat Khanum Memorial Cancer Hospital and Research Center, Pakistan

Eduardo Cazap
Professor, Medical Oncology
Editor in chief, *e*cancer, President, SLACOM
Past President, UICC
Main leader, win-win movement

Julia Sheehy-Chan
Varian Medical Systems, Siemens Healthineers

C Norman Coleman
International Cancer Expert Corps, Washington, DC, USA

David Collingridge
Editor-in-Chief, *The Lancet Oncology*
Publishing Director, *The Lancet Group*
Visiting Professor of Global Oncology, School of Cancer & Pharmaceutical Sciences, King's College London, UK

Vildane Gogu Cmega
Oncology Clinical Center, University Clinical Center of Kosovo, Pristina, Kosovo

Niloy R Datta, MD, DNB, CCST(UK)
Director-Professor & Head, Department of Radiotherapy, Mahatma Gandhi Institute of Medical Sciences, Maharashtra, India

Sneha Datta
Joint FAO/IAEA Division of Nuclear Techniques in Food and Agriculture, Department of Nuclear Sciences and Applications, International Atomic Energy Agency (IAEA), Vienna, Austria

Andres Diaz
GHC, USA

Manjit Dosanjh,
University of Oxford, Oxford, UK
and
CERN, The European Organization for Nuclear Research, Geneva, Switzerland

Ntami Echeng
GHC, USA

Ahmed Elzawawy
Professor and Chair, Alsoliman Clinical Oncology and Radiation Oncology Center, Port Said, Egypt
Clinical Oncology and Nuclear Medicine, Suez Canal University, Ismailia, Egypt and Chair, Board of directors, Global Oncology University (GO-U)
Chair, Win-Win Movement

Lara Finan
Senior Publisher, *e*cancer

Melvin Foote,
Constituency for Africa, USA

Eric Ford, PhD, FAAPM FASTRO
Professor, Director and Vice-Chair of Medical Physics, Department of Radiation Oncology, University of Washington, Seattle, USA

Katie Foxal
Head of Publishing, *e*cancer

Jessica Fricchione
IOP Publishing

Diane Gashumba
Former Minister of Health, Rwanda
Ambassador, win-win movement

Daniel Goncalves
Neopharma Lda., Maputo, Mozambique

Sir Muir Gray
The Oxford Centre for Triple Value Healthcare, Oxford, UK

Saiful M Huq
University of Pittsburgh School of Medicine, USA
Leader in win-win movement

Taofeeq A Ige
Chief Consultant Physicist / RSA / Adjunct Senior Lecturer
University of Abuja, Abuja, Nigeria

Luca Incrocci
Professor, Radiation Oncology, Erasmus MC Cancer Institute Rotterdam, The Netherlands
Ambassador, win-win movement

Omoruyi Credit Irabor
Thomas Jefferson University Hospital / Sidney Kimmel Cancer Center
Philadelphia, PA
and win-win movement

Ilir Ismaili
University Clinic for Radiotherapy and Oncology, Skopje, North Macedonia

Alexander Jenkins
University of Oxford, Oxford, UK

Sayeda Yasmin-Karim
Harvard Medical School, USA
and
GHC, win-win movement

David J Kerr
Professor of Cancer Medicine, Oxford University, UK
Main leader, win-win movement

Krystyna Kiel
Rush University Medical Center, USA

Francine Kouya
Mbingo Baptist Hospital Bamenda, Cameroon

Tibor Kovacs
Jiahui International Hospital, Breast Institute, Shanghai, China

Allison Landman
Deputy Editor, *The Lancet Oncology*

Gilberto Lopez
Editor-in-Chief, *JCO Global Oncology*
Professor Medical Oncology

André Lucas
Radiotherapy Service, Hospital Central de Maputo, Maputo, Mozambique

Alvaro Luongo-Cespedes
National Institute of Cancer (INCA), Uruguay

Suzana Manxhuka-Kërliu
University of Prishtina, Pristina, Kosovo

Kevin Massoudi
Varian Medical Systems, Siemens Healthineers

Shaban Memeti
Institute of Public Health, North Macedonia

Her Royal Highness Princess Dina Mired
Honorary Ambassador of Win-Win Movement
Immediate Past President—Union For International Cancer Control (UICC)

Paul Mobit
Cameroon Oncology Center Douala, Cameroon

Sulma Mohammed
Purdue University, USA

Manar Montasser
Clinical Oncologist, Suez Canal Authority Hospital, Ismailia, Egypt

Michele Moreau
University of Massachusetts Lowell, USA

Elizabeth Charlotte Moser
Chief Scientific Officer, Nanocan Therapeutics Corporation, Princeton, NJ, USA

Romy Mueller
Brigham and Women's Hospital, USA
and win-win movement

Pacifique Mugenzi
Rwanda Cancer Centre, Military Hospital, Kigali, Rwanda

Gazmend Nafezi,
University of Prishtina, University Clinical Center of Kosovo, Pristina, Kosovo

Sara Navarro,
Neopharma Lda., Maputo, Mozambique

Gayatri Narayan
UM-AI LCC, Delaware, USA

Kingsley Ndoh
University of Washington, USA

Habib Nehme
Executive Vice President, Japan Asia Pacific Turkey India Middle East and Africa and Chair of Commercial Board, Elekta

Iracelma Neto
Radiotherapy Service, Hospital Central de Maputo, Maputo, Mozambique

Marielle Ngamije
GHC, USA

Twalib Ngoma
Professor, Muhimbili University of Health and Allied Sciences, United Republic of Tanzania
Past President, AORTIC
and
Main leader, win-win movement

Wilfred Ngwa, PhD
Professor, Radiation Oncology, Dana Farber/Harvard Cancer Center, University of Massachusetts Lowell
and Johns Hopkins University, USA
Director, Harvard Global Health Catalysts Program
Director, win-win movement

Atara Ntekim
University of Ibadan, University College Hospital, Nigeria

Donna O'Brien
International Cancer Expert Corps, Washington, DC, USA

Kyuhak Oh
MD Anderson Cancer Center, Houston, TX
And
University of Washington, Seattle, USA

T A O Oluwasola
Department of ObGyn College of Medicine/University College Hospital, University of Ibadan, Nigeria

Dennis Palmer
Baptist Institute of Health Sciences, Mbingo Baptist Hospital Bamenda, Cameroon

David Pistenmaa
International Cancer Expert Corps, Washington, DC, USA

Miles A Pomper
International Cancer Expert Corps, Washington, DC, USA and Geneva, Switzerland

Ralf Muller-Polyzou
Dipl.-Ing., patent engineer, Head of Business Unit, LAP Laser Applikationen GmbH
PhD candidate Institute of Product and Process Innovation, Leuphana University Lüneburg, Germany

Paul Ruff
Emeritus Professor of Medical Oncology, University of Witwatersrand, Faculty of Health Sciences, Johannesburg, South Africa

Massoud Samiei
Nuclear Energy, International Atomic Energy Agency (IAEA), Vienna, Austria

Bishwambhar Sengupta
Department of Radiation Oncology, University of Washington, Seattle, USA

Fiza Shaukat
Harvard School of Public Health, USA

Mohammad Ullah Shemanto
South Asia Centre for Medical Physics and Cancer Research (SCMPCR), Alo Bhubon Trust (Alo-BT), Dhaka, Bangladesh

Valerie Sinden
Varian Medical Systems, Siemens Healthineers

Felix Sinzabakira
Rwanda Cancer Centre, Military Hospital, Kigali, Rwanda

Catarina Souto
Mercurius Health SA, Lisboa, Portugal

Richard Sullivan
Professor, Chair of Trustees, ecancer Global Foundation, UK

William Swanson
University of Massachusetts Lowell, USA
and win-win movement

Clare Thibodeaux
Vice President, Scientific Affairs, Cures Within Reach, USA

Daivi Rodima-Taylor
Boston university, USA

Ana Ugrinska
University Institute of Positron Emission Tomography, Medical Faculty, UKIM, North Macedonia

Verna Vanderpuye
Korlebu Teaching Hospital, Accra, Ghana

H.E. President, Tabaré Vázquez
Radiation Oncology, H.E. the late Tabaré Vázquez, was the immediate Past President of the Republic of Uruguay and Honorary Ambassador of Win-Win movement

Sara Velha
Radiotherapy Service, Hospital Central de Maputo, Maputo, Mozambique

Andrew Whitman
Siemens Healthineers

Dow Wilson
Former CEO and President, Varian Medical Systems, (Incorporated in Siemens Healthineers)
and
Ambassador, win-win movement

Holger Wirtz
Dipl.-Ing.,Head of Medical Physics, CTO,Lake of Constance Radiation Oncology Center, Strahlentherapie , Singen/ Friedrichshafen, Germany

Jana Wood
PharmD, Dana Farber Cancer Institute, Brigham and Women's Hospital, Boston, MA, USA
University of Veterinary Medicine and Pharmacy in Kosice, Slovakia
and win-win movement

Golam Abu Zakaria
Professor of Clinical Engineering, Anhalt University of Applied Sciences, Koethen, Germany
And
Chairman, South Asia Centre for Medical Physics and Cancer Research (SCMPCR), Bangladesh
Leader in win-win Movement

Bashkim Ziberi
University of Tetova, North Maceodnia, Havard Medical School
Leader in win-win movement

Anthony Zietman MD FRCR FASTRO
Shipley Professor of Radiation Oncology, Massachusetts General Hospital and Harvard Medical School, USA
Editor-in-Chief Emeritus *International Journal of Radiation Oncology Biology Physics*

Keynote by Her Royal Highness Princess Dina Mired

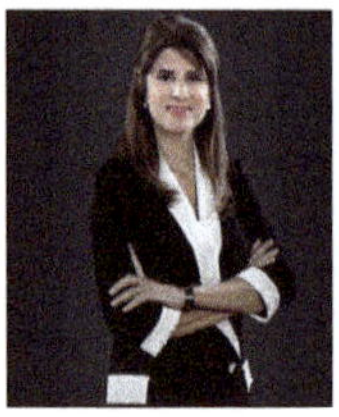

Immediate past president—Union for International Cancer Control
Honorary Ambassador of Harvard Global Health Win-Win Initiative
Patron of the International Society for Pediatric Oncology (SIOP)
Member of the WHO's Expert Group for the Elimination of Cervical Cancer
Special Envoy for NCD's for Vital Strategies
Member of the United Nations University (UNU) High-Level Advisory Committee for the Gender and Health Hub

Keynote speech by HRH Princess Dina Mired

The Harvard GHC Win-Win Initiative Keynote Speech by HRH Princess Dina Mired, President of the Union for International Cancer Control

Link to video: Global Health Catalyst Summit, HRH Princess Dina Mired, president of UICC, 24 May, 2019 at Harvard Medical School, Boston, MA, USA https://www.youtube.com/watch?v=uaUndnUMYmc&feature=youtu.be

Dear friends and colleagues, greetings from Amman.

I would like to thank the Harvard Global Health Catalyst and the Win-Win initiative team for giving me the chance to address you all. Thank you, professor Ahmed Elzawawy and professor Wil Ngwa. And I want to acknowledge here as well Dr Eduardo Cazap, our wonderful past president of UICC.

The world does not need more conferences, it needs more partnerships!

I saw that in one of your conference write-ups, and I could not agree more. With the current global burden of cancer of 18.1 million new cancer cases each year, with 9.6 million mortality, 70% in the developing world, it is very clear that no one single organization has the knowledge, capacity, or the experience to address this heavy global cancer burden alone, which is why it is so important to recognize that we need more and more impactful collaborations and partnerships across all stakeholders, all geographies, and all sectors.

Partnerships are central to the way that the Union for International Cancer Control (UICC) works. In fact, partnership is in our DNA. Our organisation brings together over 1100 members and 51 partners across 177 countries. Many of you are valued members of UICC and have been part and parcel of our work and helped us forge many meaningful collaborations all over the world.

I would like here to highlight a few win-win partnerships that UICC was part of; where these partnerships delivered the objectives, it set out for maximum impact for cancer patients.

The first one: the non-communicable Disease Alliance (NCD) Alliance

The NCD alliance partnership was spearheaded by UICC and resulted in the impactful partnership between the International Heart Federation, the International Diabetic Foundation and the International Union Against Tuberculosis and Lung Disease. This collaborative effort led the NCD community for the first time ever to the political corridors of the UN. In 2011, the NCDs were finally acknowledged at the UN high-level meeting. Thanks to this collaboration, we now have unleashed an extra 2000 organizations worldwide to fight, on behalf of all NCD patients, about the shared cancer and NCD risks, thus, enlarging our community and amplifying our voice of our shared vision of a healthier, non-toxic world. The NCD alliance is truly an example of the power and impact of the global civil society health powerhouses when they join forces and work on a shared goal.

The second example is UICC's global 'treatment for all' advocacy campaign.
'Treatment for all' is the name of an inspiring advocacy initiative run by the UICC. It calls on the worldwide cancer community to join together to advocate and address the global equity gap in access to cancer services. This is a practical campaign tapping into the potential of mentorship partnerships. Each of our civil society 'Country Champions' is paired with a mentor organization, and can access help from our Geneva team, to build and implement a national advocacy campaign to improve access to core cancer services in their country. So far, we have 17 country champions and 14 mentor organizations. This partnership is about global experience in advocacy going local.

The third is the City Cancer Challenge Initiative (CCan)
UICC established the CCAn in 2017. The City Cancer Challenge is a multi-sectoral initiative supporting cities on the ground to take the lead in the design, planning, and implementation of cancer treatment solutions over a two-year period. The UICC developed and incubated the initiative to become its own standalone Foundation 'The City Cancer Challenge Foundation', with its own board, on January 2019. Whilst we all recognize that implementation of cancer control is overwhelming, complex, and requires significant financial resources, it is not all a question of money. A big part of the problem actually stems from the lack of proper governance and management, which results in either duplication of effort (and certainly wastefulness of effort) or scarce resources. So, the CCan model's most important feature is that it prioritizes the setting up of the right managerial architecture on the ground, establishing a truly multi-sectoral city executive team, that has all the influencers of cancer control in that city. The CCan team supports the city team in developing the right governance structure that will help it to become an effective local engine that can deliver the complex long-term solutions of cancer control. This management structure looks into who should sit at the table from the city, the political will that should be present, the voice of the patients that should be represented, and the private sector partners that should be part and parcel of the solution. The City Cancer Challenge team in turn supports the executive team in the city through the managerial steps of assessment of the gaps, priority setting, action plans, and then supporting them into making a costed action plan and through to implementation. And I would like to stress here that it is **one plan** that all work on. Then, once that is finished, then all the members and partners of UICC and CCan, then look at where they can all help fill in the gaps. I have already seen first-hand during my visits to both Ascension and Cali in Colombia, Kumasi in Ghana, the small wins and big wins that were unleashed thanks to this initiative. This partnership model is an example of how a global team can partner with local team as an objective expert facilitator to implement change on the ground in a systemized and sustainable manner.

The fourth partnership model: International Cancer Control partnership (ICCP)
The ICCP was established in 2012. For the first time ever, a group of 31 key international organizations have joined together to coordinate their efforts to support countries in national cancer control plan development and implementation. The ICCP is yet another powerful example of the power of international organizations, whose members were already *individually* working to support country cancer control planning efforts, who then joined forces to work together on global cancer planning to maximize their collective resources and avoid duplication of effort. This ICCP portal is now a practical real solution to a major gap in cancer control planning services for all countries. There are many more examples, such as your win-win initiative, partners in health, and others worldwide. What is important is to draw lessons on how and why these partnerships proved to be impactful. A few insights on what can be learnt from these cited partnership models: for starters, they are real partnerships intent on going for the long haul. They are not 'hit and 'run' partnerships. They have a long-term view to solve long-term problems. This is key. These partnership models understood the untapped power of the 'numerous' as opposed to the 'single'. For many years, our global health community worked in silos. This certainly did not help scale up the global engine to face up to the overwhelming global burden of cancer. We need more partnerships that minimize the disjointedness of efforts or duplication across the global health community, across countries. And within countries, these partnership models were fed up with the usual list of 'what we don't have' in global cancer control, especially in the developing world. They understood that we all know what needs to be done, but that we now have to just get in there and get it done. So many of these partnerships started to tick the boxes of the 'have nots' and turn them into 'haves', one item at a time. In addition, some partnerships did not only focus on technical expertise, but also recognized the importance of helping to build capacity in management expertise and infrastructure. These partnerships utilized the value of mentorship. We have so many successful organizations across the cancer control spectrum whose expertise was not tapped. There is nothing more powerful than a 'show and tell' model. The value of real mentorship cannot be overemphasized.

As the saying goes: 'If you don't dip your feet in the water, you won't know if you are missing something'. So, 'putting boots on the ground' is another. Time to escalate the efforts by walking the walk of cancer patients and health workers in a low and middle-income country to understand the reality on the ground and the particular obstacles or the untapped opportunities. Last but not least, the value of performing the 'catalyst/facilitator' role, just like your organization. Corporations benefit from expert objective facilitators who help them solve problems with fresh objective eyes, why should the health communities not benefit from this valuable role and insight? There are many more learnings and many more challenges. But there is one undisputed fact: there is no time to waste! Millions of cancer patients look to us for deliverance. We owe them to organise ourselves better and build a powerful coalition of many impactful partnerships to face off with cancer!

Thank you.

Book summary

At present, around two-thirds of cancer patients worldwide have no access to any sound cancer care. Across the world, there is an increasing gap between the required cancer care services and what is available, particularly in low- and middle-income countries (LMICs). We stress the concept that the challenge of producing real and remarkable increases in the affordability of better-value cancer care is huge. So, all stakeholders and readers in the world are considered as potential contributors in this book and partners in the Win-Win Movement.

We do not claim that this book contains the whole wisdom or final solutions for the challenges posed by the question of the affordability of better-value cancer care worldwide. But we hope that it will be like a spark and a call for all to act to make a real breakthrough for the affordability of cancer care for millions more human beings in the 3rd decade of the 21st century.

Who are the target readers?

The target readers are numerous and include professionals in all modalities of care and the sciences, international organizations, members of cancer societies, all stakeholders of cancer care in the world, health industries, governments, health and cancer care policy makers, investors, NGOs, media, and interested members of the public everywhere.

When Wilfred Ngwa agreed to edit this book, we were faced with two choices: the easiest was the classical and ordinary one, to edit the usual written texts of the authors. The second is what we applied here, according to our new model 'a living book', as explained here. All readers are invited to interact and to send back their feedback and ideas to make more progress in the upcoming years. Therefore, it is not a cold book for passive reading. It is, as indicated in the term coined by Elzawawy, 'a living book'—a new model for book publications in the 3rd decade of the 21st century. All readers are invited to send feedback.

So, in some chapters of this book, we edit hot proceedings of publication panels with links to access videos. Also, other examples of this model occur where we include the edited texts and links to videos of the contributions of Her Royal Princess Dina Mired and Mr Dow Wilson (Immediate Past President of Varian Medical Systems, which has become a Siemens Healthineers company during editing).

The notion of 'a living book' as proposed by Ahmed Elzawawy:

In recent years, the classic publication of books has faced the problem that at the time of reading, i.e. after publication, some of the information has become outdated. Readers can find a lot of new published articles, as well as electronic learning, and new sorts of media offering the opportunity for interaction.

Ahmed Elzawawy coined the term 'a living book' as a proposal for a new era of book publication in the 3rd decade of the 21st century. It contains:

(a) Hard and/or electronic book copies

(b) Links to websites, videos, and YouTube videos that accompany some of the chapters and are provided in the references. This trend was started some years ago in publications.

(c) Links to locations where readers can interact after publication and send their feedback, suggestions, and ideas.

For example, in this book, there are two links that can be used to send emails containing reader feedback: http://icedoc.net/feedback.html and http://icedoc.org/feedback.html

More links will follow.

(d) The relevant feedback will be shared and discussed with the book contributors and experts.

(e) Summaries of relevant feedback and news will appear on our different websites, for example: Global Health Catalyst, ecancerforall (previously ecancer4all), http://www.icedoc.org/Books.htm and http://www.icedoc.net/Books.htm. Some of the feedback in Spanish and English will appear in the new win-win section of the website of the Latin American and Caribbean Medical Oncology Society (SLACOM) led by Professor Eduardo Cazap in partnership with the Network of Latin American Cancer Institutes (RINC).

(f) The last point is optional. As the objective of this book is huge and will need years of continuous global effort, we intend to apply this option this time. Further progress and summaries of filtered reader feedback will constitute special parts in the next editions or books by the editors or those who will follow. Hence, it will be a sort of series of living books for this decade, and all readers will have the opportunity to interact and to contribute.

Background

In 2007, the win-win initiative was proposed by Professor Ahmed Elzawawy as an initiative of ICEDOC's Experts in Cancer without Borders (ICEDOC is the International Campaign for Establishment and Development of Oncology Centers) http://www.icedoc.org/winwin.htm and http://www.icedoc.net/winwin.htm. It aims to increase the affordability of better-value cancer treatment in the world by exploring scientific approaches. This could also help to save the international health economy from collapse and benefit the businesses of pharmaceutical companies and the manufacturers of radiotherapy machines and medical devices without ruining a country or individuals' economies. It is a win-win initiative. All stakeholders would win, in particular, the millions of cancer patients and their families in the underserved regions in the world. No one would lose. The win-win initiative became a part of the Global Health Catalyst Summit at Harvard Medical School in April 2016. The initiative has grown into a Win-Win Global Health Catalyst Movement (Win-Win GHC). The director is Wilfred Ngwa, and it includes different institutions and countries such as: Harvard Medical School, Pennsylvania University, Johns Hopkins University, Oxford University (UK), the University of Heidelberg, the University of Gothenburg (Sweden), Argentina, Tanzania, Egypt and is in collaboration with different organizations, societies, institutes, individual experts, and all stakeholders who share the same objective: to narrow the big gap in access to better-value cancer care in the world. Examples of organizations are the European Societies of Surgical Oncology, the African Organization for Research and Training in Cancer (AORTIC), the Africa—Oxford–Harvard–Hopkins Cancer Research and Clinical Trials Consortium (AFROX-H2 Clinical Trials Network), and the Latin American and Caribbean Society of Medical Oncology (SLACOM).

There are two main wings of the win-win initiative: the first wing is 'to explore scientific approaches to increasing the affordability of better-value cancer care'. By 'scientific studies', we mean not only medical, clinical, pharmacological, medical physics, and innovative health industry and informatics studies, but also economic research, business model studies and all aspects that contribute to the increase of access to better-value cancer care globally. This includes ways to deliver cost-effective, resource-sparing cancer treatment and, more importantly, how to secure better-value cancer control and care for cancer patients in the world by exploring scientific approaches and win-win scenarios. **The second wing** of the win-win initiative was proposed in November 2015 and announced on 29 April, 2016 during the Global Health Catalyst Summit at Harvard Medical School, Boston, USA. This wing relates to catalytic action and professional advice to enormously increase the rate of establishment of clinical oncology services in the world, starting with the most difficult challenges in Africa. The progress of the win-win initiative now includes the participation of distinguished leaders and faculty from different institutes and experts in the USA, Europe, Africa, South America, and South Asia, and different organizations and societies in the world to form the Movement of the Win-Win Global Health Catalyst. This movement involves professional consultants, expert volunteer catalysts, and young catalysts. We are not a funding body. We are not competing with, or replacing, any society, organization, body, governmental or private effort, or individual; rather, we are complementing and completing. We are facilitators, catalysts, and a forum for all. We encourage all to do, to connect, and to communicate with each other and to collaborate or to cooperate with **one focus, which is how to increase the affordability of better-value cancer care for the underserved patients in the world**. There is a great need for the Win-Win forum and Movement. The majority of human beings with cancer in the world have no access to any sort of evidence-based cancer treatment.

This book is divided into seven parts.

Part I: The role of the Win-Win Movement in increasing the affordability of better-value cancer care in the world

Despite the different efforts, bodies, publications, conferences, and declarations in the world, the gap between what is required from cancer care and what is available has widened in the last decade. If we continue in the same way, this situation will be aggravated in upcoming years because of the skyrocketing increase in the cost of cancer care and the increase of cancer prevalence in the world. The question that we pose and face in the Win-Win Movement and this book is: shall the world, with all its bodies, continue in the same approach and path towards a known fate? Or will it respond to the challenge through scientific approaches and realistic and smart win-win scenarios focused on a global increase of the affordability of value and patient-centered cancer care for millions of underserved humans in the world? This challenge is global, with variable intensity in different parts of the world. It faces affluent countries, but offers a much more tragic picture in low- and middle-income countries (LMICs). Why do we stress win-win scenarios? In fact, without a consideration of the realistic incentives and interests of stakeholders, the objective of increasing the affordability of cancer care for millions more humans in the underserved regions in the real world will remain just talk or unrealized plans in the new decade. After the crisis of COVID-19, it should be expected that the problem of the affordability of cancer care will be exacerbated. Then, in the constructive spirit of the Win-Win Movement, we will give hints about how to turn the expected negative impacts of COVID-19 (and its sequels, which will last for years) on different aspects of cancer care into positives! This aim of this book is not to repeat details about what has already been mentioned, which is that roughly two-thirds of cancer patients have no access to cancer care. In Africa, it is known that between only 5%–7% of cancer patients have access to radiotherapy. The Win-Win Movement is a unique movement that focuses on: (1) the exploration of scientific avenues to increase better-value cancer care in the world and the consideration of different win-win scenarios that consider the interests of different stakeholders; (2) catalytic actions and consultations to increase the number and quality of clinical oncology services in the world, regardless of who will do the work; (3) advocating for a global campaign that should be dynamic, removed from bureaucracy, with a free flow of ideas; (4) being an open forum for all and not replacing any other forums or claiming top presidency or credit; (5) avoiding rivalries, but catalysing actions and encouraging all to do. (6) The saying 'it belongs to all' is not a slogan, but it is essential in win-win tactics.

The challenges are huge and increasing. This is far beyond the capabilities of any of the existing bodies, organizations, and societies. The Win-Win Movement is a forum for all and not one more competing organization. We are not challenging any, but calling for partnerships and collaboration. We are not searching for credit or glory, but what is essential to the Win-Win Movement is to see more chances of the affordability of better-value cancer to humans in the world, regardless of who the doers are. If we cite the example of clinical oncology facilities, then the lack of radiotherapy units could be roughly estimated as at least 10 000–12 000 units for the years 2021–2030. If we add this number to the usual growth and replacement, it would be much more than what all health industries are producing. With an effective campaign and the smart mobilization of resources, there would be ample spaces in the world for the products of all health industries. We tackle the essential points about the potential increase of mobilization of different resources for cancer care services in LMICs. This also includes the necessity for the increased mobilization of win-win resources coming from the diaspora.

According to the notions of the win-win modification of the blue ocean strategy that Ahmed Elzawawy proposes in this book, we stress that there is no need to cause wasteful competition among different players and between different health industries. Some of what we cite in this book relates to the need for a cost-effective, non-bureaucratic, and dynamic international campaign (and not the current dispersed efforts), a more effective mobilization of resources, multiple business models, and education and training collaborations. A cost-effective international campaign for clinical oncology care does not mean—at all—any interference with entities or the independence and internal policy of contributors or claiming any credit in place of the doers of any achievement. By 'clinical oncology care' we mean all the modalities of cancer treatment: surgery, radiation therapy, systemic medical treatment, and also diagnosis. One of the reasons that we list radiation clinical oncology units as one of the priorities in this initiative is that these are falsely attributed as being the most expensive or difficult to establish, hence, the shortage is huge. However, clinical radiation oncology is at the heart of cancer care and it could improve healthcare and the heathcare system. We recommend—as far as possible—that radiation clinical oncology units should contain, in addition to radiotherapy facilities, services for at least outpatient cancer drug therapy as a start, clinical pharmacy, data and information and communications technology (ICT), and a nucleus of scientific reporting and research connected with the international scientific community and North–South and South–South technical and scientific collaborations (mostly via ICT). It is mandatory that the clinical radiation oncology units should be connected, working and following patients alongside surgeons and referring physicians in the community. We imply that the clinical oncology care unit would not be on the top of a mountain or as an isolated island from general healthcare, but it would be in continuous connection, exchanging information with district hospitals, community health units and professionals in the community who have major roles in first seeing patients, referring patients at the appropriate time, and following up patients after clinical oncology treatment. In the Win-Win Movement, we dislike the terms 'obstacle' and 'barrier', and we prefer the terms 'opportunity' and 'solution'. So, even for the healers in some communities, every smart effort should be made in order for willing healers to contribute as a sort of partner. They would be instructed when and where to refer patients if there are suspicious symptoms and to contribute in following up patients and sending information about patients. This could even be done verbally by phone or mobile or by any type of contact. Attention should be paid to keeping the prestige of all healthcare providers as partners in overall care in front of their customers. This is not at all easy to apply in the real world; it needs a lot to make it happen, but is there another way to make a big breakthrough? Moreover, all would win!

Investment in cancer care is a very beneficial investment in the health system in general. Hence, in this way, and contrary to popular belief, in this book and according to distinguished scientists and to the notions of the Win-Win Movement, we recommend that increasing the amount and quality of clinical oncology care would improve the healthcare system in general. Hence, it should not come at the end of the list of healthcare priorities. We previously stated (Elzawawy *et al* 2008) that 'Early detection and earlier diagnosis of cancer would be frustrating to both the patients and health professionals if there is no affordable and accessible good cancer treatment for the detected cases'. (The reference and other relevant sources are cited in this book). It is frustrating to think about conducting some sorts of specific cancer management in rural health units or provisional clinical diagnosis by the family doctor in a district hospital if there is no possibility of referral to value-based modern clinical oncology care. In all campaigns directed towards the public, policy makers, and stakeholders in different communities, there should be simple but convincing messages that include the above points, among others. In order to make scientific progress focused on how to increase the affordability of better-value cancer care in the world, we need changes in the strategies and policies of scientific publications and dissemination to back this progress. The leaders of the Win-Win publication and dissemination Movement are themselves among the distinguished editors-in-chief and editors of the scientific cancer care publications in the world. This is the topic of the chapter: 'Publications and dissemination'.

List of contributors

(in alphabetical order):

- Gemma Alderton (senior editor, Science)
- Riccardo Audisio (editor-in-chief, European Journal of Surgical Oncology)
- Danny Burke (associate CEO, *e*cancer)
- Eduardo Cazap (editor-in-Chief, *e*cancer and co-editor of 'The Oncologist', global section and past president, UICC)
- David Collingridge (editor-in-chief, The Lancet Oncology)
- Jessica Fricchione (senior commissioning editor, IOP Publishing)
- David Kerr (past president ESMO, editor emeritus Annals of Oncology, founding editor, Journal of Global Oncology, Professor of Cancer Medicine, Oxford, UK)
- Gilberto Lopez (editor-in-chief, Journal of Global Oncology (issued by ASCO))
- Anthony Zietman (editor-in-chief, the 'red journal', the International Journal of Radiation Oncology, Biology, Physics)
- and Ahmed Elzawawy: initiator and coordinator

Part II: Global health catalyst win-win channels

Part II covers major channels for catalyzing win-win collaborations for high-impact global oncology in which both high-income and low-income country stakeholders win. It covers catalytic actions and volunteer consultancies, such as the Corps of Catalysts, advisers, and Win-Win consultants https://www.globalhealthcatalyst.com/, including many participants in high- and low-income countries collaborating in global oncology. It also covers scientific researches and publications (including this book). Some examples of publications and videos can be found at www.icedoc.net/winwin.htm and https://www.globalhealthcatalyst.com/. Third, it covers the Global Oncology University (GO-U) www.ghcuniversity.org, ecancerforall (previously ecancer4all) for online education plus onsite training, and the Africa—Oxford–Harvard–Hopkins Cancer Research and Clinical Trials Consortium (AFROX-H2 Clinical Trials Network) led by Prof. David Kerr, Oxford, UK. It also includes win-win ambassadors, such as Her Royal Highness Princess Dina Mired, President of the UICC and honorary ambassador of the Win-Win Movement. Part II also covers professional ambassadors, including distinguished professionals such as Professor Luca Incrocci, Radiation Oncologist, Erasmus MC Cancer Institute, Rotterdam, Netherlands and board of the faculty of Win-Win. This part ends with coverage of the Global Health Catalyst Summits. These summits are not just meetings, but summits to elaborate collaborations, partnerships, and catalytic actions to empower the realization of the objective of the Global Health Catalyst for the sake of humans with cancer with a special emphasis on Africa. Five annual summits have been held at Harvard Medical School since 2015.

Part III: Scientific resource-saving and better-value cancer treatment approaches: the first wing of the Win-Win initiative

The chapters of the 3rd part are about scientific approaches to resource saving and increasing the affordability of better-value clinical oncology care. Ahmed Elzawawy presents an overview and many examples of published studies for scientific explorations to lower the cost of systemic cancer drug therapy and radiotherapy without compromising the outcome for patients. Known experts Niloy Datta, Sneha Datta, and Massoud Sameie, the founder and former head of the Programme of Action for Cancer Therapy (PACT), the International Atomic Energy Agency (IAEA) then present strategies for how to maximize radiotherapy access in 88 countries among the LMICs in the world. Wilfred Ngwa and colleagues then present an award-winning experimental approach that uses a relatively low-cost combination of one fraction of radiotherapy with immunotherapy smart biomaterial or drone. This leads to a response due to the abscopal effect of radiotherapy on metastatic disease. James Alaro, programme director at the National Cancer Institute Center for Global Health, USA then presents the topic of research collaboration to advance cancer care and prevention in LMICs. Eric Ford presents the invention of a ring-based compensator that lowers the cost of intensity-modulated radiation therapy (IMRT). Ross Berbeco presents an innovative method to lower the cost and time of the work needed for image guidance in radiation therapy (IGRT) by low-dose megavoltage imaging cone beam computed tomography (MV-CBCT). Ahmed Elzawawy further presents an account of repurposing/repositioning drugs and their importance for cancer. Because new drug development is inadequate, there is a great need for drug repositioning, in particular, in oncology. Using scientific approaches, old, approved drugs, alone or in combination, could have new indications and therefore offer less expensive treatments. Clare Thibodeaux, director of scientific affairs at 'Cure Within Reach' presents some of the opportunities offered by the 'Cure Within Reach' foundation for repurposing research in LMICs. Finally, Elizabeth Charlotte Moser, former vice president of Elekta and founder of UM-AI Coordinator Research and colleagues present a personalized complication risk prediction tool that could improve breast cancer care coordination management using artificial intelligence-driven predictive toolkits.

Part IV: Mobilization of different resources, win-win collaborations and partnerships

The chapters of the fourth part are about the mobilization of resources, win-win collaborations, and partnerships. Among the topics in this part are collaboration and partnership with the Latin American and Caribbean Society of Medical Oncology, the European Society of Surgical Oncology, *e*cancer medical science, the Institute of South Asia for Medical Physics and Cancer Research, collaborations with governments, and perspectives from the North Macedonian and Balkan region.

Part V: Leading health industry perspectives on radiation therapy equipment, informatics systems, and the Win-Win Movement: Varian Medical Systems (Incorporated with Siemens Healthineers) and Elekta

In the chapters of the fifth part, one of the most important visions in the real world is the perspectives of leading industries in clinical oncology. Mr Dow Wilson, Immediate Past President and CEO of Varian Medical Systems (incorporated into Siemens Healthineers during the editing of this book) presents the chapter 'Increasing value-based radiotherapy in LMICs and sustainable partnerships for Africa'. The vision of Elekta Medical Systems 'We are here till cancer is not!' is presented by Mr Habib Nehme, a vice president of Elekta for emerging markets.

Part VI: Examples of Initiatives and actions

In the chapters of the 6th part, as we always say in the Win-Win Movement, we 'Don't keep talking about barriers and obstacles (that we all know about)', but instead, we focus on **opportunities, positive actions, and solutions**. Hence, the chapters present examples of initiatives and deeds: the International Cancer Expert Corps (ICEC) present a 'Win^{n}' model solution with the exponential growth necessary for global cancer care. Perspectives are presented from Georgia, Tanzania, Uruguay, Angola, Mozambique, Cameroon, Rwanda, Kenya, Pakistan, and Nigeria.

Part VII: Future directions

In the 7th part of this book, the Editors present a brief view of future directions. This includes anticipated progress on the different topics covered in the book and the Win-Win Movement. The progress of the Global Oncology University, which will be a main theme of the upcoming Global Health Catalyst summits, is covered. Upcoming summits will be hybrid meetings.

All are invited to contribute to this living book by sending their feedback, ideas and suggestions. We call upon partners, international cancer care bodies, societies, organizations, industries, and all stakeholders to crystallize and develop an effective international campaign to make a remarkable and historical increase in value-based clinical oncology units in the world in the next ten years. Moreover, the progress and new ideas that serve as the objective of this book will be one of the main themes of the next annual GHC summits.

As usual, at the end, we stress once more that Win-Win is a movement and a forum; therefore, the independence, the credit, the achievement, the internal policy of all contributors, individual experts, organizations, and societies are respected.

We look forward to your feedback and suggestions. Please send them to:

http://icedoc.net/feedback.html and http://icedoc.org/feedback.html

(More links will follow).

Ahmed Elzawawy and Wilfred Ngwa

On behalf of the Win-Win Global Health Catalyst Movement

Part I

The Win-Win Movement to increase affordability of better value cancer care in the world

Chapter 1

The needs, the objective, the notions, and approaches of the win-win movement

Ahmed Elzawawy

To meet the global need to make a big reduction in the gap between the demand and the available cancer treatment in the world, we advocate for a global win-win scientific movement and an international campaign that focuses on realizing an enormous global increase in the affordability of better-value cancer care to serve millions of underserved cancer patients who either have no access to care (for example, the majority of cancer patients in low-income countries), or patients who have variable levels of accessibility (but with a high financial and social burden on a considerable proportion of patients) in high-income countries (HICs) and middle-income countries (MICs). All stakeholders and parties, including health systems, health industries, and increasing numbers of millions of underserved human beings with cancer in the world would win. All that is cited by the win-win initiative and in this book is based on and inspired by previous and current efforts, data, publications, and the plans of all international organizations, societies, academia, and enterprises. All that we advocate for will have no value if there is no contribution from many and the gradual joining of different parties in a global win-win scientific movement and international win-win campaign. We do not see any acceptable alternative for the next ten years, particularly in the light of the sequences of the COVID-19 pandemic. Otherwise, the gap between the demand and the supply of cancer treatment will increase, and there will be an increasing risk of economic health difficulties for all, i.e. governments, health systems in rich and less affluent countries, markets of health industries, and, most important, cancer patients everywhere. The notions of the Win-Win Movement imply that it is not challenging or replacing any other organizations, but it is a forum for all and it belongs to all.

doi:10.1088/978-0-7503-3075-6ch1

1.1 Worldwide needs—in particular, those of low- and middle-income countries

Worldwide, an estimated 19.3 million new cancer cases and almost 10.0 million cancer deaths occurred in 2020. Cancer is the second leading cause of death globally and about 1 in 6 deaths is due to cancer. Approximately 70% of the deaths caused by cancer occur in low- and middle-income countries (LMICs) in Africa, Asia, and central and South America [1, 2]. The burden of cancer incidence and prevalence is growing. It is expected that there will be an increase of the incidence of cancer to 22 million new cases annually by 2030, and 81% of the new cases and almost 88% of the mortality will occur in LMICs. The predicted global burden will be about 29.4 million new cancer cases by 2040, and the greatest increase (around 67%) will be in LMICs. It is known that the prevalence of cancer and the eventual need for care will be greater than these numbers. The increase is based on demographic changes. Based on population growth and aging, the global *cancer* burden will grow to 29.4 million *cases* annually in 2040 (assuming global *rates* remain unchanged from those in 2018) [1–5].

With the skyrocketing rise in the cost of new cancer drugs and cancer treatments that are not commensurate with the improvement in outcomes, and with the increase of the global prevalence of cancer and the economic impact of following the COVID-19 pandemic, it is expected that the problem of affordability of economically sustainable value-based cancer treatment will be aggravated in the upcoming years of the 3rd decade of the 21st century. The World Health Organization's (WHO's) cancer report, 2020 [4], indicated that it is apparent that the objective of the United Nations (UN) declarations for the reduction of one-third of mortality due to noncommunicable diseases by 2030 will not be achieved, mostly due to the delay of global progress in the management of cancer [4].

The situation of all modalities of cancer care in Africa is the most tragic. Only around 5%–7% of cancer patients in Africa have access to radiotherapy. That is why the reader will notice that in the Win-Win Movement [6, 7] and also in this book, we pay more attention from the outset to the shortage of affordable clinical oncological care in LMICs, in particular, in Africa. Regarding the shortage of cancer care, Africa is the most challenging part of the globe, but our scope is global and includes all the underserved patients in the world.

Despite all the respectable efforts, declarations, plans, and good agendas of governments, international organizations such as the UN, the WHO, the International Atomic Energy Agency (IAEA) and the big non-governmental cancer societies and unions in the world, it is known that the gap between the required and the available cancer drug therapy and radiotherapy services increased in the last decade in LMICs [4, 8–11]. In 2020, the WHO issued another excellent report on cancer to promote the setting of priorities and wise investment, which was one more needed call for cancer care for all [4]. This is in addition to the previous good reports and declarations of the last three decades.

To give realistic examples of the outcome of the last ten years using published data, an article published in 2015, whose contributors were from different affiliations, including the IAEA, replied to the critical question: 'Have we made progress regarding global access to radiotherapy services in the past decade?' They stated that, in the year 2015, there remains a deficit of more than 7 000 radiotherapy machines in the world, and that the gap between the required number and the supply is rising, particularly in LMICs [8]. Radiation therapy is estimated to be required in around 50% of newly diagnosed cases. Of the 137 LMICs, 51 (37.3%) currently lack radiotherapy facilities. The remaining 86 LMICs have 5084 tele-radiotherapy units, with a gap of around 7741 units. Thus, the mean access to radiotherapy is 33%. By the year 2030, the gap will be more than 12 000 tele-radiotherapy units [9–11]. Surely, the issue is not to install a machine and be done with it; the good functioning and sustainability of the machine should be assured by adequate infrastructure and, most importantly, by professional human support.

Another example is that in May 2013, the WHO declared and published a global action plan for the prevention and control of noncommunicable diseases for the next seven years, i.e. up to the year 2020. This plan implied an 80% worldwide affordability of essential cancer drugs and medicine by the year 2020 [12]. Today, in 2021, one year after the end of the seven-year plan, it is very clear that there is no sign that there is remarkable progress in achieving this objective. We confirm our complete appreciation of all these reports and declarations. In fact, many of the contributors of this book and the author of this chapter contributed to most of them [13, 14]. But the question we pose on different occasions in this book is: 'Should the world continue with the same approaches in the upcoming years, without any addition or modification, despite the expected worsening of the huge gap between the demand and the available reasonable cancer care in the world?' [15].

1.2 Some striking examples of the lack of access to cancer care in high-income countries!

When mention 'the underserved cancer patients', we mean globally, despite the fact that this mostly affects patients in LMICs. It is not a crime to be a European or USA citizen and miss the efforts to confront the challenge of affordability of value-based cancer treatment. Surely, the problem of being underserved in Europe or the USA does not occur with the same high magnitude as in LMICs; as believed in 2017, however, less than 30% of the LMICs reported available treatment services compared with more than 90% of the HICs [14].

1.2.1 Europe: more than 25% of cancer patients in Europe do not receive the radiotherapy they need!

Although around 50% of all European cancer patients have an indication for radiotherapy at least once in the course of their disease, more than a quarter of cancer patients in Europe do not receive the radiotherapy they need. The major reasons for the suboptimal access to radiotherapy are a lack of equipment and a shortage of trained personnel. However, there are variations within European countries in available radiotherapy devices, in personnel per inhabitant or per cancer patient requiring radiotherapy, and in workload [17].

1.2.2 The United States

There are dire predictions for the future of US cancer care if there are no changes. Clifton Leaf stated in his book 'The Truth in Small Doses' that we are losing the war on cancer in the United Sates [18]. The American Society of Clinical Oncology (ASCO) describes dire directions for the future of cancer care in the US. For many Americans, access to quality cancer care in the future could be threatened, as the growing demand for services exceeds the supply of oncologists and the cost of care continues to climb. It was expected that the annual associated costs would rise from $104 billion in 2006 to more than $173 billion by 2020 and it is estimated that these costs will escalate in the upcoming years [19].

1.2.3 The expected increase in the shortage of oncologists in the USA

It is expected that the number of new cancer cases in the United States will increase by 42% by 2025. At the same time, cancer is slated to become the leading cause of death during the same period; the number of oncologists will increase by only 28%, which will lead to a projected shortage of 1487 oncologists. Although demands on oncologists will increase, many practices will be under great financial pressure. Dr Hudis stated that the expected shortage of 1487 oncologists will present challenges for patients seeking quality cancer care. An average oncologist sees around 300 new patients each year. This means that the enormous number of nearly 450,000 new patients could have difficulty getting the care they need in 2025 [19]. Among the factors contributing to the expected shortfall are the aging oncology workforce and impending retirements. Currently, one of every five oncologists is more than 64 years old; in 2008, the number of oncologists older than 64 exceeded the number younger than 40 for the first time. The projection is that this gap will widen. Dr Caroline Hendricks reported that although oncologists feel a great deal of satisfaction in taking care of cancer patients, increased workloads and administrative burdens have driven them to make decisions to leave their practices, reduce the number of hours spent in clinical care, or retire before the age of 65 [19, 20].

1.2.4 Geographic concentrations and practice closures in the USA

Dr Hendricks pointed out that one in five Americans live in rural areas, but only one in 33 oncologists are practicing in these regions. According to the report, almost 97% of physicians practice in urban areas or urban clusters. More than 70% of the counties analyzed had no medical oncologists at all. In addition, community-based oncology practices were struggling financially and were under threat of closure, according to the Community Oncology Alliance (COA) [19, 20]. Moreover, Dr Hendricks expressed frustration that she might not be able to continue because of financial pressures. A typical community cancer clinic must spend a considerable amount of money to purchase chemotherapeutic agents that are then administered on an outpatient basis. Drug costs are set by the pharmaceutical manufacturer and the wholesale distributor. She stated that the oncologists purchase the drugs on credit and then they challenge; hence, Dr Hendricks indicated the necessity for a new business model that does not depend on purchasing and billing for oncology drugs. In fact, the ASCO reports that in small towns and rural communities, smaller practices are the backbone of cancer care. They allow patients to receive high-quality personalized treatment close to home [19, 20].

1.2.5 Other examples

Another example of disparities and demographic variations in the access to treatment is that high rates of cervical cancer are also seen in medically-underserved areas because of a lack of screening and skilled providers. One such area is the Rio Grande Valley of south Texas, located along the Texan–Mexican border, where the cervical cancer incidence and mortality rates are 30% higher than in the rest of Texas [21, 22].

1.2.6 Rising costs of cancer care in the US

According to ASCO, ever-increasing costs have created a pressing need to improve the value of patient care. The American Association for Cancer Research (AACR) reported that *cancer care costs* in the *United States are projected to exceed* $245 *billion by* 2030. The mounting costs are multifactorial, affected by the price of new therapies and a healthcare system that unfortunately allows incentives to be given for the use of tests, treatments, and services that can be unnecessary, ineffective, or avoidable. The emergence of novel therapies, which are sometimes administered in combination regimens, is helping to push costs up. Many of these new therapeutics cost up to $100,000 for a course of treatment, making them prohibitively expensive, even for patients with insurance [19, 23]. The authors of a recent published study stated that, unlike the sales of refrigerators or cars, the new cancer drug prices bear no relationship to their performance or cost of production. Drug companies benefit in the world of oncology because even drugs with a marginal therapeutic advantage can find a market position or be promoted as breakthroughs, despite a lack of considerable—or even meaningful—clinical benefit [24]. A study in the Journal of the American Medical Association demonstrated that 67% of FDA drug approvals between 2008 and 2012 were made for a surrogate endpoint and that 86% of these either failed to show or had an unknown benefit for overall survival [25]. Cetuximab was promoted in non-small-cell lung cancer, when its addition to chemotherapy resulted in a 1.2-month overall survival benefit and it came with a US $80,000 price tag for an 18-week course of treatment [26]. Adjuvant neratinib, added to early breast cancer therapy, improved two-year disease-free survival by only 2.3% at an extra cost of US $125,000 per year and was accompanied by alarming rates of severe diarrhea and eventual treatment attrition [27]. Unreasonable price setting of this nature is unsustainable and affects cancer care and its practice and the health economy [24]; eventually, it will challenge the future sales of newer cancer drugs for millions of patients.

1.2.7 The Win-Win Initiative: the problem is the game and not the players!

As can be seen from the sections presented above in this chapter, the objective and goal should be focused on the point of affordability of better-value cancer care and lessening the burden and suffering of increasing numbers of millions more human beings with cancer and their families in the world before the end of this decade. Let us ask some questions in more specific words: over this decade, out of the 12,000 additional required radiotherapy units, how many thousands of services will be realized in the real world? Surely, we mean not only the installation of machines, but also good functioning and a sustainable clinical oncology service. Hence, from now until the end of the decade, how many million cancer patients will be able to get affordable, value-based systemic cancer therapy out of the 70% of cancer patients who, if we continue with the same achievement as before, would not have access to reasonable treatment?

And surely, the question about access to good surgery is essential.

We do not see the above questions as high dams or barriers, but as potential opportunities for a global win-win. The world could achieve at least a good part—if not most—of the objective. It is a huge arena for scientific works and progress. From the perspective of industry and business, there are huge potential markets. Moreover, there are benefits for all stakeholders. All would win and *most of all, the underserved cancer patients and their families.*

Shall the world continue with the same approaches used and declared previously? Or we should add more tactics?

All of the published international and organizational efforts and the reports and declarations of the key players are excellent and they are the basis of any step forward and of any hoped-for success. However, we clearly state that the problem is not in the players, but in the game [28, 29]. Hence, agreeing with what Fineberg stated in [30], we should be globally open to additional tactics and to using every science-based tool in our inbox and outbox to achieve the goal.

1.2.8 Why win-win?

The notions of the Win-Win Initiative consider the interests and incentives of all stakeholders: cancer care professionals, governments, health industries, economies, communities' welfare, all organizations and societies in the field, and above all, cancer patients everywhere. All stakeholders should be informed and convinced that their incentives will not be jeopardized. Otherwise, they will become parts of the problem and not key players or contributors to the solution.

For example, we agree with all that is published about the need for the revision and repair of payment systems for oncologists and all professional cancer care providers in every country. Without this, the notions of the win-win, reports, plans, agenda, declarations will be just aborted wishes or statistically negligible achievements in comparison to the increasing huge lack of reasonable—or should we say, value-based—cancer care in the world. There is a risk that the whole system in some countries—including affluent countries—may even shrink!

Most of the founders, leaders, and ambassadors of the Win-Win Movement either chair or have long-distinguished activities and roles in international organizations, societies, and academia. One of the tactics and notions of the Global Health Win-Win Initiative is that we are not one more challenging organization, and not replacing any, but we are a global Win-Win Movement and a forum open to all who share the same objective, so that they can contribute and lead.

One of the major tactics is to advocate for global scientific exploration, and eventually publications, for an unlimited number of scientific studies to examine the total cost of saving cancer care while not compromising—in any way—the outcome for patients. Some chapters in this book show examples of these studies.

As it is a win-win transparent movement, and as health industries are major and indispensable stakeholders, there are chapters written by the CEO and president of Varian Medical Systems (incorporated into Siemens Healthineers) and the vice president of Elekta. Catalytic actions, collaboration, and cooperation are tactics that have been adopted in different parts of the world (the reader will find chapters containing fruitful examples in this book). The win-win movement advocates for the tactics of flexibility of thought and a free stream of ideas and suggestions that could assist in achieving the objective, a global win-win campaign and forum as a sort of 'brain trust' (a term that first introduced by Franklin D Roosevelt) [28], a cost-effective campaign for the global mobilization of resources and the promotion of needs, the feasible realization of cancer care services in the world, the win-win modified blue-ocean strategy, and the 'Fourth Way' [31, 32]

We have occasion here to quote what Renzo Canetta, vice president of oncology global clinical research at Bristol Myers Squibb, stated in the USA National Cancer Policy Forum: 'there is a need to recognize that we are all in the same type of boat, even though we may have different employers. Progress is going to come only from collaboration and not from creating little parishes where we fight against each other on petty issues' [33].

1.2.9 A brief summary of the history of the Win-Win Movement

At present, the Win-Win Movement is the short title of the 'Global Health Catalyst Win-Win Movement'.

In December 2007, **The Win-Win Scientific initiative** was proposed by Professor Ahmed Elzawawy as an initiative of ICEDOC's Experts in Cancer without Borders. It is an initiative that aims to increase the affordability of better-value cancer treatment for cancer in the world by exploring scientific avenues and catalytic actions within win-win scenarios. All stakeholders—particularly cancer patients and their families—could win. This could also lead to flourishing pharmaceutical companies, manufacturers of radiotherapy equipment, and medical devices without devastating a countries' or individuals' economies. It is a Win-Win Initiative. No one would lose! [28, 34, 35].

On 29 April, 2016, The Win-Win Initiative joined Harvard Global Health Catalyst Program and became one of its activities (it was agreed by Wil Ngwa on November, 2015). Hence, in the period from April 2016 until the end of May 2019, the title of the initiative was the 'Harvard Global Health Catalyst Win-Win Initiative'.

From May 2019 until the present, with the growth and progress of the Win-Win Initiative with increasing faculty from different institutes and experts in the USA, Europe, Africa, South America, and South Asia, different organizations, and societies in the world, the initiative became the **Global Health Catalyst Win-Win Movement (Short title: The Win-Win Movement)** [6].

1.2.10 Who we are

Initially, the initiative was composed of professional consultants as well as volunteer catalysts. However, it is open to all stakeholders who share the same objective, regardless of the gains, interests, or incentives of partners and stakeholders in the real world. It is a win-win. We are not a funding body. We are not competing with, or replacing, any society, organization, body, governmental, individual, or private effort, but rather, we are facilitators and a forum for all. We complement and complete. We encourage all to do, to connect, and to communicate with each other and to collaborate or to cooperate with one focus, which is how to increase the affordability of better-value cancer care for the underserved patients in the world. There is a great need for the Win-Win forum and movement. The majority of human beings with cancer in the world have no access to any sort of scientific cancer treatment.

1.3 The two wings of the Win-Win Initiative

The first wing: relates to scientific exploration and win-win approaches to increase the affordability of *better-value* cancer care in the world. By 'scientific studies', we mean not only medical, clinical, pharmacological, cost-effective, resource-sparing cancer treatments, medical physics, and innovation in the health industry and informatics studies, but also economic research, business-model studies, and all aspects that contribute to increasing access to better-value cancer care in the world via exploring scientific approaches and win-win scenarios.

The second wing: relates to catalytic action and professional advice to enormously increase the rate of establishment of clinical oncology services for the underserved patient regions in the world, with a special stress on starting with the most difficult challenges, e.g. those in Africa. By 'clinical oncology care', we mean all the modalities of cancer treatment and diagnosis, with an emphasis on clinical radiation oncology services. This wing was proposed in November 2015 and announced on 29 April 2016 during the Harvard Global Health Catalyst Summit

1.4 The main channels and means of the Win-Win Movement

As detailed in the different parts of this book, the channels of the Win-Win Movement include:

I. Catalyst actions and volunteer consultations: the Corps of Catalysts, advisers, and Win-Win consultants. See https://www.globalhealthcatalyst.com/.
II. Scientific research and publications (including this book). Some examples of publications and videos can be found at www.icedoc.net/winwin.htm and https://www.globalhealthcatalyst.com/.

III. The Global Oncology University (GO-U), www.ghcuniversity.org, and ecancerforall (previously ecancer4all) for online education plus onsite training.
IV. The Africa–Oxford–Harvard–Johns Hopkins Cancer Research Consortium (AFROX-H) led by Professor David Kerr, Oxford, UK.
V. The Win-Win Ambassadors:

(a) The keynote of Her Royal Highness Princess Dina Mired, president of UICC and honorary ambassador of the Win-Win movement
(b) Professional ambassadors, as exemplified by a distinguished professional, Professor Luca Incrocci, Radiation Oncologist, Erasmus MC Cancer Institute, Rotterdam, Netherlands and board of the faculty of Win-Win.

The young catalysts' Win-Win Collaboration.
The Global Health Catalyst Summits. These are not just meetings, but summits to elaborate collaborations, partnerships, and catalytic actions to empower the realization of the objective of the Global Health Catalyst Win-Win movement for the sake of humans with cancer, with a special stress on Africa. Five annual summits have been held at Harvard Medical School since 2015.

1.5 What do we mean by scientific studies and approaches?

(See the summary in section 1.3., 'The first wing').

1.6 Why do we focus on cancer treatment and particularly on clinical oncology care (Global Oncology Catalysts)?

It is agreed that a balanced approach should be taken towards global cancer control. It should encompass an increase in awareness, early detection, diagnosis, cancer treatment (using different modalities), surgery, radiotherapy, cancer systemic drug therapy, supportive and palliative care, follow-up, and relevant research and studies [36]. However, to be focused, the Win-Win Movement is dedicated to the field of oncology and places more emphasis on increasing the affordability of better-value clinical oncology services for underserved cancer patients. We previously stated that campaigns and festivals to increasing the awareness of the early detection and earlier diagnosis of cancer would be not logical and would be frustrating for both patients and health professionals if there were no affordable, accessible, dignified, and good cancer treatment for the cancers detected in patients. That would be like torture! A cancer patient is not a number in statistics or registers, but a human being with a beating heart, expectations, and hopes for themselves and their families. Some of the reasons for his/her fear of being diagnosed with cancer are the fear of the lack of accessible treatment, and the financial and social burden if treatment is available [31, 37]. One of the strongest calls for patients to seek early diagnosis is associating with the experiences of others in the same community who obtained affordable value-based care that respected their financial and social dignity [37, 38].

There are several active efforts, organizations, programs, and plans that work in different fields of cancer control. So, there is no harm if we concentrate on cancer treatment. In the Win-Win Initiative, we focus more on the important fields of cancer treatment; in particular, most of our experts are in disciplines related to cancer treatment, with an emphasis on the affordability of better-value clinical oncology care.

The definition of oncology, according to Merriam-Webster is: 'A branch of medicine concerned with the prevention, diagnosis, treatment, and study of cancer' [39]. In practice, clinical oncology relates to any type of cancer treatment that is not surgical, including radiotherapy and systemic therapies. Most cancer patients have more than one method of treatment, such as surgery to remove a tumor, followed by radiotherapy and/or systemic therapy. Because of that, the Win-Win Movement considers the main three modalities of cancer treatment: surgery, radiotherapy, and cancer drug systemic therapy for clinical oncology. The curability of those cancer patients who are cured is attributed to surgery (around 49%), radiotherapy (around 40%) and systemic therapy (around 11%) [40]. **Clinical radiation oncology** services are cost-effective, despite the expensive cost of installing a unit, but a unit will serve in treating patients for at least ten years. This is in contrast to systemic cancer drugs that have skyrocketed in price [11, 35].

1.7 Will focusing on cancer treatment have positive or negative impact on health systems?

Contrary to belief, improving access to, and the value of, cancer treatment would be beneficial in enhancing health systems and programs [33]. Hence, it should be considered as one of the top priorities in both affluent and less affluent countries.

1.8 Why global?

1.8.1 What do we mean by 'global'? What do we mean by 'global' in the term 'global oncology'?

In everyday language, 'global' means worldwide, international, universal, total, overall, and large scale. Nothing indicates that it means only parts of the world. So, contrary to the wide misuse of the expression 'global', we affirm here that there is nothing in the term 'global oncology' that means that it is for LMICs only [41, 42].

The Win-Win movement is directed to the undeserved cancer patients and regions, wherever they are in the whole world even for those in affluent countries who may struggle to afford treatment. If we have more focus on the access to cancer care in LMICs, it is not entirely exclusive. The vast majority of the underserved cancer patients are in the LMICs and the magnitude of shortage in care is much higher. Moreover, the population in LMICs represents the majority in the world. The win-win model for approaching global oncology implies confronting the challenges of cancer care with a realistic, broad scope and deep studies in different communities in the whole real world [41, 42]. Otherwise, it would be called 'oncology in LMICs'. This could be a good term, but it is not exactly 'global oncology'. Doesn't that notion seem logical for global oncology?

1.8.2 Is it global or globalization?

It is global. We admit that sometimes, there is confusion between the objectives and meanings of two different terms: 'global' and 'globalization' do not mean the same thing. However, it worth noting that despite the controversies about globalization, particularly its economic impacts, as David Kerr [43] stated, we can perceive only one side of globalization that could be positive, which is about the convergence of interests. If we apply this to global oncology, then we look at cancer patients, wherever they are in the world, to drive science and medicine forward to meet their real needs.

1.8.3 In the Win-Win Movement, LMICs are parts of the global solutions and not only the challenge

Despite all the present challenges of conducting massive and valid scientific works, more effort should be made so that LMICs can be parts of the international scientific solutions—and not only part of the burden of the severe lack affordability of cancer care. This does not mean that one solution fits all, but rather that cancer care should not only be customized according to biological markers but also to the conditions of the community where patients live, their expectations, hopes, and cultures [35].

1.9 What are the potential remarkable gains for affluent countries, health industries, and LMICs of being global in the win-win scientific approaches?

We pose this question for joint consideration: are the following worth the funding of stakeholders, scientific communities, and industry and partnerships with the locals: (a) large-scale human capacity building, (b) scientific collaboration with local teams, (c) and conducting valid scientific cancer research and clinical trials in LMICs?

It is anticipated that these would reduce the total time required to conduct clinical trials, may reduce their costs, and enrich the scientific aspects with more variability; they could pave the way for the justified use and sale of newer drugs in more cost-effective ways in markets that are at risk of shrinking in the upcoming years like those of middle-income and some affluent countries. Such an approach would assist companies to streamline the development of new drugs, technologies, and equipment, while for the locals, conducting scientific research would be a source of income for oncologists, other members of the team, and scientists and a way to achieve the affordability of some expensive drugs, technologies, and investigations, and the most important element: it would improve patient care and develop more local experience in research and publications that would be used afterwards—outside the initial trials or studies—in searching for more ways of increasing access to better-value cancer care that fits their communities and patients [44, 45].

Affluent countries and international organizations should consider investing in global scientific campaigns and large-scale global capacity building and not assisting by expressing pity, via charitable donations, or very limited endeavors for years. Institutes in affluent countries could consider qualified or trained staff or scientists in LMICs as paid co-researchers or co-workers, but living and working in their countries to conduct research that concerns their country's problems. Some of the scientific outcome of this research could contribute to better care for some problems in the affluent country. It is a win-win [41, 42].

Information and communications technology (ICT) and artificial intelligence (AI) will facilitate more working together overseas in the next ten years. Moreover, this approach will increase the human capacity for research in affluent countries and prevent brain drain to the West with its demographic consequences and cultural changes, particularly in Europe. Meanwhile, for LMICs, it would be a smart way to make local scientific progress, obtain better-value cancer care, contribute to international advancement, and prevent brain drain; hence, staff in LMICS would not be isolated from scientific advances and from colleagues everywhere. Moreover, they would be well paid while they are in their home countries [29, 35, 41, 42]. The collaboration of affluent countries should not only take the form of financial support, but preferably win-win support, a durable assistance, and partnerships with rich countries, organizations, or pharmaceutical companies in the form of technical support for the local human capacity building needed for cancer care and research, including cancer care providers, laboratory staff, research coordinators, data managers, ICT, assistance with obtaining local funds or international grants, knowing how to collaborate in international work while they are in their LMICs, the financial management of research, the ethical considerations of research, and then assistance in editing for international publications and implementation [46].

We anticipate that this global movement and win-win partnership would give science, global cancer care, health economies, and health industries big jumps forward. All would win, the HICs and LMICS and above all, cancer patients and the human community. The notion of 'reverse innovation', as described in a Harvard Business review by Govindarajan and Trimble, is that affluent countries can create far from home and win everywhere. Hence, it could be pivotal for HICs as well as for LMICs [47]. Lord Nigel Crisp described a new vision for global health in the 21st century based on our rights and accountabilities as citizens in a world so interconnected and so interdependent, hence instead of talking about international development, we should tackle co-development and agree that rich countries can learn from poorer ones as well as the other way around [48]. Accordingly, we see that win-win scenarios could flourish in a pragmatic and useful way among all parties.

Finally, as we described before, this is a win-win global oncology movement with a message of scientific cooperation based on evidence, the logical working of the brain, and a love for humanity and the good side of human beings, wherever they are on our planet [35]

1.10 Affordable cancer treatment

There is no value in all the achieved and forthcoming scientific progress, inventions, new technologies, treatments, books, publications, guidelines, conferences, and organizations if that progress in treatment is not affordable for most human beings with cancer. No need to repeat that the majority of cancer patients in LMICs in the world have no available, reasonable cancer treatment, and if it were available, it would be unaffordable or only affordable with many difficulties and high financial toxicity.

As stated on many occasions, the objective of all stakeholders should be an enormous increase of the affordability of better-value cancer care for underserved patients.

In the global Win-Win movement, we extend the term 'affordability' to the whole meaning of the word 'underserved patients' in the real world. Hence, it is not only for the majority of patients in the LMICs; we also we include millions of cancer patients in HICs and some in MICs who are only able to get their prescribed treatments with a considerable financial and social burden [42, 49].

1.10.1 ASCO's second national cancer opinion survey [50]

The ASCO's Second National Cancer opinion survey in 2018 sounded a note of high alarm. It was conducted between July 10 and August 10, 2018, among 4,038 U.S. adults aged 18 and older, including 152 people who have or had cancer. An oversample of 849 adults with cancer was added to have a large enough sample size to draw conclusions about the population of people with cancer, bringing the total number of adults with cancer surveyed to 1,001.

If faced with a cancer diagnosis, 57% of Americans say they would be most concerned about either the financial impact on their families or about paying for treatment. Surprisingly, this comes before the fear of death and that of pain and suffering.

Among caregivers responsible for paying for cancer care, nearly three in four (74%) say they are concerned about affording it.

More than six in ten caregivers (61%) say they or another relative have taken an extreme step to help to pay for their loved one's care, including dipping into savings accounts (35%), working extra hours (23%), taking an early withdrawal from a retirement account or college fund (14%), postponing retirement (14%), taking out a second mortgage or another type of loan (13%), taking on an additional job (13%), or selling family inheritances (9%).

The astonishing sequel is that that four in ten Americans (40%) are convinced that alternative therapy may cure cancer better than expensive evidenced cancer treatment. This belief persists despite research showing that patients who use alternative therapies instead of standard cancer treatments have much higher mortality rates. This means that searches for scientific cancer treatments, professional oncologists, hospitals, clinics, and the use of health industry products are facing increasingly high challenges that until now have not been well considered.

The well-known information about the tragic situation of the affordability of cancer care in LMICs and the touching increased difficulties of affordability in the USA is enough for us to call for:

> The realization of an enormous increase in the *affordability* of better-value cancer care along with physical, social, and financial *dignity* for cancer patients in the world.

It is easy to say, but it needs a lot to do be realized in the next ten years. Doesn't this deserve global action to realize this objective, starting from now, rather than speaking or reporting about it?

There is a clear need for all global stakeholders to coordinate their actions in an orchestra in which all have their importance—as a global effective win-win campaign. All would win!

1.11 Better value

After 40 years of uncertainty and money spent on quality studies, there is insufficient evidence about whether or how the quality of healthcare has actually improved. Robert Brook, a pioneer quality expert, declared in 2010 [51] :

> The end of the quality movement and long live improving value!

The notions of the third and the start of the fourth revolutions in science and health have become evident. The third and fourth industrial revolutions will transform the healthcare of rich and poor countries alike [52].

In the last 50 years, terms such as effectiveness, efficiency, cost-effectiveness, quality, and safety were the dominant words in the fields of healthcare.

Value is not measured by the quality of the process of care used. Despite the fact that quality measurement, the process of its measurement, and its improvement were considered to be of extreme importance, in terms of value, these were considered to be tactics and not as objectives in themselves. Also, in terms of value, they are not substitutes for measuring outcomes and costs.

The notions of the third industrial revolution have become evident, and its implementation is growing, while the first implementations of the fourth revolution in science and health have begun. Both the third and fourth industrial revolutions will transform the healthcare of rich and poor countries alike.

The third revolution in healthcare implies the use of knowledge and informatics to obtain better outcomes centered around the customers, i.e. the patients. Hence, it implies the use of the new term 'value'.

In 2013, Sir Muir Gray and David Kerr stated that 'value' will be the predominant term for the upcoming years. It will not make the previous terms extinct, but will embrace them [54].

Value depends on results, not inputs. Value in healthcare is measured by patient-centered outcomes achieved versus total cost, not by the volume of services delivered. Shifting the focus from volume to value is a central challenge in the third revolution of healthcare. [53, 54]

Every effort should be made to reduce the gap between cancer care outcomes and requirements. According to the notion of the win-win movement, the number of cancer services should not be counted as a final objective, but the affordability of better-value cancer treatment and care [29, 44].

If we are going to succeed in achieving affordable cancer care and an affordable healthcare system, we have to focus on the total costs [35] and not on the price of a drug or a device or a technology per se. Fineberg stressed that the crisis we have reached in healthcare in the USA necessitates finding out how to provide value with better outcomes and reduced costs. There is no point in thinking about lowering costs if you do not simultaneously consider maintaining and improving the quality of care. We have to think about both [30, 33].

Economic measures, such as cost reduction without regard to the outcomes achieved, are dangerous and self-defeating, leading to false savings and potentially limiting effective care [53].

1.11.1 A note about the four industrial revolutions

1.11.1.1 The first revolution was based on common sense

It was common sense that led to the invention of spinning and weaving machines [55] and it was common sense that led to the separation of water from sewage, long before scientists discovered the bacteria that caused typhoid and cholera [56].

1.11.1.2 The second industrial revolution

The second industrial revolution was driven by science, e.g. chemists, engineers, and physicists, who developed not only planes and plastics but also chemotherapy, linear accelerators, and positron emission tomography (PET) scanning. The second healthcare revolution led to dramatic improvements in the effectiveness of care. However, the following five problems remain incompletely solved; hence, further scientific advances are needed:

(a) Unwarranted variation in quality and outcome
(b) Harm to patients
(c) Waste and failure to maximize value
(d) Health inequalities and inequities
(e) Failure to prevent disease

1.11.1.3 The third industrial revolution

The third industrial revolution is transforming every service and industry; its drivers are knowledge, the World Wide Web (the internet), and citizens. It implies that health services:

(a) have the patient at their center
(b) are safer and more effective
(c) produce greater value from the resources invested

The objective of the Win-Win Initiative coexists with the third industrial revolution 'to get affordable, evidence-based, better-value cancer care to patients in the world'.

To put it simply: value is the relationship between the outcome and the resources used. In turn, in terms of the outcome, the determination of the quality and safety of the intervention or service are important elements [54].

1.11.1.4 The fourth industrial revolution

The fourth industrial revolution has already started its implementation and thoughts for further progress: robots and artificial intelligence, nanotechnology, and quantum computing with technologies and trends such as the internet of things (IoT) and virtual reality (VR) are changing the way modern people live and work.

The fourth revolution will be beneficial to the Win-Win Movement as we advocate for all possible scientific explorations to serve the cause of increasing the affordability of value-based cancer care.

1.11.2 Defining value by its opposite—waste

There is now a broader definition of waste, which derives from the methods and culture of Japanese industry, in particular from Toyota. What the Japanese call 'muda' means waste. Hence, any activity in a process that consumes resources without adding value for the customer is a waste [57, 58]. In healthcare, just six examples of waste categories in the USA are:

(a) overtreatment
(b) failures of care coordination
(c) failures in the execution of care processes
(d) administrative complexity
(e) pricing failures
(f) fraud and abuse

The actual total waste may be far greater than 20% of the total healthcare expenditure in the USA [59].

1.11.3 Examples of value frameworks [60]

Value frameworks in cancer care are a beginning and not the solution. Peter Bach, MD, director of the Center for Health Policy and Outcomes at the Memorial Sloan Kettering Cancer Center, New York City, designed the 'drug abacus'. It is a tool that may help to determine a more appropriate price for a specific medicine, based on what experts feel are the possible components of a drug's value.

The Institute for Clinical and Economic Review (ICER), an independent, non-profit, research-based organization, released a 'value assessment framework' that is composed of a clinical care value assessment, a health system value assessment, cost modeling, and expert input.

The National Comprehensive Cancer Network (NCCN) issued its 'NCCN evidence blocks', which uses 'blocks' to visually represent five key value measures: efficacy, safety, quality of evidence, consistency of evidence, and affordability in order to provide important information about specific recommendations found in the NCCN guidelines.

ASCO has introduced its 'value framework', which defines value as a measure of clinical benefit, toxicity, and cost.

The European Society for Medical Oncology (ESMO) has issued its 'magnitude of clinical benefit scale', which seeks to 'stratify' a drug's clinically meaningful benefit and includes measures of efficacy (i.e. survival) as well as the prognosis of the condition and the toxicity of the drug.

1.11.4 Triple-value healthcare (3V)

The Oxford Centre for Triple Value Healthcare is a program that supports health systems to achieve optimal outcomes for populations and individuals given the resources available. Their mission is to support health systems to improve their triple value (population, technical, and personal) through the dissemination of knowledge, a learning and skills development program, and deploying solutions, thereby supporting health systems to measurably improve outcomes and make better use of resources [61, 62].

1.11.5 Could there be resistance to adopting values and measures that save the resources of a country and individuals?

—Yes!

One of the causes for this is resistance to change in any form, but it is not the main reason.

Conflicts of interest are an important element. As we stated on several occasions, we are with all who support the need to repair the system of payment of healthcare providers and related posts, including administrative positions [31, 32, 44].

In the real world, it is a fact that there are different degrees of corruption at all levels and in different countries. Hence, this has a much more catastrophic impact on healthcare affordability when it occurs in countries with limited or middle incomes.

This is not a theoretical description; we know of in-depth examples in certain countries. For example, in an LMIC, where, despite the fact that it was explained to the highest health authorities and leaders of health insurance that they were wasting some billions of US dollars, they insisted they were adhering to a quality system; while, at the same time, there were many uncertainties about the real wellness of the health system, the achieved outcomes, and the lack of cost-effectiveness studies before new installations or demolishments took place accompanied by many bureaucratic papers. The reason for this is clear: it is due to unlawful incentives.

We emphasize that our role is never to police and never to interfere in any internal affairs of any country.

The notions of the Win-Win Movement imply that we cooperate in a broad global campaign to promote and convince—smartly—all parties, that with scientific value-based research and implementation, all would win and the whole health system would be saved from collapse.

It is as, we say, ‘smartly and not hardly’.

1.11.6 Could high-value cancer care keep costs down? Yes, it is possible! [62, 63]

It is possible to both deliver high-value cancer care and keep costs in check. In a survey of seven US oncology practices, researchers noted several elements that were associated with high-quality, low-cost care.

The elements that set high-value practices apart from average-value ones included the following [62, 63]:

- Taking a more conservative approach to diagnostic testing;
- Early discussion with patients about the limitations and goals of cancer care;
- Early involvement of palliative care;
- Allowing staff to practice at the highest level of their license and competence; and
- Having smaller units of care delivery affiliated with a larger healthcare system

Finally to all parties, stakeholders, and readers; this could be a historic time to lessen the suffering and the physical, financial, social, psychological, and humanitarian burden of millions of cancer patients who have no affordable cancer treatment or have a considerable fear of the burden of cancer care affordability in some high-income countries.

'Knowing is not enough; we must apply. Willing is not enough; we must do.......' —Goethe

All feedback, ideas, and suggestions focused on how to increase the affordability of better-value cancer care ***are welcome and will be diffused to all.***

Please free to send them using:

http://icedoc.net/feedback.html

http://icedoc.org/feedback.html

Replies will be sent via email or via website, e.g.: www.ecancerforall, http://www.icedoc.org/Books.htm, or http://www.icedoc.net/Books.htm.

Notes from the author:

Once again, I do not deny that despite a humanitarian motivation toward all the human beings on the globe, regardless of their nationality, color, or ideology, all the proposals for global tactics that we advocate for are based on scientific explorations of win-win scientific approaches that consider the lawful incentives of all in the real world.

We would be very satisfied if our readers said something like: 'You didn't invent anything. What you presented here is in accordance with logic and sense. Parts of what is written here align with what we published, said, did, or are planning to do.' This is because it would mean that this book and the Win-Win Movement really belong to all.

In addition to all the contributors to this book and the leaders of the Win-Win Movement, with whom we share the notions, endeavors, and inspiration of many published works and initiatives, I have had the opportunity to work, to communicate, and develop the common notions of the Win-Win Movement with many others over the years. Here are examples of names, all of whom have distinguished positions and long honorable biographies that the reader can find easily:

— My mentor and professor, Alain Laugier and the late Mme Yvonne Verth Laugier, Paris, France. They inspired me in many ways since I was student in medical school in the mid-seventies, then during my postgraduate years and some years of my career in Paris, France in the eighties. Until last year, they were following what we are doing in developing the Win-Win Movement.

Then, in an arbitrary order, as we see all of the following as very precious contributors:

— Ian Magrath, founder and president of the International Network for Cancer Treatment and Research, Melissa Adde, Mark Lodge, and all the team at INCTR.

— Julie Gralow, chief medical officer, ASCO, and colleagues in the ASCO Stratified Resources Advisory Group
— Mary Gospodarowicz, Rebecca Wong, Danielle Rodin, David A Jaffray, Felicia M Knaul, Rifat Atun, Cary Adams, Michael B Barton, Michael Baumann, Yolande Lievens, Tracey Y M Lui, Julie Torode, Jacob Van Dyk, Bhadrasain Vikram and all colleagues in the Global Task Force on Radiotherapy for Cancer Control (GTFRCC), Union for International Cancer Control (UICC) and Global Impact of Radiotherapy in Oncology (GIRO).
— Douglas Pyle, Vanessa Eaton, Vanessa Sarchet, and all the team of ASCO International. An example of ASCO hosting an international working meeting for developing the Win-Win Movement took place on Saturday 30 May 2009, at Orlando, FL, USA, during the ASCO 2009 Conference http://www.icedoc.org/Docs/Minutes_Win-Win_30_May,09_F2.pdf.
— All colleagues and collaborators in the African Organization for Research and Training in Cancer (AORTIC).
— Martine Piccart, Alexendru Enui, Rosa Giuliani, Gouri Bhattacharyya, Andre Ilbawi, Gracemarie Bricalli, James Cleary, Martina Galotti, Malvika Yvas, and all my colleagues in the team at ESMO and the ESMO Global Policy Committee.
— Masoud Samei, R. Camacho, who were in PACT, the International Atomic Energy Agency (IAEA), and my colleague Eduardo Rosenblatt.
— Joe Harford, for his constructive discussion, advice, and support during the years of his direction of NCI, International Programs,USA.
— Ben Anderson and the team of the Breast Health Global Initiative. Sandra Distelhorst supported the choice of the term 'win-win' for such an initiative in 2007.
— Gabriel Hortobagyi (who, in particular, advised on the term 'economically sustainable' in the title of one of the first win-win articles and in communications)
https://www.ncbi.nlm.nih.gov/pmc/articles/PMC2931034/
— Pamela Haylock, USA, with her deep views and support along for the ICEDOC and the Win-win development from 1999 until the present; Daniel Rutz, USA with his constructive contribution since 1999; the precious views of Lowel Schnipper, USA; and Heinz Zwierzina, Austria.

It is not just an acknowledgment, but it is fair to say that this chapter, book, and the win-win initiative are the outcomes of the views, work, face-to-face and virtual discussions, publications, and contributions of many.

Finally, to all readers, stakeholders, and key players: this book belongs to all of you. We are looking forward to global implementation in the real world with your partnership, ideas, and leading contributions.

— Ahmed Elzawawy

References and further reading

[1] Sung H, Ferlay J and Siegel R L *et al* 2021 Global cancer statistics 2020: GLOBOCAN estimates of incidence and mortality worldwide for 36 cancers in 185 countries *CA Cancer J. Clin.* **71** 209–49

[2] World Health Organization (WHO) 2021 The World Health Organization Cancer fact sheets 3 March 2021

[3] Ferlay J, Ervik M, Lam F, Colombet M, Mery L and Piñeros M *et al* 2019 *Global Cancer Observatory: Cancer Tomorrow.* (Lyon: International Agency for Research on Cancer)

[4] World Health Organization (WHO) 2020 WHO report on cancer: setting priorities, investing wisely and providing care for all *World Health Organization* https://apps.who.int/iris/handle/10665/330745 License: CC BY-NC-SA 3.0 IGO

[5] Wild C P, Weiderpass E and Stewart B W (ed) 2020 World Cancer Report: cancer research for cancer prevention *World Cancer Reports.* (Lyon: International Agency for Research on Cancer)

[6] Global health catalyst win-win movement www.icedoc.net/winwin.htm and www.icedoc.org/winwin.htm

[7] Elzawawy A 2019 Keynote speech in May 24, 2019, GHC Summit at Harvard Medical School, Boston, MA, USA https://youtube.com/watch?v=gPnfjY8kqyA

[8] Zubizarreta E H, Fidarova E and Healy B *et al* 2015 Need for radiotherapy in low and middle income countries—the silent crisis continues *Clin. Oncol. (R Coll. Radiol.)* **27** 107–14

[9] Datta N, Rogers S and Bodis S 2019 Challenges and opportunities to realize 'The 2030 Agenda for Sustainable Development' By the United Nations: implications for radiation therapy infrastructure in low- and middle-income countries *Int. J. Radiat. Oncol. Biol. Phys.* **105** 918–33

[10] Rosenblatt E, Acuña O and Abdel-Wahab M 2015 The challenge of global radiation therapy: an IAEA perspective *Int. J. Radiat. Oncol. Biol. Phys.* **91** 687–9

[11] Atun R, Jaffray D A and Barton M B *et al* 2015 Expanding global access to radiotherapy *Lancet Oncol.* **16** 1153–86

[12] Collingridge D and Sullivan R 2014 Affordable cancer care: pipedream or achievable reality? *Lancet Oncol.* **15** 257–8

[13] Elzawawy A 1999 Professional education. Cancer strategies for the new millennium *World Health Organization Cancer Strategy* **1** 47

[14] Porter A, Aref A and Chodounsky Z *et al* 1999 A global strategy for radiotherapy: a WHO consultation *Clin. Oncol. (R Coll. Radiol.)* **9** 368–70

[15] Elzawawy A 2017 One more proposal to allocate resources for the win-win approaches to increase the affordability of cancer drugs and radiotherapy in the world *J. Cancer Prev. Curr. Res.* **7** 00250

[16] Ngwa W, Ngoma T and Zietman A *et al* 2016 'Closing the cancer divide through *Ubuntu*: information and communication technology-powered models for global radiation oncology.' *Int. J. Radiat. Oncol. Biol. Phys.* **94** 440–9

[17] Lievens Y, Borras J and Grau C 2020 Provision and use of radiotherapy in Europe *Mol. Oncol.* **14** 1461–9

[18] Leaf C 2013 *The Truth in Small Doses: Why We're Losing the War on Cancer and How to Win It* (New York: Simon & Schuster)

[19] ASCO makes dire predictions for the future of US cancer care – medscape – Mar 12, 2014 https://medscape.com/viewarticle/821837
[20] Cancer clinics closing: community oncology 'Near Crisis' medscape – medscape – June 27, 2013
[21] Ngwa W, Olver I and Schmeler K M 2020 The use of health-related technology to reduce the gap between developed and undeveloped regions around the globe American Society of Clinical Oncology Educational Book **40** 227–36
[22] Boom K, Lopez M and Daheri M *et al* 2019 Perspectives on cervical cancer screening and prevention: challenges faced by providers and patients along the Texas-Mexico border *Perspect Public Health.* **2019** 199–205
[23] Cancer care costs in the United States are projected to exceed $245 Billion by 2030 (June 10, 2020) American Association for Cancer Research (AACR) https://aacr.org/about-the-aacr/newsroom/news-releases/cancer-care-costs-in-the-united-states-are-projected-to-exceed-245-billion-by-2030/
[24] Hutton-Potts M and Joshua A M 2020 2017 ASCO position on the affordability of cancer drugs: arguments for a major revision *JCO Oncol. Pract.* **16** 211–14
[25] Kim C and Prasad V 2015 Cancer drugs approved on the basis of a surrogate end point and subsequent overall survival: An analysis of 5 years of US Food and Drug Administration approvals *JAMA Intern. Med.* **175** 1992–4
[26] Fojo T and Grady C 2009 How much is life worth: Cetuximab, non-small cell lung cancer, and the $440 billion question *J. Natl. Cancer Inst.* **101** 1044–8
[27] Chan A, Delaloge S and Holmes F A *et al* 2016 Neratinib after trastuzumab-based adjuvant therapy in patients with HER2-positive breast cancer (ExteNET): A multicentre, randomised, double-blind, placebo-controlled, phase 3 trial *Lancet Oncol.* **17** 367–77
[28] Elzawawy A 2008 Breast cancer systemic therapy: the need for more economically sustainable scientific strategies in the world *Breast Care (Basel).* **3** 434–8
[29] Elzawawy A 2018 GHC summit. The GHC win-win initiative, May 25, 2018, Harvard Medical School, Boston, MA, USA https://youtu.be/7R91V4CEH34
[30] Fineberg H V 2012 A successful and sustainable health system—how to get there from here *N. Engl. J. Med.* **366** 1020–7
[31] Elzawawy A 2013 The fourth way http://icedoc.org/anticancer5.htm
[32] Elzawawy A 2015 The shortage of essential cancer drugs and generics in the United States of America: global brain storming directions for the world *Int. J. Cancer Clin. Res.* **2** 016
[33] National Cancer Policy Forum; Board on Health Care Services; Institute of Medicine 2013 *Delivering Affordable Cancer Care in the 21st Century: Workshop Summary* (Washington, DC: National Academies Press)
[34] Elzawawy A 2009 The 'Win-Win' initiative: a global, scientifically based approach to resource sparing treatment for systemic breast cancer therapy *World J. Surg. Oncol.* **7** 44–5
[35] Elzawawy A 2012 Science and affordability of cancer drugs and radiotherapy in the world: win-win scenarios ed R Mohan *Advances in Cancer Management.* (Rijeka: InTech)
[36] Sikora K 1999 Developing a global strategy for cancer *Eur. J. Cancer* **35** 24–31
[37] Elzawawy A, Elbahaie A and Dawood S *et al* 2008 A delay in seeking medical advice and late presentation of female breast cancer patients in most of the world. Could we make changes? The experience of 23 years in Port Said, Egypt *Breast Care* **3** 37–41
[38] Elzawawy A November 23, 2013 How the affordability of radiotherapy and essential cancer drugs improves breast cancer control in Africa: an example from Port Said, Egypt

AORTIC 2013 Conf. (Durban, South Africa) http://icedoc.org/Docs/AORTIC2013_A.Elzawawy_Affordability%20of%20radiotherapy%20and%20cancer%20drugs&%20breast%20cancer%20control%20,Port%20Said.pdf http://icedoc.net/Docs/AORTIC2013_A.Elzawawy_Affordability%20of%20radiotherapy%20and%20cancer%20drugs&%20breast%20cancer%20control%20,Port%20Said.pdf

[39] Merriam-Webster

[40] Camacho R, Elzawawy A and Izeweska J *et al* Management and treatment *The Cancer Atlas* ed A Jemal, P Vineis, F Bray, L Torre and D Forman 2nd edn (Atlanta, Georgia, USA: The American Cancer Society) pp 76–7

[41] Elzawawy A M 2015 Could African and low- and middle-income countries contribute scientifically to global cancer care? *J. Glob. Oncol.* **1** 49–53

[42] Elzawawy A and Cazap E 2019 Global cancer care, the ecancer Global Oncology Leaders series https://ecancer.org/en/video/8112-prof-ahmed-elzawawy-on-global-cancer-control

[43] Marshall J L, Kerr D J and Mok T Jun 12, 2012 *Toward a global oncology – Medscape* – https://medscape.com/viewarticle/765329

[44] Elzawawy A 2013 Better value chemotherapy *How to Get Better Value Cancer Care* ed J A Muir Gray and D J Kerr (Oxford: Offox Press Ltd) ch 6

[45] Elzawawy A 2015 Addressing disparities in access to clinicians – *e*cancer https://youtu.be/yzJwimDJ84c

[46] Ngwa W, Olver I and Schmeler K M 2020 The use of health-related technology to reduce the gap between developed and undeveloped regions around the globe *American Society of Clinical Oncology Educational Book* **40** 227–36

[47] Govindarajan V and Trimble C 2012 *Reverse Innovation: Create Far from Home, Win Everywhere* (Brighton, MA, USA: Harvard Business Review Press)

[48] Crisp N 2011 Turning the world upside down – the search for global health in the 21st century RMS Books http://nigelcrisp.com/book.html

[49] Elzawawy A 2013 Ways of implementing affordable radiotherapy to Africa https://ecancer.org/en/video/2494-affordable-radiotherapy-and-chemotherapy-in-africa

[50] ASCO's second national cancer opinion survey results: surprising number of Americans believe alternative. ASCO Connection Jan 8, 2019 https://connection.asco.org/magazine/features/second-asco-national-cancer-opinion-survey-results

[51] Brook R H 2010 The end of the quality improvement movement: long live improving value *JAMA* **304** 1831–2

[52] Elzawawy A 2018 An introduction to affordability of better value clinical oncology.lecture: online course of global radiation oncology (CaReER 18–19), Harvard Global Health Catalyst. Global Oncology University GO-U http://icedoc.org/Docs/Elzawawy_8%20Sept.2018_GO_U.pdf and http://icedoc.net/Docs/Elzawawy_8%20Sept.2018_GO_U.pdf

[53] Porter M E 2008 What is value in health care? *N. Engl. J. Med.* **363** 2477–81

[54] Muir Gray J A and Kerr D J 2013 *How to Get Better Value Cancer Care* (Oxford: Offox Press)

[55] White L Jr 1962 *Medieval Technology and Social Change.* (Oxford: Oxford University Press)

[56] Castells M 1996 *The Rise of the Network Society: The Information Age, Economy, Society and Culture.* (Oxford: Blackwell)

[57] Morgan J M and Liker J K 2006 *The Toyota Product Development System. Integrating People, Process, and Technology.* (New York: Productivity Press)

[58] Womack J P and Jones D T 2003 *Lean Thinking. Banish Waste and Create Wealth in Your Corporation.* (London: Simon & Schuster)

[59] Berwick D M and Hackbarth A D 2012 Eliminating waste in US Healthcare *JAMA* **307** 1513–4
[60] Value frameworks in cancer care: a beginning, not the solution – Medscape – June 28, 2016
[61] The Oxford centre for triple value healthcare https://3vh.org/
[62] Jani A, Jungmann S and Gray M 2018 Feb Shifting to triple value healthcare: reflections from England *Z. Evid. Fortbild. Qual. Gesundhwes.* **130** 2–7
[63] High-value cancer care keeps costs down? Yes, it's possible! – Medscape Nov 16, 2017 https://medscape.com/viewarticle/888751?nlid=119217_2201&src=WNL_mdplsnews_171124_mscpedit_honc&uac=96841ST&spon=7&impID=1491715&faf=1
[64] Sox H and Basch E 2018 Donald Berwick 2018 strategies to achieve high-value oncology care—a beginning *JAMA Oncol.* **4** 171–2

Chapter 2

The need for a cost-effective international campaign to increase the clinical oncology services in the world

Ahmed Elzawawy

The second wing of the win-win movement advocates initiating an enormous increase of the rate of establishment of services of clinical oncology for the underserved-region patients of the world. A global campaign and forum is needed. It should be open for the leadership of all the key players in the world and for all who share the same objective. It relates (a) to global catalytic actions; (b) to the creation of global awareness among the worldwide public and stakeholders for the promotion of the needs and feasibility of clinical oncology; (c) to assisting—after arrangement with the locals—in providing business models tailored to the local conditions; (d) to providing professional consultations and technical advice from A to Z for the establishment, operation, and sustainment of clinical oncology services; (e) to coordinating educational programs and conducting relevant research; (f) to follow-up and continuous assessment to learn lessons and make more progress. All would win.

2.1 Introduction

It is unnecessary to repeat that the gap between what is required and what is available from cancer care has broadened in the last decade and will increase in the forthcoming years [1, 2]. This is not to criticize the great efforts made in the last three decades. Most of the authors of this book are involved or have had leading positions in all the endeavors, organizations, societies, and plans over the last two decades or more. We stress that there are already excellent and highly experienced players in the world, but the question is the need for win-win tactics and a global forum focused on achieving an enormous increase of better-value cancer care. All would win.

doi:10.1088/978-0-7503-3075-6ch2

As we have cited on different occasions in the Win-Win Movement and in this book, by 'clinical oncology care', we mean all modalities of cancer treatment; surgery, radiation therapy, systemic medical treatment, and also diagnosis [3].

One of the reasons that we focus on radiation clinical oncology care units is because they are commonly—and falsely—considered to be expensive services. Over the last three decades, it has been stated repeatedly and published in medical journals by many of us, by organizations, and in professional international conferences that radiotherapy of cancer is much more cost-effective than other lines of treatment, such as cancer drug therapies [4]. Despite that, such units needs a high level of primary funding for establishment, if we consider that a radiotherapy unit will work for at least ten years. Around 50%–60% of cancer patients in the world will need radiotherapy for curative or palliative reasons at least once during the course of their disease. If the need for radiotherapy could be covered by 2035, one million more lives would be saved every year worldwide, in addition to the economic gain [5, 6].

It seems as though we, i.e. clinical oncologists, international organizations, and industry, are talking to ourselves! Apart from professionals, clinical radiation oncologists and parts of the medical profession, the notions of cost-effectiveness, feasibility, how to establish clinical radiation oncology services, and the value of such services are unknown, or in the best case, not widely considered by the public and different stakeholders, including policymakers.

Should we continue with the same situation?

If we continue in the same way, the gap will increase, and there will be a lack of at least around twelve thousand radiotherapy units in the upcoming ten years globally.

From the point of view of business, there are huge inactive or even dead markets with limited opportunities for marketing and sales.

From the perspective of human challenges, governments, medicine, cancer care professionals, and all international and national organizations and cancer societies, this is a growing tragedy.

Isn't it better to search for the light at the end of the tunnel and hence, to explore scientific avenues to increase the affordability of better-value cancer care, while stressing the notion of win-win in the real world? [7, 8].

2.2 How we see the model of the clinical radiation oncology unit [7]

When, the unit is established as an initial endeavor, we recommend—as far as possible—that the unit of radiation clinical oncology should at least contain (in addition to the radiotherapy machine and the necessary devices for planning, medical physics, dosimeters, and imaging facilities), services for outpatient cancer drug therapy—if not inpatient as well—as a start, clinical pharmacy, information and communications technology (ICT), and a nucleus of scientific reporting and research connected with the international scientific community and North–South and South–South technical and scientific collaborations, mostly via ICT.

When the endeavor is in a hospital that has the space for an extension for radiation oncology, then this new unit will complete the surgical and medical diagnostic services in the hospital and share in improving the whole service and scientifically relevant cancer studies; it will be a center that serves patients and the community. This should be covered by the training and education of the radiation oncology staff.

It is recommended that clinical radiation oncology units should be connected, working and following patients with surgeons and referring physicians in the community. They should not be isolated islands, but in continuous communication, exchanging information with district hospitals, community health units, and professionals in the community who have major roles in seeing patients first, referring patients at the appropriate time and following up patients after clinical oncology treatment. All should win: the patients, the community, and medical professionals. We may suggest that some traditional healers, if convinced and (if willing) trained may have a role in refereeing and managing some of the symptoms after treatment and they could also gain. Hence, if this succeeds, some of them could support earlier treatment and not be obstacles to it.

2.3 A global win-win campaign

We emphasise the need for smart planning for an international cost-effective campaign for the effective mobilization of different resources to promote clinical radiation oncology globally, to advise on the increase of the establishment of new clinical oncology services, and to improve and expand existing services according to the real and major needs in the world [3, 7].

There is a big role for media and social media. But, it should be cost-effective and regular to promote the needs and feasibility of clinical oncology care. The messages should be short, appealing, widely and repeatedly diffused, and varied according to each potential group of audience and receiver.

Such messages should target the public and all stakeholders everywhere to convince them of the importance of clinical oncology services for millions of patients, how they are cost-effective in comparison to current medical diagnostic and treatment measures, and moreover, to show how it could be feasible to establish, run, and sustain them. It is essential that in this global campaign, the endorsement is for the treatment of cancer and is not commercial propaganda for a certain drug or named item of equipment.

Stars and celebrities in sports and the arts and known personalities in different fields could help a lot, as the message of the promotional campaign is to increase affordable better-value cancer care and not to advertise for certain commercial brands.

The technical consultations and medical advice of a big Win-Win Campaign—hopefully including most of the interested experts among our readers—could assist along the way. Some advice and technical consultations could be given by experts in different disciplines from different organizations and societies within a transparent coordination in a big win-win global campaign. Moreover, technical advice could be provided by companies who run their businesses in the early stages, assisting the locals to make radiation oncology units function in the first phase. The locals could then continue the task of serving their patients and other units as well. An example is cited in a video in the chapter about Mozambique [9]. It is not at all that we we wish to mention a certain company, but it is just an complete example, and there are several such companies in the world.

There are different business models. The choice should be one that works under local conditions for every endeavor. It could be governmental, a private–public partnership (PPP), private (e.g. with the involvement of local investors, the diaspora, or business investors from other countries), charitable, or a combination of these. Financial studies should precede any endeavor, in order that the unit, its running, sustainability, and gradual progress are assured. Getting loans and renting equipment are one of several options that could be studied to decide what could fit.

The transparent support of, continuous communication with, and the contribution of ***health industries*** in this global win-win campaign are mandatory to succeed in achieving the common objective.

2.4 A huge need for education and training

Another example that highlights the great need for an international campaign is that if we look at the staff required by 2025, if we increase the radiotherapy capacity by only 25%: 7500 radiation oncologists, 2000 radiotherapy radiographers, and 6000 medical physicists need to be trained in LMICs [5, 10].

Efforts are being made by different bodies, organizations, and academia and there are some courses here and there. Most of the programs of the different bodies are dispersed, with no relation or coordination between them in a global movement. Thus, I can pose the question: are there valid, realistic, and feasible plans to accomplish the education and training of the required number of staff?

That is one of the strong arguments supporting the need for a big 'global win-win campaign'. A feasible vision should be agreed by the many parties involved. We would encourage all educational and training programs to be announced together in more than one internet site. Gradual coordination, an increase in the number of programs, and improving and tailoring them are needed to make remarkable progress to cover the needs. It is clear that that the gap is huge, so there is ample space for all players. The current programs of all parties and organizations will have more value, without reducing any of their credit or interfering with their management. There will be great scope to involve more instructors and trainers from every possible place. ICT will help a lot [11].

Hence, a big Win-Win Global Campaign would have a big role in assisting, catalyzing, and coordinating different parties for the education and training of local staff. Once again, there are places for all to do a lot, which would result in a very big push towards achieving the common objective.

2.4.1 An example: the Global Oncology University (the GO-U) [12]

Our plan is that, apart from our courses and certificates with online education plus on-site training like the training we initiated in the first phase, such as courses in surgical oncology, clinical radiation oncology, medical physics, clinical trials, and global oncology, in the second phase, we will add announcements on the website and by email for all who would like to give information about their program in the world. We have no rivalries. We do this simply because, at present, and for the next ten years, the needs are so huge. There are places for all and coordination is greatly needed.

We stress the notion that that there is no one in the win-win movement or its campaigns who has the right to interfere with your self-management of your body or enterprise or to claim the credit that you get. We ask this of all concerned parties.

We consider what we propose here to be stimulating points that need to be crystallized and tailored by different interested parties according to real conditions. A fundamental point that we stress is that the interests and incentives of all stakeholders should be considered in the real world.

Once again, the Win-Win movement is yours and it belongs to all. So, can you do it and come together to contribute and lead in a global win-win campaign for much more productivity, more gain to you, and a well-targeted endeavor towards a common objective?

We leave the reply to all of you!

Note from the author:

This chapter was written by Ahmed Elzawawy after discussions with many colleagues and concerned persons across the world.

It reflects the notions of the whole Team of the Global Health Catalyst Win-Win Initiative:

Professors Wil Ngwa, and Paul Nugyen of Harvard Medical School; Professor Ahmed Elzawawy (chair, GHC Win-Win Initiative) and Professor David Kerr (Oxford University, UK and Win-Win), Professor Eduardo Cazap (Argentina, SLACOM and Win-Win), Professor Twalib Ngoma (Tanzania and Win-Win), Professor Stephan Avery (Radiation Physics, Pennsylvania University, USA and Win-Win), Professor Riccardo Audisio (Sweden and Win-Win), Professor Nicholas Abinya (Kenya and Win-Win), Professor Luca Incrocci (Netherlands and Win-Win), Professor Golam A Zakaria (Germany and Win-Win), Med. Phys. Holger Wirtz (Germany and Win-Win), Professor Saiful Huq (Win-Win and the president of the American Association of Physicists in Medicine (AAPM)) and Professor Bashkim Ziberi (Balkan Win-Win), Dr Manar Montasser (Win-Win) and the coordinators of the Harvard GHC programs: Dr Credit Omoruyi, Sayeda Yasmin-Karim (MD, PhD), Dr Lydia Asana, Dr Neeharika Sinha, Dr Romy Mueller, Dr Kaylie Decosmo, Dr Jana Wood, Dr Noella Bih, and Dr William Swanson.

References

[1] Yap M L, Zubizarreta E and Bray F *et al* 2015 Global access to radiotherapy services: have we made progress during the past decade? *J. Global Oncol.* **2** 207–15

[2] Elzawawy A 2017 One more proposal to allocate resources for the win-win approaches to increase the affordability of cancer drugs and radiotherapy in the world *J. Cancer Prev. Curr. Res.* **7** 00250

[3] Elzawawy A 2019 Keynote speech on May 24, 219 *GHC Summit at Harvard Medical School* Boston, MA, USA https://youtube.com/watch?v=gPnfjY8kqyA

[4] Porter A, Aref A and Chodounsky Z *et al* 1999 A global strategy for radiotherapy. A WHO consultation *Clinical Oncology* **11** 368–70

[5] Huge shortfall in radiotherapy, investment would save lives—Medscape—Sep 26, 2015

[6] 10 facts about radiotherapy—The Health Policy Partnership https://healthpolicypartnership.com/wp-content/uploads/10_facts_about_radiotherapy.pdf

[7] Elzawawy A 2018 An introduction to affordability of better value clinical oncology. *Lecture: Online Course of Global Radiation Oncology (CaReER 18–19)* Harvard Global Health Catalyst. Global Oncology University GO-U

[8] Elzawawy A 2012 Science and affordability of cancer drugs and radiotherapy in the world: Win-Win Scenarios ed R Mohan *Advances in Cancer Management.* (Rijeka: InTech) http://intechopen.com/articles/show/title/science-and-affordability-of-cancer-drugs-and-radiotherapy-in-the-world

[9] Alves F 2019 Obsession for life. Presented in Global Health Catalyst Summit Win-Win sessions at Harvard Medical School May 24, 2019 https://youtu.be/UAdj1AlePcs

[10] Atun R, Jaffray D A and Barton M B *et al* 2015 Expanding global access to radiotherapy *Lancet Oncol.* **16** 1153–86

[11] Ngwa W, Olver I and Schmeler K M 2020 The use of health-related technology to reduce the gap between developed and undeveloped regions around the globe *American Society of Clinical Oncology Educational Book* 2020 **40** 227–36

[12] The Global Oncology University (The GO-U) http://ghcuniversity.org

Chapter 3

The win-win modified blue ocean strategy

Ahmed Elzawawy

'A new type of thinking is essential if mankind is to survive and move toward higher levels' (Albert Einstein).

As a modified form of original blue ocean strategy that was introduced by W C Kim and R Mauborgne, we propose the win-win modified blue ocean strategy, which could allow an enterprise, organization, or company to grow and to gain more by opening new markets and getting new customers using a win-win strategy without destructive competition (the red ocean strategy) and without proceeding alone (the blue ocean strategy). A brief about our proposal is presented in this chapter.

3.1 Introduction

The 'win-win modified blue ocean strategy' is of one of several tactics that we propose. The blue ocean strategy, as introduced by W Chan Kim and R Mauborgne [1, 2], in their best-selling book of the same name, implies that a company, organization, or foundation creates a new uncontested market space that allows them to navigate without relevant competition, and hence to create new customers **and** new consumer value, often while decreasing costs and achieving higher profits. It is understood that this adds to the existing business and markets of an enterprise or an organization and does not reduce them.

It is called the blue ocean strategy, because the procedure focuses on the ability to create a sovereign market space and to exclude competitors from the game.

Red ocean companies try to outperform their rivals by grabbing a greater share of the existing demand. Competing in red oceans is a zero-sum game. A market competition strategy divides the existing wealth between rival companies. As bloody competition increases (which is why it is called red ocean!), the prospects for profit and growth may decline [1, 2].

doi:10.1088/978-0-7503-3075-6ch3

3.2 Blue ocean shift

C W Kim and R Mauborgne presented a way to shift to the blue ocean strategy [4, 5]. There are many successful examples of for-profit, non-profit, and governmental bodies that have shifted to a blue ocean strategy. Starbucks has been able to implement this strategy and pull in a new group of customers who were traditionally noncustomers of the industry, such as non-coffee drinkers. R Mauborgne stated that lessons can be learned from Facebook, Uber, and Amazon [4].

3.2.1 Five steps to making a blue ocean shift [6, 7]

a. Select the right scope for your blue ocean initiative and build your people's confidence.
b. Next, be very clear about the current state of play.
c. Identify the hidden constraints that you can turn into opportunities.
d. Go from the big picture to creating practical blue ocean options.
e. Launch your blue ocean move.

3.2.2 Proven steps to creating your own blue ocean strategy [8]

Step 1: Create a strategy canvas
Step 2: Raise an attribute
Step 3: Reduce an attribute.
Step 4: Eliminate an attribute
Step 5: Create an attribute.

3.3 Can a blue ocean strategy work for large, medium, and small organizations?

Blue Ocean leadership works equally for large, medium, and small organizations. In fact, one of the strengths of blue ocean leadership is its scalability—the process can be launched at all management levels or deployed at one of these levels. In the case of small companies or startups, this process can certainly be applied to the one or two management levels that are present. As long as an organization has deliverables and performance goals, blue ocean leadership has a key role to play in uplifting performance by converting disengaged employees into engaged ones and motivating people to excel and act with commitment. As blue ocean leadership allows an organization to achieve high-impact results fast and at low cost, it offers a particularly practical method for small companies to achieve rapid organizational turnarounds while saving money, given the fact that small organizations often face resource constraints [1–3, 9].

In the win-win movement, we like the three characteristics of the blue ocean strategy:

(a) Focus
(b) Divergence
(c) Compelling tag line

Also, the authors of the blue ocean strategy and the blue ocean shift stated that value innovation is important and that it is essential to consider the human factors in working; hence, it is mandatory to humanize the organization [1–3, 9].

3.4 'The win-win modified blue ocean strategy'

Ahmed Elzawawy coins a new term here, which is **'the win-win modified blue ocean strategy'**.

Despite our high admiration for, and our inspiration resulting from, the original blue ocean strategy, this strategy as presented by C W Kim and R Mauborgne implies a search for how to grow without competitors and how to open new markets [1].

My question: (1) is the big objective to move to a space without competitors? or (2) is it to open new markets, to gain more, and to make growth?

Well, we see that the reply is 'no' for the first question and 'yes' for the second.

Hence, in the win-win modification, I suggest that if more growth, opening more markets, gaining more, and getting a *wider blue ocean* imply that you move in the presence of similar activities similar to your own—considered to be external competitors outside the win-win movement—or non-similar activities that complement you, rather than navigating alone, then it would be logical to implement 'the win-win modified blue ocean strategy'.

This is not to lessen the value of the blue ocean strategy, if you find it the most suitable for your case.

In reality, in the field of clinical oncology cancer care, there **are** huge inactive or dead markets that could be potentially a great blue ocean within the forthcoming ten years. Hence, there could be places for many times (and not only double) the present products of all radiation therapy and health care industries. This win-win modified blue ocean strategy could have very ample space for all to navigate, while enormously increasing their achievements in their missions or the markets for their products. The same is true for all parties, such as cancer care professionals, all organizations, societies, and businesses as well.

Therefore, with a win-win collaboration or at least clever coordination in an effective, intense, and smart international promotion for the needs of clinical oncology care and the implementation and realization of the global campaign that we call for, all would win. The cost and effectiveness of such campaign would be reduced if one or few of the stakeholders tried to do it alone. The gain would be more in a suitable—well studied—sort of combination than if one party were to try to navigate alone.

I see that my proposal of the win-win modification for the blue ocean strategy could be also applied to similar conditions or activities in life and not only for projects for the global expansion of cancer care in the world, when there is no remarkable additional value of being alone and when you arrive at a wider ocean and more opportunities in a smart win-win forum. Also, I propose that the win-win blue ocean strategy would be a particularly suitable approach in all activities in cases (a) in which expansion needs different activities that complement each other; (b) or in which similar activities or fields are not harmed by the flourishing of these activities. Hence, the condition or the term is that there is a high potential that the strategy would result in creating a wide 'win-win blue ocean' for all.

In the fields of expansion of clinical oncology care, there are different health industries for different types of equipment, cancer drugs, providers and businesses that meet infrastructure requirements, and different stakeholders with different incentives. However, we see the importance of highlighting that we have a common focus—as you will notice on several occasions in this book—for different parties that will help a lot. It is a smart and thorough formulation of canvas in a win-win forum focused on increasing access to affordable better-value cancer care in the world to millions of human beings with approaches that consider the interests (and *les raisons d'être*) of all parties.

These different incentives are not all based on money. For example, there are legitimate economic incentives for all kinds of business—industrial, commercial, financial, and medical as they search to gain more money (otherwise they would collapse). However, for organizations, societies, educational institutions, and scientific initiatives—like ours—the incentive is to see progress in the realization of their missions.

References and further reading

[1] Kim W C and Mauborgne R 2004 *Blue Ocean Strategy: How to Create Uncontested Market Space and Make the Competition Irrelevant.* (Boston, MA: Harvard Business School Press)

[2] Kim W C and Mauborgne R 2017 *Blue Ocean Strategy with Harvard Business Review Classic Articles 'Blue Ocean Leadership' and 'Red Ocean Traps' (3 Books).* (Boston, MA: Harvard Business School Press)

[3] An introduction to 'Blue Ocean' https://youtube.com/watch?v=MXRDiYht-vE

[4] Mauborgne R 2018 On lessons from Facebook, Uber and Amazon https://youtube.com/watch?v=tRDafz8Xc-8

[5] Mauborgne R 2017 Blue ocean shift Move beyond competing https://youtube.com/watch?v=yGls0hYe9ng

[6] Kim W C 2017 On Blue ocean shift https://youtube.com/watch?v=gjsv85_v02s

[7] Kim C W and Mauborgne R Five steps to making a blue ocean shift https://blueoceanstrategy.com/blog/five-steps-making-blue-ocean-shift/

[8] Nielson J 2013 5 Proven steps to creating your own blue ocean strategy https://ignitionframework.com/blue-ocean-strategy/

[9] Mauborgne R 2020 Renée Mauborgne at Davos 2020 offering a blue ocean perspective on the next growth cycle https://youtube.com/watch?v=7NMQD0RDMV4

Chapter 4

How both high-income and low- and middle-income country institutions can win in global oncology

Omoruyi Irabor and Wilfred Ngwa

The recent World Health Organization (WHO) Cancer Report [1] describes the growing global burden of cancer as alarming, a major obstacle to human development and wellbeing, with a rising annual economic cost of over USD 2.0 trillion. The cancer burden is projected to increase dramatically in the coming years. Win-win collaborations are needed to address the growing global burden of cancer and disparities. This is particularly important because, in today's world, global health is local health and vice versa. Discoveries made in one part of the world can have tremendous benefits in other regions of the world. In this chapter, we highlight how win-win collaborations benefit high-income (HICs) and low-and-middle-income country (LMIC) institutions.

4.1 Introduction

The Executive Board of the Consortium of Universities for Global Health (CUGH) developed the following definition for global health, as published in *The Lancet* in 2009 [2]:

> Global health is an area for study, research, and practice that places a priority on improving health and achieving equity in health for all people worldwide. Global health emphasizes transnational health issues, determinants, and solutions; involves many disciplines within and beyond the health sciences and promotes interdisciplinary collaboration; and is a synthesis of population-based prevention with individual-level clinical care.

Also writing in *The Lancet* in 2010, Friedman *et al* (a working group of the Association of Schools of Public Health Global Health Committee), noted that global health is often perceived as international aid, with technologies and interventions flowing from the wealthier developed countries of the Global North to the poorer countries of the Global South. Friedman *et al* offered a more nuanced and contemporary perspective, emphasizing interdependence and recognizing the many contributions of both resource-rich and resource-poor nations. Global health is local health and can benefit both HICs and LMICs. In this chapter, we focus on highlighting how both HICs and LMICs can benefit. This can be characterized in three areas: global oncology research, education, and care/outreach.

4.2 Win-win research

Gaps in access to cancer treatment present significant challenges in resource-poor settings in HICs and LMICs. Collaborative research that develops new treatment approaches or technologies to address these gaps will indubitably benefit both HIC and LMICs. For example, the same cost-effective cancer technologies that can be beneficial in global low-resource settings can also be beneficial in underserved US populations. Although treatment approaches exist in the US for most cancers, many examples of disparities in cancer outcomes exist for certain underserved populations, in both rural and urban settings. Many factors are thought to contribute to these disparate outcomes. However, there is confidence that novel products that are affordable, portable, and whose use does not require extensive training and expertise to be deployed, can improve cancer outcomes in underserved HIC populations. Collaborative research can also help to overcome the challenges of doing research and clinical work in an international setting. Collaborations could lead to joint publications, funding, and career development for both HIC and LMIC investigators. Another potential area of win-win research collaborations is in multi-center clinical trials. Such collaborations involving both HIC and LMIC institutions could be mutually beneficial, with faster enrollment and enrollment of diverse populations needed to ensure rigor of the research outcomes.

4.3 Win-win education

In HICs such as the USA, incidence rates for all cancer sites have decreased by an average of 1.1% each year over the last ten years, but significant disparities persist in cancer incidence and mortality among certain racial and ethnic minorities and immigrant communities. The primary drivers of these disparities, such as the higher prevalence of risky behaviours, inadequate prevention and early detection, the presence of comorbidities, and poor access to treatment services also underlie the high cancer-related morbidity and mortality seen in LMICs. Global oncology collaborations that aim to address the growing scourge of cancer require human capacity and research skills for cancer care and research at the institutional level in both HIC and LMIC settings. Training to conduct investigations in global settings is limited in the U.S. and is profoundly lacking in LMICs. Researchers need training in the scientific and methodological aspects of cancer research across the cancer continuum and training to conduct research based on an understanding of the determinants - biological, social, economic—of cancer within the partner country. There is need for both HIC and LMIC training to develop the skills required to conduct international research.

Programs that support education and training in global oncology will therefore benefit both HICs and LMICs in advancing the global fight against cancer. Such programs can provide a strong foundation in collaborative culturally relevant cancer care as well as research design, methods, and analytic techniques appropriate for the proposed cancer research area, with the goal of developing independent research careers for the HIC and LMIC scientists. Education and training is crucial for filling the gap in qualified oncology health professionals in LMICs, compounded by brain drain which also benefits HICs. Training will also provide the competencies necessary for cancer research inquiries and the development of evidence-based low-cost technologies and approaches for cancer care that benefit both HICs and LMICs and reduce disparities. Such training will also help to strengthen and develop global cancer research leadership and mentorship at HIC and LMIC institutions.

4.4 Win-win care and outreach

Collaborations in global oncology care can also benefit both LMIC and HIC institutions. This is particularly crucial for LMICs, in which oncology capacity is limited. However, HICs can also benefit in learning how to provide care with limited resources and culturally relevant care for patients from different cultural backgrounds across the world.

The United States has been a world leader in global health outreach for decades; the government, academic institutions, industry, foundations, and non-profits make major investments in Africa and partner with African countries with considerable success, as seen in the President's Emergency Plan for AIDS Relief (PEPFAR) program [3, 4]. However, the African diaspora is one of the most educated in North America, and one could argue that the brain drain has benefitted the USA tremendously. This has resulted in the emergence of calls for purposeful engagement and partnership with the diaspora in global health to benefit both African LMICs and the USA. This applies to other LMICs and HICs. Greater effective engagement of the diaspora could turn brain drain and a negative history of slavery and brain drain into global health gain equality. Involvement of the diaspora in win-win collaborations can also help to overcome cultural barriers to global health and provide insights that show how HICs can better address disparities in their countries. Culture has been identified as a key challenge in global health [5].

Global health collaborations also provide major opportunities for businesses in both HICs and LMICs, whose businesses could flourish with opportunities for investment and expansion. A good example is that of HIC radiotherapy and pharmaceutical companies that are benefiting from access to new markets in LMICs. At the same time, the development of low-cost evidence-based technologies for global health will benefit both HICs and LMICs. The USA National Cancer Institute recognizes this and has launched funding opportunities for businesses to develop such technologies.

In perspective, the World Health Organization presents a model for global health collaborations in which both HIC and LMIC governments can work together to address global health challenges. The COVID-19 pandemic is an example of the benefits such collaborations can bring to both HICs and LMICs. With the rising global burden of cancer and other non-communicable diseases, there is a major win-win opportunity for collaborations at the policy level to make cancer history.

Table 4.1. Strengths in a SWOT analysis for developing a robust global oncology program done by a leading USA institution before launching their global oncology program.

Address the growing global cancer burden	Accelerate cancer research globally	Accrue benefits
• Expertise from our institution can have a major impact on the development of cancer research and clinical practice in LMICs • Our institution can help alleviate suffering, improve population health, and decrease the burden of disease • Our institution can assist with research and clinical capacity building in LMICs	• Researchers can access unique populations, molecular profiles, and phenotypes • The development of efficient technologies and modalities in LMICs can inform clinical approaches worldwide and facilitate leapfrogging (the process of skipping less efficient technologies) • The effective application of prevention and therapeutic interventions in all populations requires research be undertaken in these populations	• Increased visibility for our institution globally • Opportunity to realize our mission internationally • Support for education and training programs at our institution and abroad • Support for the career goals of our faculty and staff as well as those in LMICs • Opportunities to learn from LMICs and bring insight back to our institution • Opportunities to share expertise and break down silos within our institution

Taking into account all of the above, all institutions in HICs and LMICs are encouraged to carefully consider the benefits of global oncology. While the benefits of global oncology are readily apparent for LMICs, it is important that HIC institutions also recognize that they stand to win through greater investments in global oncology. The growing number of funding opportunities, for example, at the National Cancer Institute, are helpful in catalyzing the growth of global oncology. Table 4.1 highlights some of the benefits identified by one institution in the USA when conducting a SWOT analysis for developing a robust global oncology program.

References

[1] World Health Organization 2020 WHO report on cancer: setting priorities, investing wisely, and providing care for all (Geneva: World Health Organization) https://apps.who.int/iris/handle/10665/330745. License: CC BY-NC-SA 3.0 IGO (Accessed April 4, 2022)

[2] Koplan J P, Bond T C and Merson M H *et al* 2009 Towards a common definition of global health *Lancet* **373** 1993–5

[3] Katz I T, Bassett I V and Wright A A 2013 PEPFAR in transition—implications for HIV care in South Africa *N. Engl. J. Med.* **369** 1385–7

[4] Dzau V, Fuster V, Frazer J and Snair M 2017 Investing in global health for our future *N. Engl. J. Med.* **377** 1292–6

[5] Ngwa W and Ngoma T 2016 *Emerging Models for Global Health in Radiation Oncology.* (Bristol, UK; Philadelphia, PA: IOP Publishing)

Chapter 5

Mobilization of resources for cancer care services in low- and middle-income countries and Africa: myths, realities, and hopes

Ahmed Elzawawy

There can be no doubt that an increase in the quantity of better-value cancer care services needs resources. In this brief chapter, we present examples that show that the mobilization of resources in low- and middle-income countries (LMICs) and Africa is possible.

Introduction

In this chapter, we come to crucial questions about resources. We cite here some examples of simulating points. Hence, the reader and all stakeholders will have unlimited avenues to create more approaches for the mobilization of resources for the win-win establishment and development of clinical oncology care units in the underserved patients in the world.

It is a myth to think that there are no local resources in LMICs.

In fact, LMICs do not have limited resources, but resources that are not smartly mobilized and not utilized to serve cancer care. In fact, Africa has the curse of having a lot of resources, which is why it was colonized! (Was there another reason?)

A well-studied project with a good business model for a clinical–radiation oncology service customized to the locality could be funded by public money, by a private–public partnership, by the diaspora, or could get loans from banks or local stakeholders. Moreover, well-presented profitable value-based projects could attract local and foreign investors.

The diaspora could be asked to smartly invest and to gain from well-studied sustainable Win-Win projects. One of the aspects of well-studied projects is that the diaspora should have adequate assurance about their investment. If we consider that

doi:10.1088/978-0-7503-3075-6ch5

in 2014, the remittance from the diaspora to sub-Saharan Africa was $ 67.1 billion, we can see that this amounts to more than the total of foreign aid. So, how can we say that there are very limited resources? [1].

Annually, around $2 billion is sent from Africa to India, which is spent on cancer treatment for patients referred from Africa. If the same sum were spent annually in creating new functioning cancer care units in Africa, then in ten years, there would be a huge change. Shall we continue in the same way as before [1, 2]?

Concerning the bill for the cancer treatment of African patients from countries in West Africa treated in France, and the hope that the same sum could be spent to establish adequate modern local cancer care services in the same countries, the same question is: shall we continue as before [1, 2]?

We stress that this is not against the notion that some would gain money. We hope and we call for smart win-win, scientific approaches, hence, all would gain more than before. No one would lose. These are smart exercises in research for value-based scientific cancer care and different existing and creative business models in order to maximize the global gain and the number of winners enormously.

In a published editorial, we suggested that some of the overspending on international and regional conferences should be saved and allocated to enhance the work of increasing the number of cancer care facilities. Here, we add that it should not necessarily be spent, as we proposed in this editorial, on direct action to establish or upgrade cancer care services, but one of our proposals here is that the manufacturers of pharmaceuticals, radiation equipment, and medical devices together with international organizations and societies would contribute some of the cost of their sponsorship of conferences to the global win-win campaign and platform to promote the increase of value-based clinical oncology care. Alternatively, at least parts of these conferences should allow the presentation of studies in pragmatic and scientific ways and newer approaches to increasing the affordability of better-value cancer care within win-win settings and to increase the quality and quantity of cancer treatment care to serve millions of human beings in the world. In this way, companies and organizations would contribute to opening up huge markets in the real world and they would gain a lot! [3, 4].

Resource sparing and avoid imitating waste in overspending

As we mentioned in other parts of this book, leftover cancer drugs in vials cost around $3 billion annually in the USA. As stated in an article published in 2016, this is due to overspending driven by oversized single-dose vials of cancer drugs. Do you imagine that this waste of $3 billion could be cut down by having two or three different-sized vials for many chemodrugs and also for biologics?. Moreover, applying—whenever possible and when it is medically sound—a system of sharing the vials by pooling patients with the same infused drugs on the same day would save an expensive waste of drugs [5, 6].

If the reader asks: what are the annual worldwide sales of Varian Medical Systems (now a part of Siemens Healthineers), since it is the biggest radiotherapy equipment manufacturer? Their worldwide sales of all radiotherapy equipment, which includes accelerators, informatics, planning systems, and all of their products related to radiotherapy were equivalent to or less than $3 billion in 2019, that is to say, **equivalent to or slightly less than** the cost of the waste due to the leftovers of some cancer drugs [1, 2, 7]. The question is: do we still ask about a lack of resources? Or would it be better to speculate about the complexities behind the waste caused by overspending on unbalanced health expenditure?

When we are speaking here about the mobilization of resources, we are not particularly focused on charity. However, to be pragmatic and more effective, some of the charity funds, either from wealthy kind individuals, companies, or international or national funds should contribute to the campaign that we propose here. This is not only to teach fishing rather than to give a fish (as charity), as the Chinese wisdom implies, but also to contribute to a big cost-effective campaign that promotes and teaches how to establish sustainable projects for fishing for thousands of fishermen who will feed millions of people with the products of their projects.

There are many business models and examples for building cancer care centers. Select what works for you in a well-studied and transparent way.

In a chapter of this book, we give an example of leased equipment in a radiation oncology department in Uruguay. Moreover, as we are tackling issues in the real life, we cite here some of the financing models that have been proposed by leading radiotherapy equipment manufacturers:

(a) A five-year loan at low interest rates based on an export credit agency insuring the risk.
(b) A model of 15% downpayment, ten settlements biannually, with a six--month grace period for the first installment.
(c) Extended payment terms covered by LC 360 days. Payment for the equipment is made one year after installation, giving the clinic time to ramp up and get some income.
(d) Leased equipment with a capped lower lease price plus an additional share of income over the capped amount.
(e) Per-patient repayment of equipment, with a minimal number to be paid and additional fees for patients over the cap.
(f) Covered by a five-year extended warranty as required by the bank.
(g) Service is included in price, creating security for the end user, as the company would want the machine to work in order to get paid back.

Classic, innovative, and creative examples should be encouraged to mobilize every possible resource (financial and human resources) and to open all sorts of constructive partnerships in Win-Win scenarios that cope with the real world [7].

Note: Examples of the mobilization of human resources, education and training, win-win collaborations, and cooperation are presented in other sections of this book.

References

[1] Elzawawy A 2018 Harvard Global Health Catalyst (GHC) summit *The GHC win-win initiative* (Harvard Medical School) May 25, 2018 (Boston, MA) https://youtu.be/7R91V4CEH34

[2] Elzawawy A 2019 Keynote speech in May 24, 2019, GHC Summit at Harvard Medical School, Boston, MA, USA https://youtube.com/watch?v=gPnfjY8kqyA

[3] Elzawawy A 2017 One more proposal to allocate resources for the win-win approaches to increase the affordability of cancer drugs and radiotherapy in the world *J. Cancer Prev. Curr. Res.* **7** 00250

[4] World Health Organization (WHO) 2018 Taking up Africa cancer challenge Bulletin of World Health Organization Volume 96, Number 4, April 2018, 225-96 www.who.int/bulletin/volumes/96/4/18-020418/en/

[5] Bach P, Conti R and Muller R *et al* 2016 Overspending driven by oversized single dose vials of cancer drugs *Brit. Med. J.* **2016** 352

[6] Leftover cancer drugs in vials cost $3 billion annually—Medscape—Mar 18, 2016 http://medscape.com/viewarticle/860660?nlid=102735_2201&src=WNL_mdplsnews_160325_mscpedit_honc&uac=96841ST&spon=7&impID=1037730&faf=1

[7] Elzawawy A 2018 An introduction to affordability of better-value clinical oncology. lecture: online course of global radiation oncology (CaReER 18–19), Harvard Global Health Catalyst. Global Oncology University GO-U http://icedoc.org/Docs/Elzawawy_8%20Sept.2018_GO_U.pdf http://icedoc.net/Docs/Elzawawy_8%20Sept.2018_GO_U.pdf

IOP Publishing

Approaching Global Oncology
The win-win model
Ahmed Elzawawy and Wilfred Ngwa

Chapter 6

Top challenges in cancer care in the 3rd decade of the 21st century

Ahmed Elzawawy, Wil Ngwa, David Kerr, Twalib Ngoma, Manar Montasser and Eduardo Cazap

At the beginning of 2020, just before the wide spread of news about the COVID-19 pandemic, Professor David Collingridge, editor-in-chief of *Lancet Oncology*, and the senior editor Katherine Gourd asked some of the members of the Lancet Oncology International Advisory Board to send their thoughts, focusing on the top three challenges and opportunities in global cancer control over the next ten years. What we cite here is inspired by the reply of Ahmed Elzawawy to the request from *Lancet Oncology*.

6.1 Introduction

A general and common challenge is the lack of access and affordability of better-value cancer care and control. This lack will escalate in the next decade, particularly if we continue in the same way and with the same approaches as the ones that the world uses now. To add to the previous prediction, if the sequels of COVID-19 continue to affect economies for years and put pressure on the priorities for health expenditure, then, as we cited in in this book, these problems of affordability will be aggravated in future years more than the previous estimations suggest, unless smart and effective global actions are taken. It is time for an enormous exploration of unlimited numbers of scientific approaches and win-win scenarios that consider the interests of all stakeholders in order to tackle the global escalation of the problem [1–3].

6.2 The top three challenges and top three opportunities for global cancer control in the forthcoming decade

6.2.1 Primary prevention, early detection, and earlier diagnosis

It is known that primary prevention includes: healthy lifestyle behaviors, the avoidance of tobacco products and second-hand smoke, the minimization of alcohol intake, regular exercise, a balanced diet, and protection against ultraviolet exposure.

doi:10.1088/978-0-7503-3075-6ch6

The question is: will science in the new decade give us more precise and detailed information about the start of the formation of cancer cells and while the first colony is forming? Eventually, my second question is: would it be possible to stop cancer in these very early moments?

Very early cancer detection is still rare in the absolute sense if we consider the hidden time history from the formation of the first cancer cells until they become a macroscopic tumor. There is a wide variability in this duration for different tumors.

Taking breast cancer as an example, the current screening takes place using examinations, mammography, and other imaging procedures. Among the challenges for national screening breast cancer programs that use imaging procedures are costs, value, and feasibility at the national level in big populations.

The question here is whether we will see further development and wider application of the current blood tests for the detection of several types of cancer by looking for fragments of DNA from cancer cells within this new decade? [4].

Moreover, new opportunities are available besides blood tests. It has been shown recently that tests using saliva can detect the same conditions as blood tests without the need for an invasive blood sample. Further studies are needed [5].

The shortage of qualified pathologists is a burning challenge in many countries. There are opportunities for the further development of digital pathology in the new decade.

6.2.1.1 Information and communications technology and artificial intelligence

We stress the value of information and communications technology (ICT) and Artificial Intelligence (AI), as they could assist in the progression and facilitation of wider accessibility and the affordability of early detection, screening, and diagnosis including labs, pathology, and imaging and in better-value treatment of cancer.

In our view, there are exaggerated fears of the widespread elimination of human roles and jobs. In fact, we see these technologies as a sort of augmenting intelligence and as increasing the capabilities of human beings, as there is usually a human at the other end. Hence, this needs the preparation of human capacity for newer technologies and jobs. As a result of the estimated lack of many tens of thousands—or more—of professionals in the different technical and medical disciplines of cancer control and care in the world, particularly in low- and middle-income countries (LMICs), further development of ICT and AI would provide a big hint about lessening the burden in the new decade. This needs thorough studies of the obstacles and feasibilities and a smart presentation of the different models that could be adapted to different communities, and it should show gains for all stakeholders i.e. a win-win in the real world. The new programs of human capacity building should cope with the need for a successful implementation that increases output and expands the capabilities of the workforce of the trained human beings and not replace them, as described in some rumors. In about 20 years, 50% of all jobs will be outdated or no longer needed, and healthcare is no exception [6, 7]. AI is not meant to replace medical professionals, but those who use AI will probably replace those who do not. Hence, every healthcare provider's duty is to prepare for a future like that [7]. AI demonstrates a significant potential to improve diagnostics [8–10]; it will probably not solve the human resources crisis in healthcare, or at least it will not start with that [7]. We think that this expectation is very probable unless global changes and the continuous adaption of the training of healthcare professions is considered.

With smart and flexible approaches, the chances of improving the medical job environment and the conditions of practice could be improved, which would eventually lead to a general improvement in the quality of care. Hence, regarding cancer treatment and care (the next section of this chapter), AI would be able to take over important tasks from medical professionals. With innovative vision, AI might even bring forward a renaissance in the doctor–patient relationship [7].

This is why Elzawawy suggested using terms such as 'augmenting intelligence' or 'assisted intelligence' (both could be called AI too!) rather than the commonly used term 'artificial intelligence'. In fact, we think that developing more global programs of human capacity building that are needed to cope with the new era could make humans master the procedures with which to make unprecedented progress. In all cases, AI consists of human-made devices or programs that marvelously augment the scope and execution of what was mostly planned also by humans [1]. If they do not keep to this notion, we think that global human communities will enter circles of uncertainty and uncontrolled chaos.

6.2.2 Cancer treatment

In the last decade and despite all the declarations, commissions, conferences, and publications of international organizations and societies, the gap has widened between what is required and what is available in terms of cancer care in the world. The problem is global and affects the rich as well as LMICS, but with wide variability of the degree of accessibility and affordability.

Due to the skyrocketing rise in the costs of cancer treatment and technology and the expected increase of the prevalence of cancer, in particular in LMICs, the gap will be increased in the next decade if we continue tackling the problem in the same way [11–13].

Hence, once again, we stress the need for what we emphasized above about scientific approaches and Win-Win scenarios.

In fact, the two wings of the Win-Win initiative [3] are:

The first wing of the Win-Win is to increase the affordability of value-based cancer care in different communities in the world via scientific approaches and Win-Win scenarios that consider the interests of stakeholders in the real world.

The objective is not necessarily to decrease the price of a drug or item of equipment per se, but to achieve a scientifically-based reduction of the total cost of treatment without compromising the outcome for patients [11, 12].

In an *e*cancer video for world cancer leaders published on 12 July 2019 [10], one of the points I raised was a new proposal for the definition of the term 'top science'. I think that 'top science', in particular, in medicine, is not just a breakthrough discovery that is great in itself; it may need further scientific research, work, exploration, and perhaps innovation for this discovery to become applicable and implemented (with variability in different communities) and on how to make it accessible. That is the case if a discovery does not meet these criteria from the start [14]. There is a need to further exploit—in a positive and constructive sense—the contributions of LMICs to such challenges [15].

Also, we hope that the newly formed 'Lancet Oncology Commission for sub-Saharan Africa' will provide more clues to scientific approaches that will serve to increase the affordability of better-value cancer control and care in Africa and eventually for the world and not only report problems.

The second wing of the Win-Win relates to catalytic action and professional advice to enormously increase the rate of establishment of clinical and surgical oncology services in the world, starting with the difficult challenges in LMICs, including Africa.

For example, for radiation oncology, we—in the Win-Win movement—stress the need for an international campaign to promote radiotherapy, how it is cost-effective, how many business and financing models could be provided, how we catalyze the development of human capacities, education, and training, volunteer professional consultations, and advice from A to Z. That is to say: from the idea and the layout to the installation and running. Examples are the Global Health Catalyst Win-Win Movement initiatives: www.ecancerforall.com [16] and Global Oncology University (GO-U) www.ghcuniversity.org [17].

Industry should contribute to this campaign, not with propaganda for their machines, but promoting radiotherapy in general in the world. There should be innovative approaches to the public everywhere using short messages, not costly but effective messages using social media and other methods, and not only the classic messages to governments.

Bearing in mind the present shortage, then, over the next decade, it may be roughly estimated that there is a need for at least ten thousand radiotherapy units more than the usual rate of increase of clinical oncology services in the world.

We call on big industries and all stakeholders to make the move and to change strategies to scientific Win-Win approaches and our modification of the Blue Ocean Strategy for cancer care. All would win! (see chapter 3 'The win-win modified blue ocean strategy').

The 'Blue Ocean Strategy' is a method for creating a business strategy for an enterprise or organization, which was first described in a 2004 book by W. Chan Kim and Renee Mauborgne. Blue Ocean Strategy is based on the idea that every enterprise can achieve higher profit by turning non-customers or potential customers into customers, based on value innovation and creating new demand in non-competitive markets (the so-called Blue Ocean). This approach to profit is much easier than rivalry with the competition in existing markets [18].

As cited in the chapter 'The win-win modified blue ocean strategy', what the proposal of Ahmed Elzawawy adds is that in the original blue ocean strategy, when you create new markets from those previously considered as non-customers, then you gain a market without rivalry, you swim alone! But in the win-win modified blue ocean strategy, my view is that the potential markets for clinical oncology care and radiotherapy, for example, constitute the majority of the population of our planet. Hence, after making an effective campaign of intelligent, innovative marketing, mobilizing of resources, providing different business models that can be sustained in different communities, using all possible collaborations, partnerships, and ICT to fill the big gap in qualified staff, creating interest, and considering the incentives of all possible stakeholders, (just the essential elements of what we call for), the potential radiotherapy market will exceed the usual sales by some thousands of items of equipment. It is equivalent to the amount of equipment currently manufactured by all companies multiplied by at least three or four. Hence, the point that you navigate alone in a blue ocean is not an issue. The blue ocean would be so wide that there would be no problem if other manufacturers swim as well!

Also, Elzawawy's modification may conform more to reality and what I call the psychology of business, or the behaviors of humans and business, because if you open a new market, you can't guarantee that others will come to it as well. Hence, this is not exactly the original hypothesis of the Blue Ocean Strategy, but it is based on the original one. We advocate for a broad effective global campaign, to which many could contribute, that would open eventually huge potential markets of radiotherapy, clinical oncology, and cancer care. Therefore, there will be ample space in the blue ocean, bigger than the amount that all manufacturers and companies together can fill at present.

6.2.3 Supportive, palliative care, and rehabilitation

There is no doubt that these fields are in a serious shortage in most of the world, in particular, in LMICs.

Needless to say, facilities (adequate facilities) and drugs are needed—which surely include pain and symptomatic medications, along with human capacity building, education, and training. We emphasize the high importance of what we call 'care for professional cancer care givers'. How can one expect adequate general supportive and palliative care, when the professional palliative and supportive care givers are in need of a broader experience of care. This includes covering the financial needs of life, scientific and careers support, prestige, appreciation, work conditions, vacations, and reducing burnout.

Once again, ICT and AI could help, as cited previously in this chapter. There are specialized internet website services in the world. Some new examples of this use of ICT are initiatives of The Global Health Catalyst Win-Win Initiative: the GO-U www.ghcuniversity.org and www.ecancerforall.com [16, 17]. They provide free programs and services for all. They are in need of more development, partnership, and collaborations.

What I propose here is the formation of a Virtual International Forum for Supportive and Palliative Care that would provide an open platform for willing institutes, experts, organizations, and societies, which would be composed of many parts of the world, connected to each other and to a virtual global university. They would provide educational programs and practical advice around the clock to staff wherever they are in the world via all ICTs, including mobile phones.

6.3 Feedback from Wilfred Ngwa on the same question

The top three challenges and top three opportunities are for global cancer control in the forthcoming decade [1]:

- The *Challenge* of funding for global oncology, which remains limited. *Opportunities:* this may be alleviated by greater win-win engagement of other stakeholders, such as industry, the diaspora, etc.
- The *Challenge* of distance and time barriers. *Opportunities:* this can be alleviated somewhat by the increased use of ICT and artificial intelligence, as for the GO-U (www.ghcuniversity.org) and www.ecancerforall.com [16, 17].
- *Challenge:* Cultural barriers. *Opportunities:* this can be alleviated by greater engagement of the diaspora with a greater appreciation of the cultures of both sending and receiving countries and with the potential to change the brain drain into a global health gain through such engagement and even participation via ICT-based oncology activities [10].

References

[1] Elzawawy A 2020 Top challenges and opportunities of cancer control in the new decade. Report for the editors of *Lancet Oncology* (unpublished)

[2] Elzawawy A 2008 Breast care systemic therapy: the need for more economically sustainable scientific strategies in the world *Breast Care* **3** 434–38

[3] The Win-Win Initiative www.icedoc.org/winwin.htm and www.icedoc.net/winwin.htm

[4] Johns Hopkins Medicine 2019 New blood test uses DNA ‘packaging’ patterns to detect multiple cancer types *ScienceDaily.* [Online] May 29, 2019. [Cited: September 7, 2020.] www.sciencedaily.com/releases/2019/05/190529131206.htm

[5] Lawless K 2019 [Online] August 7, 2019 Is genetic testing with saliva the best method for risk-based breast cancer screening? DNA Genotek https://blog.dnagenotek.com/is-genetic-testing-with-saliva-the-best-method-for-risk-based-breast-cancer-screening

[6] Frey C B and Osborne M 2013 The future of employment: how susceptible are jobs to computerisation? Oxford Martin School, University of Oxford, September 1, 2013 https://oxfordmartin.ox.ac.uk/publications/the-future-of-employment/#:~:text=Carl%20Benedikt%20Frey%20%26%20Michael%20Osborne&text=According%20to%20their%20estimates%2C%20about,an%20occupation’s%20probability%20of%20computerisation

[7] Mesko B *et al* 2018 Will artificial intelligence solve the human resource crisis in healthcare? *BMC Health Serv. Res.* **18** 545

[8] Teare P, Fishman M, Benzaquen O, Toledano E and Elnekave E 2017 Malignancy detection on mammography using dual deep convolutional neural networks and genetically discovered false color input enhancement *J. Digit. Imaging* **30** 499–505

[9] Ehteshami Bejnordi B, Veta M, Johannes van Diest P, van Ginneken B, Karssemeijer N and Litjens G *et al* Diagnostic assessment of deep learning algorithms for detection of lymph node metastases in women with breast cancer *JAMA* **318** 2199–210

[10] Ngwa W, Olver I and Schmeler K 2020 The use of health-related technology to reduce the gap between developed and undeveloped regions around the globe. www.ascopubs.org. March 31, 2020

[11] Elzawawy A 2012 Science and affordability of cancer drugs and radiotherapy in the world—win-win scenarios *intechopen* January 27, 2012 https://intechopen.com/books/advances-in-cancer-management/science-and-affordability-of-cancer-drugs-and-radiotherapy-in-the-world

[12] Elzawawy A 2013 *How to Get Better-Value Cancer Care: Better-Value Chemotherapy.* ed J A Muir Gray and D J Kerr (Oxford, UK: Offox Press Ltd)

[13] Elzawawy A 2015 The shortage of essential cancer drugs and generics in the united states of america. global brain storming directions for the world *ClinMed Int. Lib.* April 15, 2015 https://clinmedjournals.org/articles/ijccr/ijccr-2–016.php?jid=ijccr

[14] Elzawawy A 2019 ecancer video online July 12, 2019 https://ecancer.org/video/8112/prof-ahmed-elzawawy-on-global-cancer-control.php

[15] Elzawawy A 2013 Could African and low- and middle-income countries contribute scientifically to global cancer care? *J. Global Oncol.* **1** 49–53

[16] https://www.ghcuniversity.org/

[17] The Global Oncology University GO-U www.ghcuniversity.org

[18] Chan Kim W and Mauborgne R 2004 *Blue Ocean Strategy.* (Boston, MA: Harvard Business Review)

Chapter 7

Turning the impact of COVID-19 on cancer care into a positive

Eduardo Cazap, Ahmed Elzawawy, David Kerr, Wil Ngwa, Twalib Ngoma, Manar Montasser and Tabaré Vázquez[1]

A light in the dark: turning the current and expected negative impact of the COVID-19 pandemic on cancer care into a positive—the view of the Win-Win movement.

Going with the notion of the win-win model, thinking positively, smartly, and globally in order to learn from the COVID-19 pandemic could lead to reshaping (for the better) value-based cancer care, telemedicine, virtual and hybrid education, cancer research, clinical trials, and conferences in the direction of increased access to better global outcomes for cancer patients in the coming years.

7.1 Introduction

We see that the change has begun, and it will accelerate after the crisis of COVID-19 pandemic. The economy, in terms of systems, notions, and in many other ways, will not be the same as before. Hence, it is expected that the problem of lack of affordability of better-value cancer care will be aggravated in the upcoming years, i.e. more than previously estimated, because of the impact of the COVID-19 pandemic, or at least, this is the widely spread gloomy rumour. But, as we are in the Win-Win movement, we are on the side of searching for global improvement and not surrendering to the dismal estimation, even though it might well be true without smart global scientific action. Hence, we are in favor of the concept inspired by the recent article 'A Flower Blooms in the Bitter Soil of the Covid-19 Crisis' [1]. Many lessons could be extracted and many developments during the COVID-19 crisis could be of use in facing the increasing lack of affordability of better-value cancer care in the upcoming years.

According to the win-win notions, we advocate turning the sequels of a crisis into opportunities to modify, to improve, and to make advances. It brings to mind phrases

[1] Past President of the Republic of Uruguay deceased on December 6, 2020 after his contribution in this chapter.

doi:10.1088/978-0-7503-3075-6ch7

from a song of Madonna! 'Not everyone is going to the future … Not everyone is learning from the past!' [2, 3] Even though we are not at all sure what is behind the messages in Madonna's song, contemplating the title and lyrics of this song while reading this section about the possible future after COVID-19 is not contraindicated—on the contrary, it helps! In fact, for us it is a useful reminder that to go to the future, we should learn from the current crisis of the COVID-19 pandemic.

In fact, in the Win-Win movement, we are exploring and collaborating together to pave the way for our younger generation everywhere in the new decade.

In this short section, we give some examples of many expected changes and how we see that the sequels of COVID-19 could precipitate modifications and advances in the upcoming years.

7.2 The rate of innovation in healthcare during the COVID-19 crisis has been astonishing

As an example of a leading affluent country, the drivers that have enabled rapid innovation in the USA are [1]:

- Urgency: there has been urgency and a common enemy that mobilized and united efforts. In the USA, this resulted in the urgent implementation of unprecedented public health measures that resulted in 95% of Americans being subject to stay-at-home orders.
- Flexibility: the massive infusion of flexibility into the traditionally rigid healthcare system and the reimbursement and healthcare industry diminished barriers to innovation and increased tolerance towards creative solutions. Entrepreneurs encourage principles such as 'test and learn' and 'fail fast' to stimulate creativity and speed, yet we rarely see these principles invoked on such a large scale and with such high stakes as we have seen during the COVID-19 crisis.
- Collaboration and partnerships: the collaborations that spring to mind are those between healthcare authorities, scientists, governments, and organizations. However, an amazing example of collaboration occurred when New York essentially merged all 200 hospitals in the state into a single operating body to enable supplies and capacity to be rationally and skilfully allocated.

  While the absence of systems-based thinking among stakeholders in the industry has stalled progress in the past, during this crisis, we have seen remarkable examples of competitors who are now collaborating, such as Apple and Google combining forces to develop a contact-tracing platform.
- Focus on the whole population: we have been forced to think about the needs of the whole population more than ever before, which has drawn attention to these issues and developed the jargon with which to discuss them.

7.3 Current and prospective changes in oncology care, education and training, research, and conferences

7.3.1 Cancer care and telemedicine

In the USA, the percentage of physicians using telehealth has risen from less than 20% two years ago to almost 50% in April 2020 [4], and an estimated one billion visits will occur virtually this year [5]. We think that patients enjoy telemedicine; many doctors have now learned the technology and will most likely not go back to the same level of seeing patients physically. In the USA, past resistance to telemedicine has been due to insurance companies not wanting to reimburse its costs. They have now been forced to do so, and we hope it stays.

The situation from a Latin American perspective:

The most urgent changes that were required in various countries of the region before the SARS-Cov2 pandemic, based on expert groups and civil society opinions, were divided into four areas: medical, epidemiological, economic, and public policy. The group chaired by Edurado Cazap will produce a report together with Dr Tabaré Vázquez, immediate past president of the republic of Uruguay; that report will be directly related to the capacity of the system to adequately respond to cancer and chronic non-communicable diseases. The recommendations of the report can be summarized as follows: legislative modifications that ensure the right to health; increase public spending on health to at least 6% of the gross domestic product; strengthen a care model based on a primary healthcare (PHC) strategy and increase financing for the first level of care. It is also desirable, following the WHO recommendation, to create an 'integrated health system' that improves the current inequitable segmentation and fragmentation of the health system in many countries of the region [6]. The proposals for the time after the pandemic provided by a Latin American group of cancer experts from nine countries are:

Table I.

What happened during the pandemic?
• **Clinical practice:** a sharp drop in cancer prevention and screening, consultations, and follow-up.
• **Policy**: the development of guidelines and recommendations for cancer care during the crisis.
• **System-level changes**: specific protocols for cancer prevention, diagnosis, care and palliation, sometimes different from the ones established by the NCCP.

Table II.

Positive aspects to keep
• **Telemedicine**: remote consultations, online medical prescriptions, scheduling of appointments, etc.
• Home-based chemotherapy.
• Hypofractionated radiotherapy—short courses.
• Public communication of health issues, population awareness.

Table III.

Main Recommendations
• **Personal**: maintain prevention and follow-up. Avoid cancer treatment discontinuation. Ask your doctor.
• **Medical**: answer patients about what can be delayed, which decisions have options, and what must be done, even during the crisis.
• **Health Systems**: keep healthcare systems functional and operative for cancer patients. Avoid an excessive focus only on the COVID epidemic. Aim for resilient health systems.
• **Public Policy**: preserve NCCP operations and funding.

Table IV.

Challenges
• The role of cancer and non-communicable diseases (NCDs) in the post-pandemic environment.
• How governments and health systems will address the number of delayed patients together with the usual volume in the post-pandemic period.
• The estimated increased number of late diagnoses and later-stage patients.

Reference : Latin American Report on Cancer post-COVID19 (unpublished) [7]

7.3.2 Education and training

In the last two decades, there has been a slowly growing trend for virtual education and training in the world. In the fall of 2017, we in the Global Health Catalyst (GHC) Win-Win movement launched Global Oncology University (GO-U) to provide virtual education in the fields of the clinical care of cancer, i.e. surgical, radiation, and medical oncology, global oncology, medical radiation physics and a course on clinical research and cancer trials [8]. We also launched ecancerforall as a comprehensive cancer centre in the cloud for consultation, education, training, and research [9]. In fact, when Wilfred Ngwa raised the idea, the staff and faculty of the GHC Win-Win Movement supported it, as we expect that there is a real need for it now and more in the future. However, one could not have predicted the occurrence of the COVID-19 pandemic and its impact on virtual education and webinars.

Harvard, like other institutions, has transitioned completely to online learning, and some universities are considering this in 2020. Professors are learning the technology and better ways to communicate via online learning. This is one of the things we now want to leverage for our GO-U platform. We just completed a survey of Kenya and African centers to assess their readiness and should begin online training this summer. This is a good opportunity for GO-U to help, and such online learning may be more widely adopted after COVID-19. Hopefully, we can also potentiate a partnership with *e*cancer led by Eduardo Cazap, who stressed the importance of this issue.

7.3.3 Research

Eduardo Cazap, editor-in-chief of *ecancermedicalscience* and a leader in the GHC Win-Win Movement has stated that *e*cancer has developed a fast-track for submissions related to cancer and COVID-19. As soon as we receive the submission, we make the first evaluation on the same day; if it is ready for review, the reviewers have two days for the review and, if accepted, the paper is published the next Friday. The average time for approval is close to 1 week, which is very different from the previous review process.

As we always say in the win-win movement, there are unlimited scientific topics for research that could contribute to an increase in the affordability of better cancer care in the world. One of the issues that we raised in the Africa–Oxford–Harvard Cancer Research consortium is that the COVID-19 pandemic will force research into/adoption of some areas such as hypofractionated radiotherapy. This is actually one of the clinical trials we would like to start in Africa. Wilfred Ngwa stated that our recent paper on hypofractionated Radiotherapy [10] establishes this as definitely part of the win-win. Also, biomaterial drone studies would allow for one fraction of radiotherapy instead of the conventional 35–40 fractions in combination with an immune-adjuvant for metastatic prostate cancer and pancreas cancer [11].

In the USA, hypofractionated radiotherapy has also been adopted slowly because of insurance. During the COVID-19 pandemic crisis, hypofractionated radiotherapy was recommended by ASTRO to minimize the exposure of patients to COVID-19 [12]. The same fractionation is recommended in the UK [13].

Shorter radiotherapy treatments are an excellent option, but for years there has been reluctance from our radiotherapy colleagues to adopt these techniques widely. They are reimbursed by fraction, so shorter techniques are not economically viable, and it would be necessary to adapt the reimbursement modalities to facilitate shorter treatments.

The experiences gained from the shift to oral chemotherapy and outpatient chemotherapy infusion and the avoidance of chemotherapy protocols that necessitate hospitalization during the COVID-19 pandemic are some of the many approaches that we have highlighted in several win-win publications since 2007 to increase access to cancer treatment [14, 15].

The risk–benefit ratio for clinical trial participation has become hidden during the COVID-19 pandemic. Conversely, in some studies, patients with cancer who are enrolled in clinical trials have expressed a strong interest in continuing trial participation, despite the intensified risk [16].

Some of the positive points that could learned from the lessons of the COVID-19 pandemic that could improve clinical trials after the crisis are [17]:

- **Increase the value of trials**: resources must be assigned wisely to optimize the value of clinical trials and prevent a slowdown of this critical aspect of cancer research.
- **Raising the bar in clinical research:** the scientific community must share its collective insight to raise the bar in order to conduct the clinical trials that have the greatest potential for yielding meaningful outcomes, supported by

strong biological hypotheses that go with patients in the communities of studies of and guided by validated biomarkers.

- **Re-establishing clinical trial design to increase efficiency:** invalid substitute endpoints should not replace overall survival and quality of life as the most relevant outcomes in randomized clinical trials [18].
- **Avoiding waste:** the sharing of trial protocols within the research community will reduce dismissals and should be possible in the pre-competitive and post-competitive stages of drug development. Attention should be paid to discouraging the testing of drug combinations that do not have a clear track to improving the therapeutic index.
- **Addressing relevant questions:** particularly with the notions of win-win movement, i.e. that research and trials could lead to resource-sparing cancer treatment, increase its value, and contribute to increasing the affordability of proven-value care. Some examples are cited in this book [4, 15], such as repurposing drugs, different radiation therapy technologies and fractionations, decreasing the unproven duration of courses of drugs and upcoming trials such as drones of immunotherapy, and the use of smart biomaterials accompanied by a single fraction of radiotherapy in metastatic prostate carcinoma [11].
- **Rethinking clinical trial dogmas:** in order to increase transparency, maximize data accuracy, and ensure pharmacovigilance; clinical trial operations have become progressively more complicated. Despite the incorporation of modern tools, such as web-based data sharing and capture platforms, trials remain heavily bureaucratic.

The COVID-19 pandemic has steered us to reconsider the value of some practices that were supposed to be obligatory: (a) the wet-ink signatures required for trial documents that should be reduced, or even better, replaced by electronic signatures; (b) duplicate requests by different sponsors for investigator credentials, site feasibility, and declarations of conflict may be replaced by an open online database containing the available information for all; (c) the value of excessive serial physical examinations in asymptomatic patients is a subject of inquiry [19]. However, care must be taken to not to omit physical examinations, as this will compromise vigilance; (d) for laboratory tests, mobile or internet appointments for tests in local laboratories and imaging departments may be sufficient, negating safety concerns and potentially saving time and resources; (e) eligibility criteria of unproven value should be removed from protocols; (f) there are opportunities to decentralize and to create frameworks for scientific studies and research; (g) future frameworks could facilitate tissue diagnosis, molecular characterization, and staging locally, while virtual tumor boards and discussions could be regularly conducted; (h) the administration of drug infusions in local satellite centers has also been explored [20].

7.3.4 Conferences

Back in March 2017, in an editorial based on the notions of the win-win initiative, Ahmed Elzawawy presented a proposal as part of brainstorming. The objective is to save most of the expenses of the majority—but not all—of the conferences paid for by pharmaceuticals and radiotherapy manufacturers so that oncologists can travel from LMICs to attend international conferences. The saved sum could be one of the resources used to increase the access to cancer care in some underserved regions. It is not a call to stop all support for attendance or travel but to limit it.

One of our suggestions in this editorial was that information communications technology (ICT) could allow wider participation from LMICs, while saving the expenses of travel, airlines, and accommodation to be used for increasing the access to cancer services in underserved regions. Also, we suggest that companies will pay fees to societies and organizers to allow access for individuals and virtual group participation by universities or hospitals, while saving travel expenses and onco-tourism! Hence, societies would not lose the fees from registrations, but potentially registration, interactive participation, and the audience could be augmented [21].

Three years from the above-cited editorial, in March–April, 2020, with the appearance of the COVID-19 crisis, there are other reasons to think about virtual conferences. The title of a recent Medscape article was clear enough to say 'Medical Meetings May Be Forever Changed'. The reader can access hot comments at the end of this online article [22].

We advocate reason and moderation in the coming years. This does not mean—in any way—that we are calling for a complete cancellation of face-to-face summits or the main big conferences, or that we completely ignore the value of face-to-face meetings, but it would give them more importance and increased registration—after reducing some hundreds of conferences in the world to being virtual—and would increase the audience if online participation were added to the face-to-face on-site attendance.

Face-to-face meetings, with their value, will be restored after the COVID-19 pandemic, but we hope that they will be fewer in number and they could be hybrid meetings, i.e. face-to-face plus a virtual meeting.

For example, the upcoming GHC Win-Win annual summit in May 2021 will be either hybrid or virtual, according to the state of the COVID-19 pandemic.

Companies could invest the saved funds in a global campaign that could establish at least ten units of clinical oncology in LMICs yearly using this funding. That is more than the total that is accomplished at present by all international organizations, including the International Atomic Energy Agency and all other initiatives together. Moreover, as we cited in other parts of this book, we stress the great need to fund an effective campaign to promote the establishment of clinical oncology and the running of value-based services. This is not intended to compete with any initiative, but to complement, potentiate, and partner with all the current efforts. These clinical oncology units would treat patients and create jobs, training, and collaborative relevant research. Moreover, they will assist in paving the way for more establishments, the running of clinical oncology units, and more marketing for the sales of cancer treatment drugs and equipment.

Are all these reasons not sufficiently convincing?

We do not claim that the abovementioned way of saving some funds will solve all problems of affordability, but it is just a small contribution. It is one of many win-win calls to search together for several ideas for solutions, instead of complaining. The implementation of this proposal and its sustainability depends on its win-win for all!

On the other hand, we need to consider several other aspects that are part of the process, not only the simple educational ones. Pharmaceutical companies, convention centers, societies and organizations, private meeting organizers, airlines, hotels, etc. are also parts of the equation, and in the post-COVID world, the economy will urgently need to continue with personal meetings or hybrid approaches for economic reasons.

We do not claim that this proposal is ideal and should be applied as-is in the real world; however, this crisis is also an opportunity to be flexible and alert to making the necessary changes and adaptations.

7.4 Concluding note

Learning from the experiences gained during—and hopefully after—the COVID-19 pandemic, and going with the notions of the Win-Win movement, we can say that we should move globally in order to let beautiful flowers blossom from the bitter soil of both the lack of affordability of better-value cancer care and the impacts of COVID-19 on the health system, economy, and spending, including that of cancer care. Hence, we stress once more the concept of using all the possible smart approaches in order to turn a crisis into a constructive step forward.

References

[1] Ryu J, Russell K and Shrank W 2020 A flower blooms in the bitter soil of the Covid-19 crisis *NEJM Catalyst.* https://catalyst.nejm.org/doi/full/10.1056/CAT.20.0321?cid=DM97637_Catalyst_registered_users_HMO_HOC_HOO_HOU_HSM_LTC_MSP_OTH_PHC_PHO_PRS_REA_COL_ANC_COR_PTR_AMC&bid=247866169

[2] Madonna, quavo—future (lyrics). *Youtube* May 17, 2019 https://youtube.com/watch?v=E7mJtN75NiM

[3] Marshall Q K *et al* Madonna future song lyrics. *Google.* [Online] universal Music Publishing Group, Warner Chappell Music, Inc., Kobalt Music Publishing Ltd https://google.com/search?q=madonna+future+song+lyrics&rlz=1C1JZAP_enEG883EG883&oq=madonna+future+song+lyrics&aqs=chrome..69i57.17751j0j4&sourceid=chrome&i.e.=UTF-8

[4] Dallas T X 2020 Merritt Hawkins April 22, 2020 https://merritthawkins.com/news-and-insights/media-room/press/-Physician-Practice-Patterns-Changing-as-a-Result-of-COVID-19/

[5] Becker J and Trzcinski A U S 2020 April 10, 2020 Virtual care visits to soar to more than 1 billion. Forrester.

[6] Cazap E The situation from a Latin American perspective. Personal communication

[7] Latin American Report on Cancer post-COVID19. Unpublished data

[8] Global Oncology University (GO-U) www.ghcuniversity.org

[9] ecancerforall www.ecancerforall.com

[10] Irabor O C *et al* 2019 Expanding global access to breast and prostate radiotherapy through evidence-based hypofractionation techniques *Int. J. Radiat. Oncol. Biol. Phys.* **105** E12

[11] Ngwa W *et al* 2018 Using immunotherapy to boost the abscopal effect *Nat. Rev./Cancer.* **18** 313–22

[12] ASTRO-COVID-19 recommendations and information-summary https://astro.org/Daily-Practice/COVID-19-Recommendations-and-Information/Summary

[13] 2020 Nice Guideline. COVID-19 rapid guideline: delivery of radiotherapy NICE guideline. Published 28 March 2020 https://nice.org.uk/guidance/ng162/resources/covid19-rapid-guideline-delivery-of-radiotherapy-pdf-66141897390277

[14] Elzawawy A 2012 Science and affordability of cancer drugs and radiotherapy in the world: win-win scenarios ed R Mohan *Advances in Cancer Management.* (Rijeka: InTech) http://intechopen.com/articles/show/title/science-and-affordability-of-cancer-drugs-and-radiotherapy-in-the-world

[15] Elzawawy A 2013 Better value chemotherapy *How to Get Better Value Cancer Care* ed J A Muir Gray and D J Kerr (Oxford, UK: Offox Press Ltd)

[16] Sidaway P 2020 COVID-19 and cancer: what we know so far. *Nat Rev Clin Oncol.* **17** 336

[17] Araujo D V, Watson G A and Siu L L 2020 The day after COVID-19—time to rethink oncology clinical research *JAMA Oncol.* **7** 23–4

[18] Prasad V, Kim C, Burotto M and Vandross A 2015 The strength of association between surrogate end points and survival in oncology: a systematic review of trial-level meta-analyses *JAMA Intern Med.* **175** 1389–98

[19] Mehrotra A and Prochazka A 2015 Improving value in health care—against the annual physical *N. Engl. J. Med.* **373** 1485–87

[20] Cinar P, Kubal T and Freifeld A *et al* 2020 Safety at the time of the COVID-19 pandemic: how to keep our oncology patients and healthcare workers safe *J. Natl. Compr. Cancer Netw.* **18** 504–9

[21] Elzawawy A 2017 One more proposal to allocate resources for the win-win approaches to increase the affordability of cancer drugs and radiotherapy in the World 2017 *J. Cancer Prev. Curr. Res.* **7** 00250

[22] Mulcahy N 2020 Medical meetings may be forever changed Medscape Med. News. https://medscape.com/viewarticle/927626

Chapter 8

Main global health catalyst networks and means

Wilfred Ngwa and Ahmed Elzawawy

(On behalf all the leaders, ambassadors, faculty, and colleagues in the GHC Win-Win Movement)

In this chapter, we present the main means and channels of the Global Health Catalyst (GHC) Win-Win Movement and initiatives (GHC Win-Win): the Corps of Catalysts, advisers, and Win-Win consultants; scientific research and publications (including this book); the Global Oncology University (GO-U) www.ghcuniversity.org for online education plus onsite training; ecancerforall (previously ecancer4all); the Africa–Oxford–Harvard Cancer Research Consortium (AFROX-H); the corps of the honorary and Win-Win distinguished ambassadors; the Young Catalysts' Win-Win Collaboration; and the Global Health Catalyst Summits.

8.1 Introduction

As mentioned before, the Win-Win initiative was proposed by Ahmed Elzawawy in December 2007, and its two wings are described in chapter 1. The development of channels took place after the adoption of Win-Win Initiative in April 2016 by the Global Health Catalyst, directed by Wilfred Ngwa, Harvard University, USA. Partnerships and collaborations with many distinguished contributors are the basis of the hand-in-hand spirit of the Win-Win Movement of GHC.

Hence, up to the fall of 2019, it was named the Harvard GHC Win-Win. Starting from the year 2020, as a result of broader partnerships and leaderships, GHC Win-Win took the name of the Global Health Catalyst Win-Win Movement (GHC Win-Win), directed by Wilfred Ngwa, with activities initiated and led by colleagues at Harvard University (Johns Hopkins University and the Dana-Farber/Cancer Institute are the main coordination sites), the University of Pennsylvania, Oxford University, Argentina, Sweden, Heidelberg University in Germany, Tanzania, Egypt, the South Asia Institute of Physics and Cancer Research, and others. As a principle, partnerships are open to all organizations, institutes, societies and individuals, experts and stakeholders who share our common objective of increasing the affordability of better-

doi:10.1088/978-0-7503-3075-6ch8

value cancer care in the world via scientific and practical approaches. In the coming years, Professor Wilfred Ngwa will help to direct the whole Global Health Win-Win initiative and channels, with the main hub at Johns Hopkins University in collaboration with other leading institutions: Harvard, UPENN, and Heidelberg, with different partners and collaborators around the world.

As we explained in chapter 1, we started the Win-Win movement with its channels as a result of evident needs before the COVID-19 crisis, but in the world after the crisis, it becomes a must.

The main channels of the GHC Win-Win Movement are:

1. The Corps of Catalysts, advisers, and Win-Win consultants.
2. Scientific research and publications (including this book).
3. The Global Oncology University (GO-U) www.ghcuniversity.org for online education plus onsite training and ecancerforall (previously ecancer4all).
4. The Africa–Oxford–Harvard Cancer Research Consortium (AFROX-H).
5. The corps of the honorary and Win-Win distinguished ambassadors.
6. The young catalysts' Win-Win collaboration.
7. The Global Health Catalyst Summits.

Note about ecancerforall

ecancerforall (previously ecancer4all) was established by Harvard GHC and its Win-Win Initiative (see https://www.ghcuniversity.org/).

- The premier Comprehensive Cancer Center in the Cloud (C4), which exists to dramatically increase access to cancer care, research, and education

Service offerings:

(a) CARE: tele-oncology: e-consultation, second opinion, e-contouring, remote treatment planning and quality assurance support, plus other Win-Win advice to establish more clinical oncology–radiotherapy services. These are offered by the Corps of Catalysts, advisers, and Win-Win consultants.
(b) EDUCATION: online learning, with tutorials to complement workshops. A Part of GO-U.
(c) RESEARCH: multicenter clinical trials, implementation research, AFROX-H clinical trial network including new drones technology combining radiotherapy with immunotherapy
(d) Outreach: diaspora, industry, government, e.g. *IBM partnership for artificial intelligence* in chemotherapy to assist doctors to use appropriate treatment guidelines

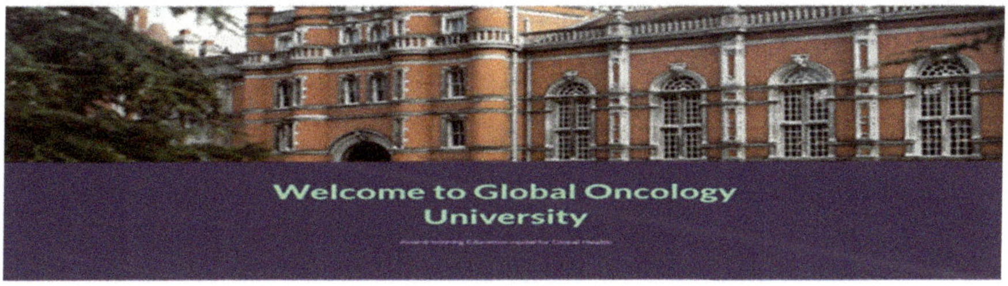

Global Oncology University (GO-U) provides access from any country to the same world-class education and training as that available at the world's best universities and medical schools. See https://www.ghcuniversity.org/ and https://www.ghcuniversity.org/faculty https://www.ghcuniversity.org/academics.

Academic excellence with high impact: GO University is dedicated to being the leading high-impact global oncology university in the world. It is founded on an Excellence in Education Award-winning collaborative global health training model; hence, academic excellence is at the very core of everything at this university. Our faculty is amongst the best and includes members from Harvard University (USA), Johns Hopkins University (USA), the University of Pennsylvania (USA), the University of Massachusetts (USA), Oxford University (UK), the University of Heidelberg (Germany), the University of Gothenburg (Sweden), and experienced faculty from all over the world. Moreover, there are open contributions from a global health consortium including professional societies (including international, high-income, and LMIC societies such as FAMPO and AORTIC) and growing partnerships including industry, and health ministries of different countries aiming to build crucial human capacity to strengthen healthcare systems.

GO-U empowers a crucial global workforce, building on an award-winning collaborative education model with online lectures accessible from any country, and practical/clinical training in local/regional credentialed sites across the globe.

GO-U is a premier University that offers continuous medical education, degrees (Master, PhD) and clinical MMed, and residency training in clinical oncology (radiation and medical oncology) with the vision of eliminating global cancer health disparities.

It also includes the courses and training in surgical oncology, clinical trials … research, artificial intelligence, medical physics, imaging, clinical pathology, and global oncology.

The world has already webinars and online courses. The peculiarity of the GO-U online courses, programs, and training is that we are not only providing students with classical information, knowledge, skills, and competency, but also tackling the most urgent yet affordable issues in clinical cancer treatment that can be tailored to different communities. An important flavour is that as far as possible, faculty and trainers present different scientific options for the management and treatment of cancer and not just one guideline; hence, candidates do their best on a scientific basis to provide best-value patient-centered cancer care that fits local communities and to increase its affordability in the real world.

Moreover, as we expressed clearly to the Harvard GHC Win-Win initiative and partners, what is peculiar to the GO-U is that 'We are not preparing the students for the present only, but supply them with skills and brainstorming to remarkably improve the availability and affordability of value-based cancer treatment and relevant research in their own countries. We are also keen for the GO-U to have the special flavor of not only making candidates ready for the present, but giving them tools that are 'wings to fly' for the near future and what we may predict or not for the future.

Hence, as a result of its distinguished faculty and partnerships and by the formation of competent human scientific capabilities in the world, the GO-U can contribute to improving the present and preparing for more prospective advances in cancer treatment and care.

Interactive discussions with students are encouraged so that they can suggest and present proposals to solve their local problems as useful exercises. In the GO-U postgraduate and continuous education courses, the students are also taught the principles of how to establish their services and how to update existing services.

Practical information about different business models, the running of services, and the realistic management of the daily problems of operations and maintenance is provided. That is why the faculty are not only from universities and institutes, but also from industry as well, as their active contribution to the schedule of the GO-U is essential to management in the real world. The involvement of personalities from big societies, organizations, and initiatives is considered in order to give students information on how to be connected and how to benefit from the international community and be a part of it. In the win-win initiative, there are no rivalries with any, but we are complementing all. The information and skills about how to perform relevant research and how to be connected to international scientific communities are considered in the schedule by experts in research and trials. Moreover, lectures and useful information will be presented by the editors of high-impact journals and of ecancer articles and videos. A clever approach to reality and giving patients the most accessible better-value care in the present will be accompanied by continuously updated information, preparing the students for new developments in artificial intelligence, the use of robots in cancer diagnosis and treatment, digital radiology, and digital pathology. All the above points are just a part of what I mean by the special flavor of the GO-U, which contributes to its success and support.

So, we are asking the entire distinguished and cherished faculty to contribute their input and thoughts to making this specific flavor for the GO-U that belongs to all of you, as it is driven by your GHC Win-Win initiative.

Finally, all we have done and are doing is teamwork that is progressing in very friendly and constructive ambiance. We are looking forward to seeing further contributions from the distinguished faculty and collaboration with different organizations and institutes to make remarkable progress and move together.

Note about the honorary and distinguished ambassadors of the Harvard Global Health Catalyst Win-Win Initiative

Background: it is known that there is a great need to enhance effective efforts to fill the huge gaps in value-based clinical oncology care worldwide!

The Harvard GHC Win-Win Initiative adopts scientific approaches and Win-Win scenarios that consider all stakeholders. We also emphasize that we are catalysts, consultants, and advisers. We are not competing with, or replacing any others, but we are complementing, empowering, and positive mediators and open to all partnership and collaboration. We are not a funding body.

Moreover, to achieve a remarkable increase in clinical oncology and radiotherapy services, broad advocacy is needed at all levels globally.

The required roles of the honorary and distinguished Win-Win ambassadors:

- They are kindly asked to be high representatives, advocates, and voices for the cause of the initiative at different levels and on international and national occasions.

For the distinguished ambassadors (who are usually professionals and experts in fields related to cancer):

- They are volunteer experts who can advise and act as catalysts for the establishment and development of clinical oncology–radiotherapy services. We are NOT marketing certain devices or drugs and are not agents for any company, but we can offer technical and medical advice about radiotherapy-clinical oncology projects from A to Z, i.e. from the idea until the service is operational and for years afterward. Our GO-U and ecancerforall (previously ecancer4all) can help.
- Some of the Willing Win-Win ambassadors could help by advising and mentoring the Harvard GHC Win-Win young ambassadors. ecancerforall provides an e-platform (we are one initiative, with one focused objective).

The corps of the Harvard GHC Win-Win young catalysts:
There are increasing numbers of hundreds of young volunteers from different countries who join the corps of the Win-Win young ambassadors. They will form the corps of different activities of the initiative. This helps in the present, and it also assures sustainability and their future progress.

AFRICA OXFORD HARVARD JOHNS HOPKINS CANCER RESEARCH and CLINICAL TRIALS CONSORTIUM (AFROX-H Trials Network)

AIMS: The aims of the AFROX-H Network are to:

- Create a clinical trials network, supported by Oxford and Harvard, with the capacity to undertake proof-of-principle phase II and large-scale phase III studies incorporating the leading African comprehensive cancer centres
- Conduct multicenter clinical trials and scientific studies. This could leverage information and communications technologies and artificial intelligence
- Provide education and training to build the sustained human capacity needed to support the network
- Partner with governments, international organizations, NGOs, research institutions, and industry to support the network

The Global Health Catalyst summits
The summits, initiated and directed by Wil Ngwa and colleagues are not just meetings, directed by Wil Ngwa and colleagues, but summits to elaborate collaborations, partnerships, and catalytic actions to empower the realization of the objective of Global Health Catalyst Win-Win movement for the sake of humans with cancer, with a special focus on Africa. Five annual summits have been held at Harvard Medical School since 2015.

This book, which describes the different topics of the win-win movement will be the main theme of the upcoming Global Health Catalyst summits (which will be hybrid). All are invited to contribute to this living book by sending their feedback, ideas, and suggestions. From now until the Summit, we call on partners, international cancer care bodies, societies, organizations, industries, and all stakeholders to crystallize and develop an international effective campaign to make a remarkable and historical global increase in value-based clinical oncology units in the next ten years. Moreover, the progress and new ideas that serve as the objective of this book will be one of the main themes of the next five annual GHC summits.

Chapter 9

Publications and dissemination

Ahmed Elzawawy, Eduardo Cazap, David Kerr, Wilfred Ngwa, with contributors: Gemma Alderton, Riccardo Audisio, Danny Burke, David Collingridge, Jessica Fricchione, Allison Landman, Gilberto Lopez, Richard Sullivan and Anthony Zietman

With contributions from:
The contributors in the panel and follow up are among the distinguished leaders of cancer care publications in the world (in alphabetical order):

- **Gemma Alderton (senior editor, *Science*)**
- **Riccardo Audisio (editor-in-chief, *European Journal of Surgical Oncology*)**
- **Danny Burke (associate CEO, *e*cancer)**
- **Eduardo Cazap (editor-in-chief, *e*cancer, co-editor of the global section of *The Oncologist*, and past president, the Union for International Cancer Control (UICC))**
- **David Collingridge (editor-in-chief, *The Lancet Oncology*)**
- **Jessica Fricchione (senior commissioning editor, Institute of Physics (IOP) Publishing)**
- **David Kerr (past president of the European Society for Medical Oncology (ESMO), editor emeritus of the *Annals of Oncology*, founding editor of the *Journal of Global Oncology*, professor of cancer medicine, Oxford, UK)**
- **Allison Landman (deputy editor, *The Lancet Oncology*)**
- **Gilberto Lopez (editor-in-chief, *Journal of Global Oncology* (issued by the American Society of Clinical Oncology (ASCO)))**
- **Richard Sullivan (chair of the trustees, *e*cancer Global Foundation, UK)**
- **Anthony Zietman (editor-in-chief, the 'Red Journal' or *International Journal of Radiation Oncology, Biology, Physics*)**

—**Discussants: Sarwat Hussain** (professor of radiology at the University of Massachusetts and the editor-in-chief of the *Journal of Global Radiology*), **Twalib Ngoma** (a professor and clinical oncologist, Tanzania, a leader in the GHC Win-Win

Initiative, vice chancellor of Global Oncology University GO-U, and past president of AORTIC), **Biatrice Wiafe Addai** (breast surgeon, Ghana, president-elect of AORTIC), **Elizabeth Charlotte Mosser** (a radiation oncologist and Chief Scientific Officer, Nanocan Therapeutics), **Eric Ford** (a professor of radiation oncology and a medical physicist, Seattle, Washington, USA), Cristina Stefan (past President, AORTIC), Rose Anorlu (President, AORTIC) and Miriam Mutebi (President Elect, AORTIC). (The Editors welcomed feedback and discussions from many colleagues and will continue to receive openly from all after publication of this book.)
—Contributors to progress and early outcome: Richard Sullivan (chair of the trustees, *e*cancer global Foundation, UK), **Allison Landman** (deputy editor, *The Lancet Oncology*).
—Coordinators of follow up: Ahmed Elzawawy, Eduardo Cazap, David Kerr and Wilfred Ngwa.

This chapter has three sections: section 9.1 is based on Ahmed Elzawawy's notes sent to contributors and on discussions with the panelists—contributors in the weeks before the Global Health Catalyst (GHC) Summit on May 25, 2019. It therefore reflects their common ideas and not a single view. The aim was for the Summit to crystallize—together—a call for a global scientific win-win movement and therefore also for publications focused on a common objective, which is how to remarkably increase the affordability of value-based cancer treatment in the world, in both affluent and less affluent countries. Section 9.2 is the summary of the minutes of the session 'Publications and Dissemination' held on May 25, 2019 during the GHC Summit at Harvard Medical School, Boston, MA, USA. The following is a link to the session: https://www.youtube.com/watch?v=r0v1nJISLuM&feature=youtu.be. Section 9.3 is a brief about the early outcomes and perspectives.

9.1 Section 1: Ahmed Elzawawy

An introduction

We will avoid a long introduction and background, as we are all deeply aware of the skyrocketing rise of the cost of cancer treatment and that there is an increasing crisis in its affordability. The continuous rise in the cost of treatment is not commensurate with the increase in value-based outcomes. This problem is increasingly manifested in high-income countries (HICs) and to a greater extent in low- and middle-income countries (LMICs). Despite the endeavors of all, i.e. organizations, societies, publications, conferences, and commissions, the gap between what is required and available cancer treatment services in LMICs has broadened in the last ten years! If we continue in the same way, then this situation will be further aggravated [1].

Hence, there can be no doubt that there is a need for lot of relevant research and publications of strong evidence, which includes fields of scientific exploration, win-win scenarios, ideas, thoughts, and efforts. This win-win scientific movement could lead to the achievement of the common objective, which is to fill the huge gaps in the affordability of better-value cancer care, particularly for the underserved patients in the whole world (referred to in the text as the 'objective'). The goal is that cancer patients in the world should get their value-based treatment with dignity (referred to in the text as the 'goal'). In the win-win movement, we see that a human who has dignity has essential components: at a minimum, the financial, physical, and social aspects of dignity. The focus here is: 'how can a movement aiming to increase publications in high-impact journals, ecancer publications, and videos serve the common objective and the goal via scientific approaches and Win-Win scenarios?' In addition to the present large roles played by high-impact journals, ecancer publications, and publishers in serving this cause, we suggest the devotion of larger tracks and permanent sections in journals and ecancer publications to encourage authors from everywhere to publish scientific studies, trials, reports, editorials, and ideas focused on scientific approaches to increasing the affordability of better-value care in the world (the aim). Our real success will be measured by achieving a remarkable increase in the affordability of better-value cancer treatment in the world (the objective) and not just the number of publications, conferences, and commissions.

We present here a sort of brainstorm in the form of questions and answers that summarize points as seen by the Win-Win initiative

Q1: Who will gain?
Answer: All would win. As we know, in most cases, good ideas, suggestions, scientific findings, or inventions are treated as if they never existed if they are not published.

The win-win scientific publication movement acts as a stimulator and it would smartly serve all parties in the real world i.e. the progress of science, in particular, 'human-being-centered sciences', cancer patient care in both rich and less affluent countries, improve the outcomes of the practice of oncology, widen the fields of research and publications for cancer scientists, and lessen the burden on governments.

The increase in affordability for millions more cancer patients would decrease the risk of systemic economic collapse. It may boost the medical device and pharmaceutical industries by increasing their consumers and expanding their markets. To avoid any confusion about boosting industries in the last sentence, disclosure of any conflict of interest should be applied as standard.

Q2: What is the gain for journals, in particular, high-impact publications and ecancer publications?
Answer: The movement could enrich the flow of submitted articles meeting the common objective of this meeting. This is aligned with the general missions and objectives of journals.

Q3: Does this mean accepting articles with reduced scientific quality in these sections?
Answer: No.

In addition, this raises the issue of 'what is high-quality published science?' that Ahmed Elzawawy mentioned in ecancer video interviews with Eduardo Cazap as a part of series focusing on visionary global oncology leaders [2]. High-quality published science could consist of excellent discoveries. However, there is also a great need for research and studies to describe how to use, how to implement, and how to make cancer care affordable for human beings in the real world via scientific approaches. In addition, there is an increasing demand to define, using scientific and patient-centered bases, which diagnostic tests, treatments, and care would be of real value for patients in different communities in the real world.

Moreover, we emphasize the value of North-South and South-South scientific collaborations in joint research that provide technical and scientific assistance, starting with the design of studies, protocols, and projects, tests, data management, the interpretation of findings, and assisting in the revision of texts, all published in publications that would include the names of all the authors of the combined work. All would win [2–5].

Q4: Does 'in these tracks in journals or sections' mean that articles would only be accepted from or about LMICs?
Answer: No.

Articles will be accepted from everywhere in the world; from affluent and less affluent countries, provided that they are of good scientific quality and that they serve the objective. In some articles and ecancer videos [3, 6], we have cited some examples of how LMICs could contribute scientifically to the progress of cancer care, both in their countries and in the world. What would count is that the articles accepted for publication are scientifically sound explorations or research related to increasing the value and/or affordability of a treatment or diagnostic methods [7–9].

Q5: Is the concern regarding scientific approaches to value-based cancer treatment and the affordability due to financial reasons?
Answer: No.

What ultimately counts is that the patients can receive their value-based treatment without many difficulties in obtaining their care. The reasons for difficulties are variable. Hence, the fields of study are open to any who can realize greater availability of care.

One example is the problem of shortage of essential cancer drugs and generics in the USA. We have tackled this problem in some of our publications [10, 11], based on many important studies in the USA [10, 11]. In one of these articles (which is open access) the reader can find a brainstorm that aims to effectively lessen the problem in the USA while thinking globally [11].

Q6: Does this mean global health or global oncology? If so, then what would this movement add?
Answer: Global oncology and global health are broad terms that include many items, including the present topic [12]. However, global oncology is more specific to our area.

In perspective, this movement particularly focuses on the publication of articles and videos about scientific exploration for solutions or ideas that could lead to an increase in the affordability of and/or better-value cancer treatment in different communities. Hence, it is not duplicating or challenging many good works about global public health issues that provide precious information about the magnitude of the problems, recommendations, and plans. The world is still in need of thousands of publications focused on scientific solutions or at least potential solutions to realize the common objective and goal, as stated in the meeting and in this chapter. All fields of science could be tackled, e.g. pharmacokinetics, pharmacodynamics, pharmacogenomics, clinical trials, and studies of resource-sparing cancer care that could lead to a decrease in the total cost of a treatment or drug without compromising its outcome. Moreover, studies about human capacity building in all disciplines of cancer care and research, programs of education and training in all modalities of cancer care, medical physics, relevant economic studies, and business models are recommended. In addition, all the relevant practical approaches and implementation research that could lead to an increase in the value and potential affordability of cancer care in the world should be encouraged [2, 7, 9]. Many scientific examples are cited in different chapters in this book.

Hence, this could be the start of a big movement led by the panelists and all the distinguished leaders of the scientific cancer community. To be realistic and achieve a smooth outcome from this win-win publication movement, we emphasize the that issue of its adoption (or otherwise) and the details of its implementation will be according to the internal policy and affairs of each journal. Finally, we hope that this publication movement will be translated into our common goal which is: 'Millions more cancer patients will get their better-value treatment with dignity in the upcoming years in the real world.'

9.2 Section 2: all panelists and contributors

Here is a summary of the minutes of the session 'Publications and Dissemination', May 25, 2019, GHC Summit at Harvard Medical School, Boston, MA, USA. It is written in the form of a panel discussion. The reader can find a link to its video at the end of this section. As this is a living book, readers can join in extended participation whenever they like after the publication of the book. They can send further points and constructive suggestions using the feedback link at the end of this chapter and at different points in this book.

Panel Moderator: Ahmed Elzawawy

Introduction

I hope that this session with the distinguished panelists and all participants will be the start of a big change for the better. It was preceded by our preparatory meeting and the notes to contributors (as shown in the first section of this chapter). This will continue as a growing Win-Win Movement by all of you.

An increasing problem that we are confronting everywhere in the world, both rich and poor, is the affordability of better-value cancer treatment with dignity, i.e. social, financial, and physical dignity. Our meeting is not a talk of politicians, it is not a talk of general public health, but the issue is at the heart of global oncology and as a part of global health. It concerns what we work for as doctors, scientists, physicists, and chemists. Science can give us unlimited solutions. However, publications will not do everything. There are duties for all organizations and all societies. In the Global Health Catalyst Win-Win Initiative, a part of our task is to encourage and to catalyze explorations of scientific approaches to increasing the affordability of better-value cancer treatments. We don't talk about begging, pity, weeping, the magnitude of the problem, or tragic situations. But we focus on how science could find solutions. Scientific approaches are unlimited. They could comprise radiology, radiotherapy, clinical trials, and surgical oncology. They also include, among others, conducting pharmacokinetic, pharmacodynamic, pharmacogenomic, biological, and clinical studies and selecting which patient will benefit from this drug and which patient will not benefit, searching for more indications and uses for certain treatments or newer combinations of repurposed drugs, radiology, radiotherapy, and all relevant fields.

We are not calling for publications to accept articles at less than scientific levels. When we say 'patient centered', we are not leaving science, this is science. The third and fourth revolutions in healthcare and science imply being 'patient centered'. Among the elements of the fourth revolution are artificial intelligence, big data, and advances in computing. So, we are not at all leaving science.

We are confronted with skyrocketing costs and—eventually—difficulties with the affordability of cancer care. In a recent ASCO survey [13] in the USA, around 40% of cancer patients abandoned oncologists and oncological medicine. The primary cause of their fear of cancer is due to the cost of treatment. Hence, we can imagine what is going on in developing countries. Last month, the FDA announced a pilot study to recycle the oral pills used in cancer immunotherapy. Some patients die with expensive oral drugs left over; other patients can use these drugs. These are real examples that show how there is a crisis in the USA; one can then envisage what could be the case be for millions of patients in underserved regions of the world.

This is just a short introduction. But, with all of you, I hope for this to be the start of a big movement for the sake of all stakeholders. As we say always, it is win-win.

David Collingridge, panelist

The issue of global health and the publishing aspect of global health is extremely important. I have two roles at The Lancet Group, as both Editor-in-Chief of *The Lancet Oncology* and as the Publishing Director for our specialty journals. I often say to all editors to keep an open mind whenever they are reviewing new submissions. It is very easy to look at a paper with your PhD hat on and find a problem with anything. But, you need to ask yourself, 'is it the best data on this issue?'. 'Is this the best information we have got on this problem?' If it is, perhaps we should proceed with it, regardless of the faults. *The Lancet Oncology* approaches this type of dilemma in many ways, which I mentioned in my talk. With Commissions, for example, we want to challenge a community to find new data. Last week, I was in Montevideo and I was talking to one of the government ministers. It is always interesting to see how much information governments are sitting on—and how rarely it is widely published. That real-world data can be incredibly useful: if you look at breast cancer survival in Uruguay, it is approaching 85%. This is the same as Western Europe and Northern America. But would you have thought that would be the case in Latin America, from Uruguay? Clearly, that is the case, but little of that data is published in the global literature. It is the job of an editor to encourage publication of this data. It is very easy for a journal like mine to receive the big ground-breaking clinical studies, phase two or three trials, but we know these contain restricted numbers of patients. So, real-world validation that these treatments work in the wider community is incredibly important. It goes beyond that, though; it's about providing the evidence to inform policy and health policy. We all talk about evidence-based medicine, but we really should be shouting about evidence-based policy and dissecting policy from politics. I think journals and magazines have an important role in informing and educating everyone in this area, but also uncovering new data and bringing this information to light.

Anthony Ziteman, panelist

I am the editor-in-chief of the 'red journal', the *International Journal of Radiation Oncology, Biology, Physics*. The thing that always snuggles me in this world of Instagram and Google is that they still exist, and they bind us together. Radiation oncologists in Peru or Boston or Bogata or Botswana will all read the red journal. That is an incredible opportunity; it is an opportunity to publish good and relevant science. If I feel that a particular piece of clinical science has good relevance outside the usual confines of Northern Europe or the United States, I will actually solicit a commentary, an editorial, to highlight that fact. But, the one thing we have found that has been the base of community binding is: every second edition, we invite someone from a particular nation around the globe to write their experience of the practice of oncology in their own country. I don't want to know what's similar between Uruguay and the United States; I want to know what's different. I want them to bring out cultural differences and I want them to bring out their local solutions. We have some marvelous examples of this. Just hearing from Japan, another high-tech nation, but it is a nation that has a terrible relationship with radiation, think Hiroshima, think Fukushima. So, they have big problems essentially persuading patients to have lifesaving therapy. In Iran, one of the problems is essential; it is a problem to get radioactive materials for the treatment of cervical cancer. The Philippines is a nation of seven thousand islands; all of the radiotherapy is concentrated on one of them that is in a city, Manila, with the worst traffic problem in the world. So, that's the problem that they have to solve. Another good example is also from the Philippines: their great resourcefulness, in which the immobilization devices that hold patients still for radiotherapy are very expensive. So, they went to their local mattress manufacturers, and they got something called Chemical A and Chemical B. When you mix the two together you get a fabulous material for holding heads still for the radiation beam. These are little examples for local solutions that can be propagated throughout journals. So, the journals are places for good science, and you have to highlight that, but they are also opportunities for us to showcase the innovations that people developed for their own environments.

Gemma Alderton, panelist

I am the senior editor at *Science Magazine*. I commission and edit reviews of the journals. I don't handle research manuscripts. *Science* is a broad, multidisciplinary journal; it is not necessarily a clinical journal, but we are very much interested in clinical problems and global health. Its global health coverage has predominantly been in infectious disease. So, I attended the Global Health Catalyst to learn more about the issues being discussed at this meeting, to meet people, and tell us that they are here and want to hear from us. *Science* is not just a research journal, there are lots of parts of the journal for commentary and policy forums as well, to try to help crystallize key ideas in important areas. I emphasize that participants are very happy to talk to us and hopefully find some ways to raise awareness of the topics that are being discussed at the Global Health Catalyst.

Riccardo Audisio, panelist

I am the editor-in-chief of the *European Journal of Surgical Oncology*. I start by disputing some of the words. I am very critical of science. Science should not only be based on clinical trials that suit new drugs of pharmaceutical companies. But, they have no adequate outcome data. I think the scientific approach is a work in progress. So, that is: you pretend something which is good, just aiming for the next step. We do want outcome data, as David Collingridge mentioned before. An example is that since total meso-rectal excision was introduced for rectal adenocarcinoma, ten years later, we have a national database. All Scandinavian countries, all Dutch people enjoyed the 15%–18% gain that was supposed to be achieved, that's the whole country saying so, and we don't need a trial for that. Therefore, I am a little bit reluctant in setting rigid guidelines. Within the global perspective, I think we need to be respectful of what our scientists have been producing and very much so encourage them to do more. But, I cannot see economically advanced countries imposing or bullying low- to middle-income countries because their standards are not achieved. Wouldn't it be interesting to look at the opportunity of critically accessing how much of the standard is really feasible? I think this is a great opportunity that you are offering here.

Danny Burke, panelist

I am the CEO of *e*cancermedicalscience. *E*cancer is an education platform for the global oncology community. We deliver education in multiple formats. We have about 7000 education videos, and we are still filming some at this conference with the experts discussing their topics. We also developed e-learning as a continuous medical education platform. We publish news from all the leading conferences as well. The relevance for the topic is that they have a journal that they publish. They are all about breaking down barriers to education on a global level. One of the barriers to journal publishing can be cost, so we operate at a pay what you can afford model. Over 90% of the authors don't pay anything; they have specific grants, so they contribute in that way. Everything that they produce, everything across the platform is totally open access, so there is no delay in access to the information. Anyone across the world can access it as soon as it is published. We are looking into what more they can do. We have a team of about 20 based in an office in the UK. We have teams going to various different meetings across the world on a weekly basis looking at what we can do to really support the global oncology community, educating healthcare professionals so that patients can receive the best care possible.

Jessica Fricchione, panelist

I am from IOP Publishing which is based out of Bristol, UK. I work remotely in New Jersey. Of the five Global Catalyst Summits, this is my fourth one. What an honor to come and see how it has grown. A lot of the work they are doing is in collaboration with Dr Wil Ngwa to try to disseminate this information that comes out of these rooms to a broad and wide audience. I had authors there to work with people in the rooms. I do something different—books. It is a different medium than journals, different audience, different structure, but a lot of it is the same. Some of the challenges are the same, that is, getting information out to the widest audience that we can. One of the things we have been doing at IOP is working with governments, so we have collaborations with the Egyptian knowledge bank and the Minister of Education in Egypt. So, every person in Egypt, no matter what institute they are at, private or public, and all of the libraries in Egypt have access to the IOP journals and all of the e-books. Those are the types of things we are doing as a company to try to work with funders and governments to get access to as many people as possible. It was a pleasure to be here and I liked what my fellow panelist David Collingridge said about keeping an open mind and tying in the commission strategies and really trying to separate the policy from politics. I specify that as something that really resonated with me and publications binding everyone together. There are other platforms; they have electronic platforms and other mediums. I am happy to work with anyone who has any questions to see how we can better disseminate information.

David Kerr: professor at Oxford University (email contribution)

David Kerr is one of the pillars of the Harvard Global Health Catalyst Win-Win Initiative, a professor at Oxford, and editor emeritus of the Annals of Oncology (ESMO) and the founding editor of JCO Global Oncology issued by ASCO.

I am certain that this excellent panel will devise a strategy to promote publication, dissemination, and wider engagement with the concept of better-value cancer care. We must find a way to communicate to our colleagues, patients, and their families that better value does not in any way equate to poor care, but rather strives to achieve a greater degree of equity without sacrificing major health benefits.

Q: Can our journals define the enemies of better-value cancer care?

Answer by David Kerr:

- Unwarranted variation in quality and patient experience
- Patient harm, even when quality is high
- Waste, namely the consumption of resources which do not add value for patients
- Inequities and inequalities in care
- Inadequate focus on prevention

Q: Can we explore need and demand?

Answer by David Kerr:

- Increasing need—our Western populations are aging and cancer is, predominantly, a disease of the elderly.

- Increasing demand—each modest advance is hailed as a 'breakthrough', further increasing demand for marginally effective treatments or unnecessary scans or ever-more aggressive surgery.

Gilberto Lopes, editor-in-chief of JCO Global Oncology

I am very supportive, and I am with you hand in hand. It is a start, and we will do this change. I would like to send everyone the draft of the proposal, and it's the people who will make the movements that will be for the good of all: patients, science, industry, and all.

Eduardo Cazap, panelist

I want to be clear about what we are doing here today and what the objectives are. Usually, the contributions of the journals are mainly devoted to research and the dissemination of scientific information. So, I think the point made by Professor Audisio and his dispute is really useful in this regard. What is science? Science is the application of the realistic in health, realistic possibilities, to as many as possible of the population. If we have science for the elite of a people, we don't have science, we have a gap between reality and a few selected beneficiaries of science.

So, I think there is need to explain that in addition to basic, clinical, and translational research into cancer, there is a need for more types of research. Of course, we are not denying science, but we need to have a wider interpretation and more collaboration of science for better cancer control. Also, we need to include cancer policy research. We expressed this clearly with the relevant editorial world of cancer. Moreover, we need to include implementation research, because science in a lab or in a clinic without applicability to real populations is not really fair to our patients.

It is not only for the patients, since one of the mistakes of our work is that we need to work with healthy populations. One of the problems in the community today is that our universities in most countries (not all) are preparing doctors only for the sick people. Our Ministers of Health are actually Ministers of Disease.

We need to widen the concept of publications for research and science to publications for better cancer control that include information, education, and the important component of research, but with objectives that are not only for peer research and their success with a publication, but research that means benefit of some kind for populations, systems, or the globe in general.

I think that one of the reasons for the invitation of the important people today is to share the way in which publications in a proactive way (not only by receiving their submissions), can promote a better understanding of the way in which we can overcome the situation in which cancer research is dominated by central countries. An example, if you consider the International Agency for Research on Cancer (IARC) (not sure if you know the constitution of IRAC), it is a part of the United Nations System, so they have representatives from the different countries of the world. There were no Latin American countries until there was some work done with Brazil and Argentina, and now there is one seat in IARC from all the Latin American regions and that is Brazil. So, can you imagine that the directions of the main agency for epidemiology and research are missing the objectives of some countries of the world?

The amount of information that we have (including in the guidelines) in the so-called evidence-based medicine by organizations and societies is barely provided by patients that comprise 5%–8% of the world population. So, that's the reason we were discussing together just before this meeting; in which way can we deliberate together about how to contribute to really widening the information and the science in a proactive way and try to include information from sources from different parts of the world?

In my country, Argentina, there are huge databases; one includes seven million people, the retired. Nobody knows the information that is in that database. I asked for some contribution to the National Cancer Institute in an official way; it was impossible. I think that, for example, asking for better availability of the existing information from important publications in the world can contribute a lot in order to have information from sources that are not accessible.

In summary, I think the idea of a win-win publications and dissemination movement, as expressed by Ahmed Elzawawy, is to try to share a way of understanding that the research and publications of international literature can contribute in some way to the populations that are really exposed to cancer in many regions of the world. At present, there is a real distance between the types of information from high-level resources and application to real big real populations in real life. This distance is actually astronomical. Many of the people present here today know that.

I would really like to have the input of the panelists on how they see their journals. If the journal is doing this already, that's great, but if not, how do you see that you can contribute to produce some type of agreement to be more proactive in collecting information from sources that are not today the usual sources of data?

David Collingridge, panelist

I'll answer this from my own experience in terms my travels around the world talking to government ministers and various agencies—there is a huge amount of data that has not been surfaced, agreeing with Eduardo Cazap. A huge amount of very valuable data: but if you don't ask, you will never get. And, whenever I have asked whether this data could be published, recognizing I come from a privileged position working at *The Lancet*, but whenever I've asked a Minister to publish data, quite often they are very open to that. So, I strongly believe editors have a galvanizing, catalytic ability to bring data into the open, and I would encourage others to ask more often.

Anthony Ziteman, panelist

I add that we are beyond the age of the randomized trial being the only thing that could ever get published. There are so many data sources out there; there are so many innovative people who are able to look into it, that even the junior doctors commonly look up public databases. And then there must be equivalents around the globe; any new source of information, we have been incredibly receptive to.

That it's about the authors; ultimately, we can only publish what the authors provide. So it is about working with organizations such as AORTIC, UICC, and SLACOM, and other organizations that represent different parts of the world to encourage people to submit their data or their research or findings or whatever it may be, then there is a chance to publish it. That is because without the authors, there is no chance of publishing it at all.

Ahmed Elzawawy, moderator

What we have commenced today in meeting with the leading contributors and with the panel and the discussion that was preceded by our preparation together for this meeting, will not be the ended by this session; it is just the start. The success of this publications and dissemination movement depends on all of you and your continuous input. The world is in need of an unlimited number of scientific works to find solutions to accessing better-value cancer care.

Sarwat Hussain, participant

I am a professor of radiology from the University of Massachusetts. I am the editor-in-chief of the *Journal of Global Radiology* that was instituted in 2015. One of the difficulties of publishing in the western English-speaking journals is that most of the world or most of the people who do research in the world are not very good at English. Then the world ends up in a regional newspaper. Because of this problem, sometimes authors do not attempt to send their work to the English-speaking journals, even though their research can be real time and reflect the reality on the ground.

What we have done in our journal is scholar twinning. It means, let us say, there is an article from a non-English-speaking country like Iraq, and they have written it up and done good research, but the language is not suitable for an English-speaking journal. So, we twin the non-English-speaking scholar with someone in our department or the US who will take the data, the local indigenous data and write it up in such a way that it is of the standard that can be accepted in a Western English-speaking journal. Then we have the original researcher as the first author, and the rewriter as the second author. In that way, we are able to get the real data from the ground, rather than government cooked up, as we know from the developing world.

Ahmed Elzawawy, moderator

- This comment about the quality of scientific writing and editing in the English language and scholar twining is extremely important.
- I completely agree that tackling the issue directly with your colleagues everywhere would bring real data and scientific outcomes, rather than asking ministers in LMICs to issue some governmental reports. These reports should not be considered as absolutely scientifically valid information. But these reports are useful in preparing work and not necessary to publish in every case or to enter into political embarrassments, but they would serve in

our comparison and verification of different data. Anyway, science is a continuous and endless search for the truth!

Biatrice Wiafe Addai, participant

I am from Ghana and I am President-elect of AORTIC. I always say that we cannot work in oncology without the media. What advice has been planned on the ground has to go to the people, but a lot of attention has been placed on communicable diseases, infections, HIV, tuberculosis. But when we look at Africa and the developing world, cancer is catching up. So, we need to do more than what is happening, we need to engage more. A lot of scientists in Africa are overwhelmed by the media. They come in to assess people to know how to put their thoughts in writing; if we don't do that, we expect them to write. Sometimes their publications will come and you will refuse them, you won't accept them. So, somebody sends a publication two, three times; it's refused. The person then reclines. Please let us engage more. There is a lot of work to be done. Change policy, direct attention in the right way.

Ahmed Elzawawy, moderator

I agree. There is a lot to be done. Once again, it is just the start of the movement of publications and dissemination. So, please keep presenting input, suggestions, and contribution.

Comments sent by the audience

Cannabis medicine has a growing importance and it should take more space in cancer research and journals.

Another comment from the audience: it will be helpful to indicate what we mean by publishable? Because there was a workshop in Nigeria last year, a colleague did a survey and a study, and she is actually looking to publish. We were participating in that. Would you consider that publishable? Also is it a challenge for journals to find reviewers who can properly assess that this has an impact? Because that is also another big part too, people might not even be aware of the challenges when someone is reviewing something that maybe they are not qualified to do.

David Collingridge, panelist

It all comes down to the quality of the research; ultimately, for any peer-reviewed journal, we are interested in quality research. So, when talking about data that can be published, there are levels of quality. Survey data is qualitative and there are journals that publish a lot of qualitative data. There is a special methodology for that, and there are very well qualified referees out there who are well adapted to critique qualitative work. So, yes, there is probably a venue for a large survey that will have the specialist knowledge and expertise to look after it appropriately.

Elizabeth Charlotte Mosser, participant

I am a radiation oncologist and I am vice president of clinical development at Galera Therapeutics.

The dissemination of knowledge is not only by journals, it is also by congresses; as mentioned, there are meetings of ESMO, ASCO, ASTRO, and the ESTRO. So, we are much narrowed in those dissemination places, which are very Western dominated as well because of the language barrier. The other side is when you have a meeting in Uruguay or even in Brazil and have people there to speak; I cannot accept those invitations all the time, it is traveling, it is intensive. So, to have a quality meeting elsewhere or in different audiences is not easy. My question is: can we be more innovative there? Can we use those meetings that are more local so we can have the AORTIC example which is always in places difficult to me to travel to? Could that be a form? However, from people speaking, it can be kind of a reporting journal or a special edition afterward to help the spread, the dissemination side of that meeting, so it can have a larger reach.

Updated comment on this point from the editors

After the Summit, during the COVID-19 pandemic, virtual meetings and information and communications technology (ICT) have become common. In fact, this step was proposed by many—including us—in the last decade, but the pandemic accelerated the global adoption of virtual conferences and eLearning in medical consultations and many aspects of work and life. This will continue.

Danny Burke, panelist

I answer by saying that as *e*cancer, we have been to the last five to six AORTIC meetings; we interviewed the key speakers there. We in *e*cancer make the videos available for free so that people who cannot travel to all the meetings can have access. They are normally published within the week. That is exactly what we are about as an organization, because people cannot travel to every meeting. We'll go to the ASCO annual conference next week and have expressed how we are going to do 60–80 interviews with the key speakers there. We also are going to be going to AORTIC in November 2019, and we run educational events in Latin America and India. Another point in reference to the questions: *e*cancermedicalscience works with authors, so we are publishing a special article from Africa at the moment, pointing out some of the authors are actually in the room. Peter Boyle is the key author on that. A lot of the papers submitted are not of the standard that would normally be accepted by the Western journals, so we work with authors to bring everything up to the standard that is required to be published in a Western journal. As an organization, that is what we are all about, bringing in information from different parts of the world to the global oncology community with a view to improving patient care.

Twalib Ngoma, participant

I am a professor, a clinical oncologist from Tanzania, a leader in the GHC Win-Win initiative, vice chancellor of the Global Oncology University (GO-U) and past president of AORTIC,

How it is a pleasure to have editors-in-chief of the high-impact journals present. The rejection rate from the high-impact journals is quite high. Something I think is that there is a feeling that whenever there is a journal article from Africa, there is some bias to start with. English is not our mother tongue. So, there will always be a problem with language. I would like to have a situation like the *e*cancer journal, where randomized clinical trials were mentioned, but we might not be doing that. But, what if the editors-in-chief were going to be helpful like the *e*cancer journal. I was involved in an *e*cancer control series. They sent it to us and then they reviewed it, with very positive reviews, and then they worked on that to help bring the standard of the articles to the standard of the *e*cancer.

But sometimes people are in a situation, even the reviewers, when they review the journals, they come back and you look at them. Then, you don't agree with what the reviewers want you to do. The editor-in-chief doesn't need to take everything the reviewers say, but if the editor-in-chief isn't going to be helpful then it becomes a problem. So, we would like to ask editors-in-chief to help so that they can bring the standard if there is good data that can be reportable, because some articles are being refused by one journal and then sent to another journal with the same impact factor and then they are acceptable. I ask what the basis is. For example, if *Lancet Oncology* refuses that article, then the *Red Journal* accepts it, what is the explanation?

Ahmed Elzawawy, moderator

I would like to add something. I say that this current or movement is the start of something, and should be joined with other things. One of the things is that we should raise the levels of scientific research in developing countries. This is not a call to accept a paper that is away from science or away from sense; that is why I do appreciate the feedback about scholar twining a lot. Hence, it helps in editing before publication and then you add a second colleague from Harvard, or from Pennsylvania or from Oxford or other institutes as a second author. Why not? It is a win-win.

That is why yesterday we spoke about the global oncology university GO-U, a virtual university. You are all welcome to join, to teach online—investigators, young investigators to incorporate with them, to help them to do good research design, to revise their data, to revise their statistics, to edit with them, and to publish with them. Also, there could be connections with other institutes.

As I mentioned before, a researcher or a professor at Harvard, Pennsylvania, Oxford, or wherever could get benefits from involving investigators, researchers, clinicians, or radiologists in Tanzania, in Egypt, in Latin America, or wherever in LMICs in being co-authors. All would gain. The locals from anywhere in the LMICs would be good collaborators in research. This may diminish brain drain, as the locals would be part of the international scientific community while they practice and gain in their own countries. The world is in need of such a big win-win scientific publication movement concentrated on real aspects and solving local and global challenges.

Gemma Alderton, panelist

Science—as a journal—has a very low acceptance rate of about 7% of all submissions. But, we travel to try to educate people about what they are looking for and how things work. Like *Lancet Oncology*, it works with authors to developmentally edit their work so that they communicate as clearly as they possibly can. Just by the way, after a few minutes I'll start my session which is all about how science works, what editors are looking for, how reviews work, the entire editorial process behind the scenes and how to communicate your work. So, it is all about the problem that is being talked about.

Anthony Ziteman, panelist

The concerns raised by Twalib Ngoma that there may be bias against a paper that comes from a developing country is serious. My journal—as well as a number of other journals—has instituted double-blind reviews. So, the viewer has no idea where the paper came from, no idea who the authors are. That has been very reassuring for our authors.

Eric Ford, participant

I am a professor of Radiation Oncology, Medical Physics, Seattle, Washington, USA.

I also appreciate double-blind reviews as a reviewer too. I want to make the comment/question related to everything. What he has noticed is an issue much later upstream, so in the study design and the conception of the research. There has been a lot of discussion around the language and the presentation around a study that is already done. The twinning model was very interesting, but that happens much later and if you do not have a good study design from the beginning, it is really hard to get it up to that level. I then ask if anybody has experience around this. I have been struggling with this with my collaborators and I have been trying to assist in any ways that I can. It is quite challenging.

David Collingridge, panelist

It is something we are working on quite strongly in The Lancet Group. *The Lancet Oncology* runs publishing workshops and one-to-one sessions frequently, and many of my colleagues on the other Lancet journals do so as well. One of the key interests when running these workshops is protocol design, study design, and data analysis. These are fundamental barriers to publication, and have been so for many years. So, a lot of the work done in these events is about interrogating what a researcher is aiming to get from the study, and how those objectives inform study design. Coming to the point of assistance, there is a program called 'Publishers Without Borders'. In that program, editors and publishers help regional in-country journals; for example, if they need help on how to set up an editorial board, how to get registered in PubMed, or how to set up peer review systems; there is a lot of cross-learning that can be of help there. Our parent company, Elsevier, runs a specific initiative in this area and *The Lancet* participates frequently.

Anthony Zietman, panelist

It's not necessarily blind to the nation, but it is blind to the authors. If it is important that it is research that is done in Kenya, then it has to be explicitly stated in the data, that information is not redacted. So the double-blind review is really a way of reducing the bias that reducers may or may not have against authors who they may consider to be from lesser universities, unconsciously.

A comment from the audience

A lot of my peers used to follow the *Journal of Negative Results*. They mentioned that it really taught them about the type of research that they should not do and not waste their resources and time on. So how important is it to publish negative results in journals?

Antony Zietman, panelist

Negative results are very important. A well done negative study is a huge contribution.

Eduardo Cazap, panelist

Perfect is against the good! I want to summarize in a simple way, if possible, some core concepts and take-home messages:

- The idea is that the journals can collaborate in promoting good study design and methodology. Without a good design and methodology, a publication is impossible.
- To write editorials at oncology journals and sites to tackle this win-win publications and dissemination movement, its objective, this meeting, and the further progress.
- Reviewers should not only have the science and the knowledge but also understanding of the global issues in order to be fair with their scientific evaluations.
- If necessary, the journals may help with proper native English editing.
- The idea expressed by the panel is basically to expand science, knowledge, and data to more countries and populations as well as to improve the quality of the publications worldwide, which is something that is very basic.
- To include scientific research on cancer treatments, more information about different aspects of cancer control in the real world.

I tried to summarize in a few points the main issues during this debate. Perhaps there are more points, but the minutes of this important stimulating meeting will be summarized and published, as Ahmed Elzawawy described, to be available for all.

Ahmed Elzawawy, moderator

At the end of this meeting, we consider this to be the start of the 'Publications and Dissemination Movement'. As a win-win initiative of the Global Health Catalyst, we are extremely glad that we prepared and catalyzed for it. It is conducted by distinguished editors and scientists. Moreover, it welcomes all editors and publishers. The only way to make progress is with all of your contributions. Within the notion of the win-win, it belongs to all. Its progress is measured by the increase in the publication and dissemination of scientific cancer care and control relevant to the world's population. However, its achievement will take place when scientific works and approaches translate into an increase in the affordability of better-value cancer care and control for the majority of the population in the real world.

On behalf of all my colleagues in the Win-Win initiative, I thank you all. 'We are partners, and with you all, something big could be done'.

The link [14] to the video of the Global Health Catalyst Summit Publications and Dissemination session, May 25, 2019 at Harvard Medical School, Boston, MA, USA is: https://www.youtube.com/watch?v=r0v1nJISLuM&feature=youtu.be.

9.3 Section 3: early outcomes and prospective developments

By: Wilfred Ngwa, Eduardo Cazap, David Kerr, Richard Sullivan, Alison Landman, Gliberto Lopez, Gemma Alderton, and Ahmed Elzawawy

We do not claim any credit or that this meeting is the sole cause of any positive outcome, but our aim is to share the stimulation and the call for a win-win publication movement. Many think that there is a great need for it and that the time is ripe for it. As we always emphasize, praise is for the doers and many of those who will realize the implementation and progress.

We present here what the editors already see as early outcomes from the win-win session. We expect this to be amplified in the coming years and we will continue to grow this movement in the forthcoming Global Health Catalyst summits and beyond.

After the 2019 Global Health Catalyst summit at Harvard Medical School, Richard Sullivan, chair of trustees for the *e*cancer global foundation and Eduardo Cazap (editor-in-chief, *e*cancer and president of SLACOM) discussed the new strategic direction for *ecancermedicalscience*—focusing on supporting cancer care in under-resourced settings. The journal planned to change its submission criteria from 21st September 2020 to exclusively publish articles that feature at least one author from an LMIC or which have a significant impact on under-resourced settings. They issued that change because of the rising flow of cancer cases in LMICs. *ecancermedicalscience* is well placed to support authors and readers to publish and read the latest cancer information free of charge [15].

The Lancet Oncology also commissioned a Lancet Oncology Commission for Sub-Saharan Africa chaired by Wilfred Ngwa, Beatrice Addai, and David Kerr with the Lancet Oncology deputy editor, Ali Landman.

Science editor Gemma Alderton has also published a number of articles on Africa, including the following articles:

- Hosny A and Aerts H 2019 Artificial intelligence for global health *Science* **366** 955–956.
- Rebbeck T R 2020 Cancer in sub-Saharan Africa *Science* **367** 27–28.
- Addai B W and Ngwa W 2021 COVID-19 and cancer in Africa *Science* **371** 25–27.

A number of articles have also been published in the *Red Journal* and the *ASCO Journal of Global Oncology*, which could be considered outcomes of the win-win session on scientific approaches to increase access to better-value care. IOP Publishing has also commissioned and published a number of e-books on global oncology and continues to do so. This appears to just be the beginning and more is expected in the upcoming Global Health Catalyst summits, where we will continue to engage high-impact journal editors to get involved in the goals of this win-win movement

Note from the Editors:

As we stated before, this book belongs to all readers. So, after publication, all can still send feedback, input, and suggestions to http://icedoc.net/feedback.html and http://icedoc.org/feedback.html. We will forward the feedback to the distinguished panel members, who have kindly agreed to reply.

We are just starting. The editors of journals and books, scientists, and all readers will contribute to the progress of the movement for the sake of cancer patients everywhere and for science. All stakeholders would win.

References

[1] Yap M L, Zubizarreta E and Bray F *et al* 2015 Global access to radiotherapy services: have we made progress during the past decade? *J. Global Oncol.* **2** 207–15

[2] Elzawawy A 2019 ecancer video July 12, 2019 https://ecancer.org/video/8112/prof-ahmed-elzawawy-on-global-cancer-control

[3] Elzawawy A M 2015 Could African and low- and middle-income countries contribute scientifically to global cancer care? *J. Glob. Oncol.* **1** 49–53

[4] Crisp N 2011 *Turning the World Upside Down – The Search for Global Health in the 21st Century*. RMS Books http://nigelcrisp.com/turning-the-world-upside-down/

[5] Govindarajan V and Trimble C 2012 *Reverse Innovation: Create Far from Home, Win Eerywhere* (Brighton, MA: Harvard Business Review Press)

[6] Elzawawy 2013 ecancer video. Affordable radiotherapy and chemotherapy in Africa http://ecancer.org/conference/349-aortic-2013/video/2494/affordable-radiotherapy-and-chemotherapy-in-africa.php

[7] Elzawawy A 2012 Science and affordability of cancer drugs and radiotherapy in the world: win-win scenarios *Advances in Cancer Management* ed R Mohan (Rijeka: InTech)

[8] Cazap E, Magrath I, Peter Kingham T and Elzawawy A 2016 Structural barriers to diagnosis and treatment of cancer in low- and middle-income countries: the urgent need for scaling up *J. Clin. Oncol.* **34** 14–9

[9] Muir Gray J A and Kerr D J (ed) 2013 *How to Get Better Value Cancer Care* (Oxford, UK: Offox Press Ltd)

[10] Elzawawy A and Kerr D 2013 Variation in the availability of cancer drug generics in the United States of America *Ann. Oncol.* **24** 17–22

[11] Elzawawy A 2015 The shortage of essential cancer drugs and generics in the United States of America: global brain storming directions for the world *Int. J. Cancer Clin. Res.* **2** 016

[12] Cazap E and Anderson B 2016 Vision for the Global Health and Cancer section *Oncologist* **21** 521–2

[13] ASCO's Second National Cancer Opinion Survey results: surprising number of Americans believe alternative therapies can cure cancer. ASCO Connection Jan 08, 2019 https://connection.asco.org/magazine/features/second-asco-national-cancer-opinion-survey-results

[14] Session global health catalyst summit. Publications and dissemination session, 25 May 2019, Harvard Medical School, Boston, MA, USA https://youtube.com/watch?v=r0v1nJISLuM&feature=youtu.be

[15] Sullivan R and Cazap E 2020 New strategy for *ecancermedicalscience*: supporting publications in in under-resourced settings https://ecancer.org/en/video/9149-new-strategy-for-ecancermedicalscience-supporting-publications-in-under-resourced-settings?utm_campaign=automated-emails&utm_source=siteupdates-en-html&utm_medium=email

Part II

Global Health Catalyst win-win channels

Chapter 10

Ecancer for all and the Global Oncology University (the GO-U)

Wilfred Ngwa, Ahmed Elzawawy, Stephen Avery, David Kerr, Eduardo Cazap, Riccardo Audisio, Golam Abo Zakaria, Bashkim Zeberi, Nicholas Abinya, Luca Incrocci, Lydia Asana, William Swanson, Omoruyi Irabor, Saiful M Huq and Twalib Ngoma

Note from the Editors:

Parts of this chapter are adapted from: Lydia Asana, Credit Irabor, Samuel Seppo, Chrystelle Jean, Twalib Ngoma, Ahmed Elzawawy and Wilfred Ngwa (2021), 'Using advanced information and communication technologies to advance oncology education in Africa'—ecancer

https://ecancer.org/en/journal/article/1211-using-advanced-information-and-communication-technologies-to-advance-oncology-education-in-africa
https://doi.org/10.3332/ecancer.2021.1211

This chapter covers the comprehensive cancer center in the cloud (C4) or ecancerforall initiative, one component of which is the award-winning Global Oncology University (GO-U). ecancerforall is an initiative of the Global Health Catalyst (GHC) win-win movement, established to reduce global cancer health disparities, which includes filling a major void in the education and training of oncology healthcare professionals in low- and middle-income countries (LMICs), while also training the next generation of global health professionals from high-income countries (HICs). ecancerforall's vision is to provide access to cancer care, research, and education from anywhere in the world with access to the internet or Wi-Fi. GO-U provides access from anywhere in the world to the same excellent education and training as that available at the world's best universities and medical schools. The University was collaboratively founded and funded by faculty from the University of Pennsylvania USA, Harvard University USA, the Africa–Oxford (AFROX) Foundation, the University of Heidelberg (Germany), the University of

doi:10.1088/978-0-7503-3075-6ch10

Massachusetts and a growing global health consortium including professional societies (e.g. FAMPO, AORTIC) and partnerships between industry, diaspora organizations (looking to turn brain drain into global health gain), and health ministries in different countries working to build crucial human capacity to strengthen healthcare systems. GO-U builds on an award-winning collaborative learning model, offering online lectures accessible from any country and practical/clinical training in local/regional credentialed sites. GO-U is the premier university that offers both continuous medical education, degrees (Master, PhD), and clinical MD residency training in oncology, with the vision of eliminating global cancer health disparities. Online classes begin in the fall of each year with planned complementary practical training in a number of credentialed LMIC partner institutions. Workshops and short-term education exchanges between LMIC and HIC institutions augment practical training. GO-U is complemented by the yearly Global Health Catalyst summits organized at Harvard and around the world, which have the goal of educating as well as initiating and strengthening collaborations for high-impact global health outcomes. GO-U has a high level of commitment to excellence that translates into highly effective health benefits around the globe. Its outstanding faculty, together with its collaborative education and training model make GO-U one of the leading global oncology education and training platforms available.

10.1 ecancerforall a.k.a comprehensive cancer center in the cloud (C4)

In the USA, approximately 250,000 patients each year receive their cancer diagnosis at an NCI-designated cancer center. An even larger number of patients are treated for cancer at these centers each year, and thousands of patients are enrolled in cancer clinical trials at NCI-designated cancer centers. These centers also provide public education and outreach programs on the topics of cancer prevention and screening, as well as patient education that gives special attention to the needs of underserved populations. The rapid pace of discovery and the improved cancer treatments that the NCI-designated cancer centers have helped pioneer have contributed substantially to increasing the number of cancer survivors in the United States, as well as to the quality of their lives. C4 is designed to extend this model globally, beginning in Africa, in a powerful initiative expected to benefit millions of cancer patients in the coming years.

C4 was seed-funded as part of the Global Health Catalyst Win-Win Initiative following major preliminary work and assessment in Africa. The Global Health Catalyst is a leader in information and communications technology (ICT)-powered global health, leveraging unprecedented diaspora engagement. C4 has four components: care, research, education and outreach. The care component includes e-consultations (including second opinions), online tumor boards, remote treatment planning, and quality assurance support. In the research component, the C4 builds on the infrastructure and model of the NIH-funded Quality Assurance and Review Center (QARC) which offers institutions credentials for participation in clinical trials, writes protocols in preparation for Cancer Therapy Evaluation Program (CTEP) reviews, manages data acquisition for protocol quality assurance, and participates in outcome evaluation. QARC currently houses more than 1,000,000 images of 80,000 patients treated using more than 450 protocols. With this tremendous amount of data, which includes growing amounts from the global health work, the C4 envisions becoming the premier ICT-powered comprehensive online cancer enterprise in the world. The Africa–Oxford–Harvard Clinical Trials Network has been established as one of the multi-center clinical trials networks for high-impact global oncology. This includes cancer centers in Nigeria, Kenya, Cameroon, Tanzania, Ghana, and South Africa, with plans to extend to other developing countries. In the education component, the C4 is focused on the Global Oncology University, as described below. By taking the successful Comprehensive Cancer Center (C3) Dana-Farber/Harvard Cancer Center model to the next level, the cloud (C4) ensures that anyone with access to the internet or a phone can access the same world-class care as that offered at the Dana-Farber/Harvard Cancer Center. The C4 provides a platform for all to participate, regardless of geographic barriers. Doctors and retirees with only 15 min a week to spare can pool that time (like a car pool) to provide services. C4 is committed to maximizing the impact of its work for cancer patients and ultimately realizing a world where everyone can access quality cancer care research and education.

10.2. The Global Oncology University model

The global burden of cancer is projected to continue growing in the coming years in LMICs, with survival rates that are amongst the lowest relative to HICs [1]. This is exacerbated by the dearth of oncology health professionals. The limited capacity with which to train oncology professionals is a major contributory factor to the shortfall in human resources which stymies local control efforts in LMICs [1]. Consequently, concerted efforts are taking place to increase the cancer health workforce and promote an equitable distribution of resources. Such a development requires proactive efforts in each country through the provision of oncology education, training, and mentorship opportunities for current and future cancer workers [1]. As LMICs face a shortage of oncology mentors, collaborative educational initiatives with mentors and trainers within and outside the continent are essential [1, 2]. A few initiatives, such as the Global Health Service Partnership, employ traditional face-to-face education and training options. However, this often necessitates extended travel and disruption to work, generating time and financial expenses that could be prohibitive or impractical for trainers in some regions [1].

In response to these challenges, virtual oncology education and training have been suggested as tools for workforce development [1, 3, 4]. Virtual education, also known as electronic learning (e-learning), refers to instruction in a learning environment where the trainer and the trainee are separated by time or space, or both, and where the trainer provides course content through an ICT platform that utilizes course management applications, multimedia modules, the internet, videoconferencing, etc. Rather than replacing traditional training, e-learning may be blended with traditional training, serving as a complementary mechanism for remote oncology education and instructional contents prepared by experts. However, given the obstacles encountered in accessing internet services in many

LMICs, including the low levels of computer literacy, inadequate infrastructure, and the high costs of internet bandwidth, there are concerns that oncology trainees may lack the capacity and skill base required for internet-based training [1, 5]. For example, while internet connectivity has grown by more than 8500% since 2000, Africa's internet penetration was still as low as 31.2% in 2017, below the global average of 51.7% and reflecting an inner digital divide that ranges from 4.3% in Niger to 89% in Kenya [5].

Besides the connectivity issues, virtual oncology training in LMICs is possible only with cultural acceptance and the availability of other ICT infrastructural and managerial support systems, such as electricity, e-learning software and hardware, personnel to manage access to learning materials, technical standardization, and a framework to review learning resources [6]. During the Global Health Catalyst summit of 2018, the Global Oncology University (GO-U) initiative was launched to provide a platform for collaborative education that integrates the best of face-to-face training and virtual education. GO-U builds on an award-winning collaborative learning model with online lectures that are accessible from any country, and practical/clinical training in local/regional credentialed sites. The online classes are provided by the best faculty in the world and accessible from anywhere using a collaborative approach in which the faculty pool their time with that of other experts. Practical training at local credentialed sites allows trainees to get credit for practical experience locally without the need to travel outside their regions. GO-U has already trained over 1000 trainees from LMICs in Africa and Eurasia. The use of ICTs and online learning has also grown significantly in the advent of the COVID-19 pandemic, leading to increase utilization of online learning in LMICs, with now great opportunity to maximize the impact of GO-U and the C4.

10.3 Educational needs

In an effort to optimize the learning experience for oncology training, educational needs assessment and e-learning readiness studies were conducted among oncology healthcare professionals as part of the Global Oncology University initiative. The investigation sought to identify and document gaps and potential challenges that might arise from implementing e-learning. Potential solutions for remedying gaps either before implementation, during the implementation process, or as part of continuous improvement were also explored.

Oncology professionals responded from 22 African countries, including Algeria, Botswana, Burkina Faso, Burundi, Cape Verde, Chad, Congo, Gabon, Kenya, Malawi, Mali, Morocco, Niger, Nigeria, Rwanda, Seychelles, South Africa, Tanzania, Togo, Tunisia, Uganda, and Zambia. Participants were part of the oncology workforce in a total of 40 institutions: 13 were universities, eight were national teaching hospitals, five were cancer institutes, eight were organizational or NGO-sponsored training centres, three were other hospitals (including private healthcare facilities), and three were institutions outside of Africa (excluded from the analysis). Overall, more oncology health professionals (67.3%) felt confident

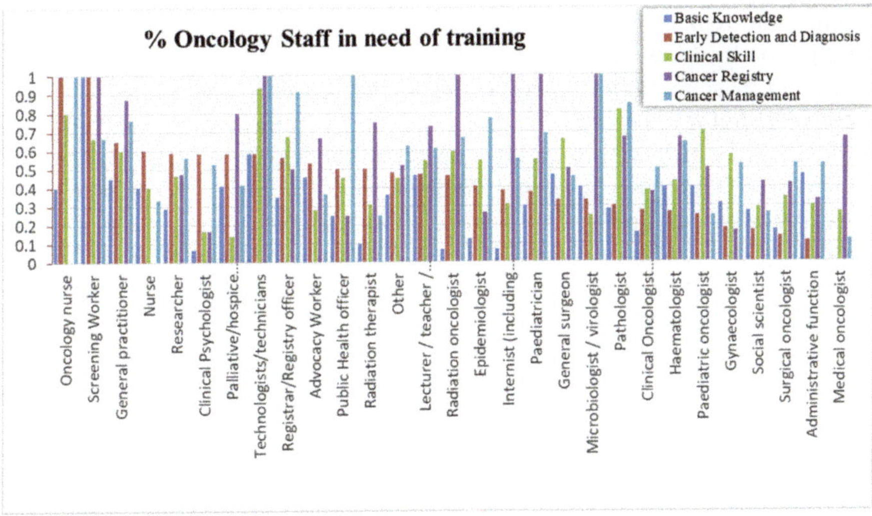

Figure 10.1. Overview of educational needs among oncology health professional study participants.

about their basic medical knowledge, 56.4% felt adequately prepared for the early detection and diagnosis of cancer, 52.1% were satisfied with their clinical skills, 43.9% were prepared for work in cancer data registry, and only 41.6% felt adequately prepared for their role in cancer management. Consequently, 33%, 44%, 48%, 58% and 60% of all felt they needed further training in the areas of basic knowledge, early detection and diagnosis, clinical skill, cancer data registry, and cancer management, respectively. The areas of strength and weakness differed for each specific profession (see figure 10.1); however, medical oncologists were consistently at the higher end, while oncology nurses and general practitioners were consistently at the lower end of self-confidence, except for cancer registration, in which all oncology nurses felt adequately trained.

10.4 Assessing the readiness and prospects of web-based oncology education

Readiness denotes mental or physical preparedness for some experience or action. Experts in the field have developed many models to assess e-learning readiness for institutions, trainers, and learners. In assessing readiness, e-learning readiness for trainees only was assessed using the most frequently utilized components of known reference models identified in the literature. The questions used for assessment focused on the five most commonly used elements across all models, including: (i) access to technology, (ii) technological skills/competence, (iii) capacity for self-directed learning, (iv) confidence in other prerequisite skills, and (v) motivation [7].

Access to technology refers to the need for trainees to either have the necessary technological devices or have access to them [7]. Participants were asked to indicate whether they had personal computers or any smart device meeting a minimum e-learning requirement. The minimum computer requirements for e-learning vary according to the Course/Content Management System (CMS) or Learning Management System that is used to deliver the course materials. However, the minimum technology required for this study is the minimum necessary for Skype communication, which is a computer or smart device with at least a 1 GHz processor and 256MB of RAM installed. Respondents were also asked to indicate whether they had or could afford internet connectivity for an online course. A 56Kbps connection speed was deemed feasible for asynchronous virtual oncology education and a minimum of a 1 Mbps broadband connection speed was deemed necessary for synchronous visual/audio learning.

Technological skills/competence signifies the trainee's efficacy in using a computer, the internet, and other smart devices [7]. Survey respondents were asked to indicate whether they were confident in using computers or smart technologies, and if they could efficiently utilize the internet and software for virtual learning. Each further stated whether they would be comfortable using a computer or device several times a week to participate in an online course.

Capacity for self-directed learning entails a process in which individuals take the initiative, with or without the help of others, in diagnosing their learning needs, formulating learning goals, identifying human and material resources for learning, choosing and implementing appropriate learning strategies, and evaluating learning outcomes. Respondents were asked to indicate whether they had all the computer literacy skills needed to find learning sources, determine which strategies they should employ, evaluate themselves, and navigate online learning platforms and processes for themselves. Respondents were asked to indicate the availability of trained teaching and ICT personnel in their institutions who could assist them should they be unable to self-direct.

Motivation is the students' willingness and eagerness to attend classes via online or electronic methods [7]. Motivation was gauged by comparing their preference for e-learning modalities versus face-to-face learning. Respondents were further prompted to indicate whether they had ever taken an online course. Estimations for motivation were based on the percentage of respondents who had completed courses.

Confidence in prerequisite skills and yourself is a combined component, which comprises one's own trust in the skills required to be successful in e-learning and towards oneself.[7] Respondents were asked to indicate whether they felt they were confident in their capacity to communicate effectively and at pace with course participants and instructors (both in writing and speaking) via an online platform.

Among the respondents, 110 out of 128 had personal computers that met the minimum specification, 86 had computers in their workplace, and 95 had other technological devices, such as tablets and phones, that could adequately support e-learning. All respondents had internet connectivity, but only 20 (15.7%) had a quality connection with more than than 1 Mbps of bandwidth speed capable of supporting synchronous e-learning; 113 of 127 respondents had the necessary skills to operate a computer or smart device for e-learning. The same number felt capable of navigating the internet in support of learning activities, such as research, assignments, and accessing online libraries, while 101 respondents felt comfortable using the internet several times a week for an online course. Although 113 thought that they had the necessary computer skills, only 47 of 128 respondents felt they had all the computer literacy skills needed to function as independent learners. However, 48 indicated they could easily access technical support provided by their institutions when required, and 56 reported they could seek administrative help from e-learning experts. This makes synchronous self-directed learning feasible for 48 respondents and asynchronous self-directed learning possible for 107. Only 43 (33.5%) of oncology staff preferred e-learning over the traditional face-to-face training modality. Although 25 participants worked or were trained in schools that were supportive of online courses, only eleven (11) participants indicated that they had ever taken an online-based course. All eleven candidates completed their courses. All courses blended face-to-face and e-learning and none (0) were strictly online oncology courses. A hundred and one participants indicated confidence in their ability to communicate effectively with course participants and instructors (both in writing and speaking) via an online platform. Based on these responses, the weighted averages for technological access, technological skill and competence, capacity for self-directed learning, motivation, and confidence in other prerequisite skills were 69%, 86%, 51% 42%, and 80%, respectively (see figure 10.2).

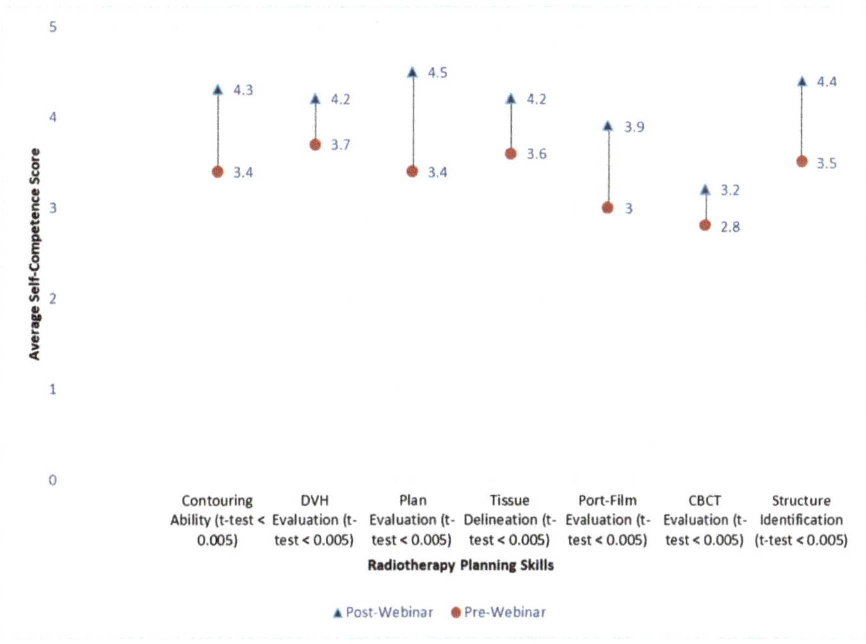

Figure 10.2. Difference in competence scores before and after an online training session on radiotherapy contouring. A score of five signifies full competence in the prerequisite contouring skill and one denotes complete incompetence. Study participants rated themselves using pre- and post-class questionnaires.

Table 10.1. Results of readiness assessment survey [9].

Area	Survey quesetion	Number out of 128
Technological access	Own a personal computer that can adequately support videos and other software for e-learning	110
	Have access to computers (not personally owned)	86
	Own another technological device that can adequately support videos and other software for e-learning	95
	Access to internet connectivity to complete an online course	127
	I have and can afford internet quality of ⩾1 Mbps *(for real-time synchronous e-learning)*	20
Technological skills/ competence	Have the basic skills to operate a computer or technological device for e-learning (e.g., saving files, creating folders etc).	113
	Capable of navigating the internet (for example, using search engines and library database)	113
	Comfortable with using a computer or device several times a week to participate in a course.	101
Capacity for self-directed e-learning	Have all the computer literacy skills needed for online self-learning without assistance; i.e. capable of functioning independently (requires advanced skills, such as software installation and the ability to perform online research using various search engines and library databases)	47
	Feasibility of self-directed learning with synchronous virtual learning (e.g. through GoToMeeting, Skype, and other standard synchronous e-learning interfaces)	68
	Feasibility of self-directed learning with an asynchronous virtual learning modality (e.g. CD-ROM, etc.)	107
	Can easily access technical support provided by work/ training institution when needed (information and technology personnel)	48
	Can easily access administrative support provided by work/training institution when needed (trained e-learning personnel and managers)	56
Motivation	Prefer e-learning modalities over face-to-face learning	43
	Have ever taken an online course	11
	Completed online course they took	11
	Comfortable with using a computer or device several times a week to participate in a course.	101
Confidence in other prerequisite skills	Capable of communicating effectively and at pace with course participants and instructors (both in writing and speaking) via an online platform.	101

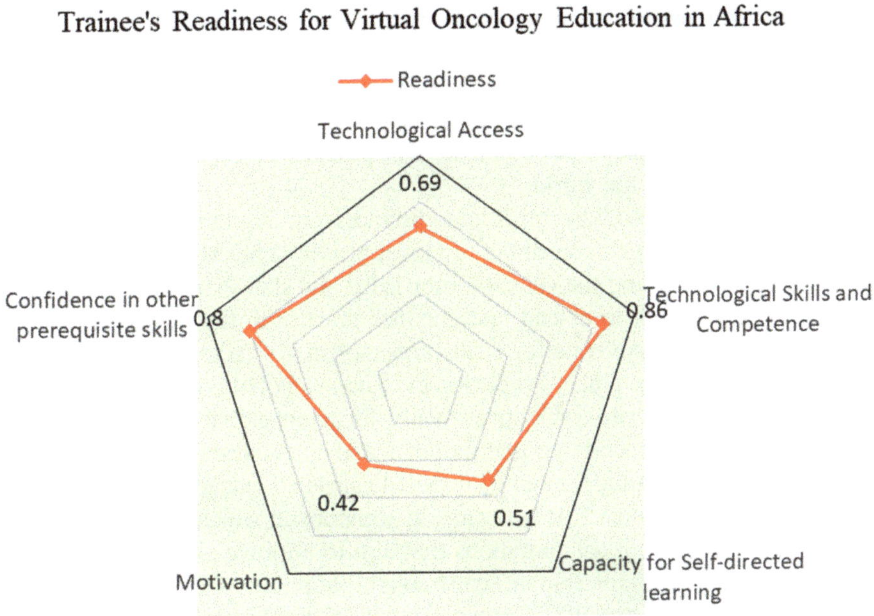

10.5 Radiotherapy training experience at the Global Oncology University

Radiotherapy is employed in the treatment of over 50% of cancer patients. Following the assessment of readiness, a radiation oncology training program was implemented via the Global Oncology University training platform. A survey assessing participants' confidence in the necessary skills needed to contour a treatment plan was administered before and after training in contouring. Self-confidence on each skill was self-reported on a scale of one to five. A general average score for each component was calculated as the sum of the scores divided by the total number of respondents. There was a marked improvement in self-confidence in contouring after a single one-hour webinar session (figure 10.2). While this is simply an indication of potential, the results of this assessment suggest the value that virtual education and training can bring to the transfer of knowledge, skills, abilities, and even perception in oncology education and training. In the case of the GO-U contour training example, participants' perceptions of their own abilities were positively affected after a one-hour webinar, which could lead to a greater openness to additional training opportunities, combating some of the hesitation towards e-learning identified in other assessments.

10.6 Global Oncology University impact

The challenges posed by the exponentially growing cancer burden in LMICs are both daunting and urgent. GO-U offers opportunities to make strides in education and training for health professionals in low-resource countries. Studies have shown that the key elements are in place for this collaborative education platform to enable high-impact collaborations in response to the growing global cancer burden. This can be particularly useful in radiation oncology, in which partners from different nations with diverse backgrounds can cooperate to bridge the chasm that currently exists in the availability of safe, effective radiation therapies as an accessible cancer treatment option for LMICs [8]. For clinicians, researchers, educators, and advocates who give of their time and talents to make these services possible through GO-U, ICT provides an opportunity to change the world without traversing the world.

Former barriers imposed by time and distances are no longer an excuse (albeit legitimate) for an inability to contribute to global health gains. Many seasoned scholars and practitioners understand the value of knowledge and skill sharing as a responsibility and a gesture of goodwill to extend and enhance practice in the professions they hold dear. GO-U provides an avenue for such professionals to make a meaningful impact worldwide, while leaving a philanthropic legacy. Finally, global populations are afforded the opportunity to make profitable investments, focus on global policies that promote national priorities, and encourage international and intercultural exchanges that ultimately foster goodwill, setting the stage for global gains that extend beyond global health gains. There are opportunities for win-win-win scenarios in which all stakeholders both contribute and benefit from collaborations that aim to improve global oncology efforts.

The GO-U is an example of a global health collaboration *par excellence* and has already resulted in the training of over 1000 oncology health professionals in LMICs over a two-year period. Following the success of this approach, GO-U is now ready to scale up its impact as one of the leading win-win collaborative education approaches across the world. So, while needs abound and resources are limited, cancer education and training for LMICs now has unprecedented opportunities for human resource development in cancer education and training via GO-U. This could include the participation of diaspora oncology health professionals, turning brain drain into a global health gain.

References

[1] Irabor O C, Kerry V B, Matton J and Ngwa W 2017 Leveraging the global health service partnership model for workforce development in global radiation oncology *J. Global Oncol.* **4** 1–8

[2] Morhason-Bello I O *et al* 2013 Challenges and opportunities in cancer control in Africa: a perspective from the African Organisation for Research and Training in Cancer *Lancet Oncol.* **14** e142–51

[3] Ngwa W *et al* 2015 Potential for information and communication technologies to catalyze global collaborations in radiation oncology *Int. J. Radiat. Oncol. Biol. Phys.* **91** 444–7

[4] Ngwa W *et al* 2017 Potential role of the quality assurance review center platform in global radiation oncology *Int. J. Radiat. Oncol. Biol. Phys.* **99** 956–62

[5] Anon. https://www.internetworldstats.com/stats1.htm (Accessed April 4, 2022)

[6] Ruiz J G, Mintzer M J and Leipzig R M 2006 The impact of e-learning in medical education *Acad. Med.* **81** 207–12

[7] Demir Ö and Yurdugül H 2015 The exploration of models regarding e-learning readiness: reference model suggestions *Int. J. Prog. Educ.* **11** 173–94 https://ijpe.inased.org/makale/2420

[8] Ngwa W *et al* 2016 *HHS Public Access.* **91** 444–47

[9] Asana L, Irabor C, Seppo S, Jean C, Ngoma T, Elzawawy A and Ngwa W 2021 Using advanced information and communication technologies to advance oncology education in Africa *Ecancermedicalscience* **15** 1211

Chapter 11

Africa–Oxford–Harvard/Hopkins Cancer Research and Clinical trials Consortium (AFROX-H2 Clinical Trials Network)

David Kerr, Twalib Ngoma, Wil Ngwa, Ahmed Elzawawy, Dennis Palmer, Francine Kouya, Paul Mobit, Verna Vanderpuye, N A Othieno-Abinya, Atara Ntekim and Paul Ruff

Link to Video: Kerr D, the GHC Win-Win Initiative, May 24, 2019, Harvard Medical School, Boston, MA, USA. https://youtu.be/qpHZ2pIUsQQ

The AFROX-H2 Network (Africa–Oxford–Harvard/Hopkins cancer research and clinical trials Consortium) is the brainchild of Professor David Kerr at Oxford University, who is world renowned for his efforts to heal the whole world of cancer. He has built clinical trial networks across many countries, including some in Asia. This chapter covers such a network for Africa, which includes cancer centers from different African countries with support from Oxford University and colleagues at Harvard and Johns Hopkins. A first AFROX-H2 clinical trial is in motion, with a focus on hypofractionated radiotherapy, and will be followed by trials using biomaterial drone technology developed at Harvard. This network is a great epitome of the win-win scientific initiative.

11.1 Introduction

Cancer accounts for almost 13% of all deaths globally per year, equating to around eight million people. This is greater than the combined number of deaths due to HIV/AIDS, tuberculosis (TB), and malaria. Although the world is rightly focused on controlling the spread of acute diseases such as these, the lack of focus on cancer is a matter of great concern; it is a chronic disease which is a great source of suffering in developing nations such as those in Africa, where resources for treatment and prevention are limited or nonexistent.

The challenges facing researchers in low- and middle-income countries (LMICs) are formidable; 90% of global health research expenditure is directed at diseases that affect 10% of the world's population; of 1223 new drugs developed between 1975 and 1997, only

doi:10.1088/978-0-7503-3075-6ch11

13% were directed at tropical diseases; sub-Saharan Africa bears 24% of the global burden of disease, has 3% of the health workforce and less than 1% of the financial commitment to healthcare; the imbalance in the global health workforce is exacerbated by the massive emigration of trained professionals from Africa to North America and Europe.

The key challenges facing cancer researchers in Africa are as follows:

- Lack of infrastructure, funding, and human resources
- Lack of reliable data, poor quality, and a lack of standardized medical records, deficient registration of the causes of death (as most deaths occur at home),
- Almost no public–private partnership
- Cancer is not yet a priority on the African and global health agendas
- Relative lack of available scientific and technical opportunities
- Feasibility and cost-effectiveness of research
- Lack of training and partnership opportunities

In addition to the abovementioned known challenges, in the Global Health Catalyst Win-Win Movement, as shown in different parts of this book, we emphasize that scientific explorations and clinical trials are essential approaches to increasing the affordability of better-value cancer in Africa and also the world within the win-win global scope. The adoption of the win-win scientific notion and objectives and the encouragement and motivation of all stakeholders could considerably lessen the challenges facing research in Africa and LMICs in the real world. Conducting clinical trials is a means and not an objective in itself.

Despite the significant barriers facing African clinical researchers, it is apparent that there is an eagerness to contribute to better understanding the natural history and biology of African cancer patients and to conduct trials of novel therapeutic approaches in these populations. This hunger to contribute knowledge for the benefit of African citizens and perhaps the wider African diaspora includes established, clinical leaders and the new generation of trainees who see the extraordinary levels of research being undertaken with predominantly Caucasian cancer patients and question whether the results of those clinical trials can automatically be applied to the patients they treat within their own clinical practices. Remember that there is no more highly selected patient group than those entering any cancer trial, given the long list of inclusion and exclusion criteria, raising questions about the generalisability of the results, regardless of ethnicity.

11.2 Establishing the Africa—Oxford–Harvard–Hopkins Cancer Research and Clinical Trials Consortium (AFROX-H2 Clinical Trials Network)

We define a clinical network as a geographically disparate group who share a common aim; in our case, it is to improve the quality and duration of every cancer patient's life. Networks may be born out of necessity; if certain elements of care can only be accessed from certain sites, then a tertiary or even quaternary referral system becomes the norm. This may be true of specialised services, such as radiotherapy, bone marrow transplantation, liver resection/ablation of hepatic metastases, complex surgery for certain tumour types (pancreas, sarcoma, head and neck etc.), for which relatively limited resources and expertise are concentrated in a finite number of clinical centres. We will develop this philosophy to create a trials network supported by expertise in Oxford and Harvard, but which will be based on and driven by the top comprehensive cancer centres and colleges in Africa; their functions are described in the following sections.

11.3 African leadership

- We have formed a network of the top comprehensive cancer centres in Africa, and Professor Twalib Ngoma, Muhimbili University of Health and Allied Sciences, United Republic of Tanzania has been elected as the Network Coordinator, providing national leadership and the dominant liaison point with Oxford/Harvard/Johns Hopkins.
- Each of the centres will be supported by a grant for staff (clinicians, nurses, and data managers) and infrastructural support (remote data entry systems, etc).
- Staff training programmes will be jointly undertaken by Oxford/Harvard/Hopkins–Africa to promulgate good clinical practice (GCP), standard operating policies (SOPs) etc using on line continued medical education (CME) programmes.
- Centres that wish to participate in phase 1 (which will be the first to undertake human studies) will be offered a face-to-face training programme for Fellows in the Phase 1 Trials Unit in Oxford.
- Patient recruitment commitments for early-phase and randomised trials will be made by each centre.
- Steps will be taken to ensure protection of intellectual property rights (IPR) for novel agents.
- Comprehensive cancer centres in the network include the following hospitals and university centres:

Professor Twalib Ngoma
Professor of oncology
Muhimbili University of Health and Allied Sciences, United Republic of Tanzania
Professor Ahmed Elzawawy
General director, South and East Mediterranean College of Oncology (SEMCO) and professor of clinical oncology, Suez Canal University, Egypt
Professor Dennis Palmer
Dean, Baptist Institute of Health Sciences, Mbingo Baptist Hospital
Bamenda, Cameroon
Dr Francine Kouya
Chief oncologist,
Mbingo Baptist Hospital
Professor Paul Mobit
CEO of Cameroon Oncology Center
Douala, Cameroon

Dr Verna Vanderpuye, MD
Korlebu Teaching Hospital, Accra, Ghana
Professor N A Othieno-Abinya
Department of Oncology, University of Nairobi, Kenya
Dr Atara Ntekim, MD
Department of Oncology, University of Ibadan/University College Hospital
Professor Paul Ruff, MD
Department of Oncology, University of Witwatersrand, Johannesburg, South Africa

11.4 Oxford and Harvard support

- Trials coordination office (https://www.oncology.ox.ac.uk/research/srf/oncology-clinical-trials-office-octo) with responsibility for statistics, programming, remote data entry, generation of standard operating policies, staff training, monitoring and maintenance of quality standards of the Food and Drug Administration (FDA) and European Medicines Agency EMA)
- Establishing a single-nucleotide polymorphisms (SNP) based pharmacogenetics and bioinformatics service to determine the correlation between germline polymorphisms in metabolic enzymes and target pathways in Africa
- Clinical support for phase II (led by Professor Mark Middleton and Harvard colleagues) and phase III trials portfolio (led by Professor David Kerr and Harvard colleagues) with guaranteed slots and recruitment commitments for industrial trials.
- Partner with BIO Ventures for Global Health (https://bvgh.org/) to survey African institutions' clinical trial capabilities—with a focus on cancer. The results of each institution's survey have been condensed into an online profile, which will be published on our publicly-accessible website. This website, and the profiles contained therein, will be promoted to pharmaceutical and biotechnology companies, academic researchers, and oncology experts to encourage those organizations to conduct clinical trials of their innovative cancer products at one or more of the profiled African institutions. The following fields are covered in this survey:

- Previous clinical trials experience—especially in phase 3 and epidemiological studies
- Personnel—clinical, data collection, and specialist nursing support
- Diagnostic facilities and equipment—imaging endpoints are an essential of most cancer trials
- Laboratory equipment and techniques—increasing use of molecular diagnostics to select patients for particular drugs means that we may ask centres to collect and store samples for central molecular analyses
- Cancer treatment facilities—surgery, radiotherapy, and chemotherapy delivery
- Pharmacy processes—to ensure appropriate drug accountability
- Systems and data management—to ensure high-quality data collection
- Local research ethics review board

Partnerships and collaborations with organizations: one example is the South and East Mediterranean College of Oncology (SEMCO) [1, 2]. The faculty of SEMCO from different countries and collaborators will contribute to education and training to build human capacity in cancer researchers in addition to consultancy during the studies and follow-up. In the upcoming period, courses and webinars will be mostly online until the end of travel restrictions, which will hopefully take place after the termination of COVID-19 pandemic in order to restore onsite and face-to-face modalities in addition to virtual meetings.

The Management Board: In addition to the above list of African leadership, the Management Board comprising the PIs from each of the network centres, will provide leadership within their individual centres and ensure systematic communication and collaboration within the new consortium by providing mechanisms that facilitate communication, training, and education:

- rolling programmes of multi-disciplinary seminars, workshops, and courses supported through the collaborative communication strategy.
- rolling programmes allowing sharing and cross-training.
- support will be provided by developing an interactive presence on a dedicated website. The website will form a key plank of the consortium's communication programme.

The primary function of The Steering Committee will be to provide strategic oversight and set research directions, review research infrastructure development proposals and work programmes, review the consortium's progress in meeting its objectives, and guide the relationship of the consortium with its principal research partners.

The consortium will be managed according to the principles of good governance and internal control to help ensure clarity of vision and common understanding of purpose.

11.5 What will the AFROX-H2 network deliver?

I. The scientific contribution of Africa to studies and trials that could lead to increased access to cancer care and palliation [2, 3].

AFROX-H2 is already starting to discuss some relevant proposals. One phase 1/2 clinical trial will focus on combining radiotherapy and immunotherapy using smart delivery technology (biomaterial drones), with an initial focus on pancreatic and metastatic castration-resistant prostate cancer, which disproportionally affects African populations. Recent work indicates that the use of a single fraction of radiotherapy in combination with immunotherapy can significantly boost both local and metastatic tumour kill with a major increase in survival and the development of immune memory. The smart delivery approach could also significantly reduce systemic/overlapping toxicities. This innovative scientific treatment approach is expected to result in potentially better outcomes, increased access to care, a major reduction in cost, and enhanced convenience for patients (see https://www.ncbi.nlm.nih.gov/pmc/articles/PMC7193821/).

Another potential phase 2/3 trial involves the use of cannabinoids to manage the side-effects of chemotherapy/radiotherapy and the management of cancer pain instead of opioids.

II. The scientific contribution of Africa in the era of personalized medicine.

Clearly, we can set a number of deliverables, milestones, and metrics for conventional trial endpoints, e.g. recruitment times, data quality audits, etc., but we are aiming to establish a network which embraces this era of personalized medicine in which treatment selection for each cancer patient might become individualized or customized. This is possible because of advances in molecular profiling, a technique whereby each cancer might be typed according to the pattern of gene and protein expression and correlated with the cancer stage, prognosis, and natural history. There is worldwide acceptance that such molecular profiling, facilitating the targeting and customization of treatments, represents the next leap forward in improving the quality of care of cancer patients.

The expansion of our knowledge of cancer biology is creating molecular profiling options for many tumor types and there is now the possibility that we can achieve the long-sought-after goal of selective and specific personalised treatment. However, there are consequences that come with tumor subtyping and highly targeted treatment. Older classes of drugs, such as non-specific cytotoxic chemotherapeutic agents, target a very broad spectrum of tumour types and hence can be widely used. In contrast, highly targeted therapies will be restricted in application to a subset of patients whose tumors display the required expression of a biologic or genetic abnormality. Given that cancer is such a heterogeneous disease, it is likely that a very large number of targeted therapies will be required to treat the diversity of tumors.

Nick la Thangue and Rachel (Midgley) Kerr [4] stated in 2013 that despite the fact that the focus is on biomarkers, we consider the proposal of Elzawawy, 2012 [5] that the terms 'personalized' or 'customized' should be extended to include more aspects of human host variability in pharmacogenomics, pharmacodynamics, and pharmacokinetics for different drugs, as well as other personal variations in human beings, such as their socioeconomic aspects and expectations. Therefore, the term 'personalized treatment' will evolve from 'the mechanics' of hitting one target in the tumor to the broader concept and vision of medicine that considers the integration of biological tumor issues, human aspects, and medical wisdom to enhance the overall outcome for individual patients

11.6 Challenges to the conventional drug development paradigm

Drug development is a long-term, high-risk, and very expensive undertaking with a well-recognized high rate of attrition. The cost of bringing a new medicine to market is spiraling and is now estimated to range from \$800 million to as much as \$1.7 billion per drug. One of the factors that contributes to these enormous costs is the high attrition/failure rate of drugs as they progress through the development pipeline (currently, after pre-clinical studies, a drug passes through three phases of clinical trials: phase I looks at toxicity, phase II looks at efficacy, and phase III assesses the drug in a large population to gain statistically significant data). The drug candidates that survive a decade or more of pre-clinical development and enter phase I testing have only an 8% chance of reaching the public in the form of a marketed product, and the success rate is even lower in oncology (~5%). Improving the efficiency of drug development through lower attrition rates or faster development times would have a major impact on the cost of new drug development.

Currently, there are over 600 new anticancer agents in development, and it is to be expected that the portfolio/pipeline of therapeutic candidates for cancer created by basic science laboratories and seeking clinical validation will increase significantly over the next ten years. With such a strong pipeline, the challenge now facing the industry is how to prioritise the large and growing list of candidates and select for further investment those that have the highest probability of successfully completing clinical development and achieving commercial success. Drug developers are constantly trying to seek ways of identifying candidates that are unlikely to succeed early in the drug development process, so that they can make 'go/no-go' decisions early and redirect resources as appropriate. However, making such decisions early in the drug development process is very difficult, unless developers have access to the sort of biomarker analytical and pharmacokinetic modeling expertise which we will build into our trials network, which gives us the opportunity to accelerate the development of pharmacy and biotech drug development programmes.

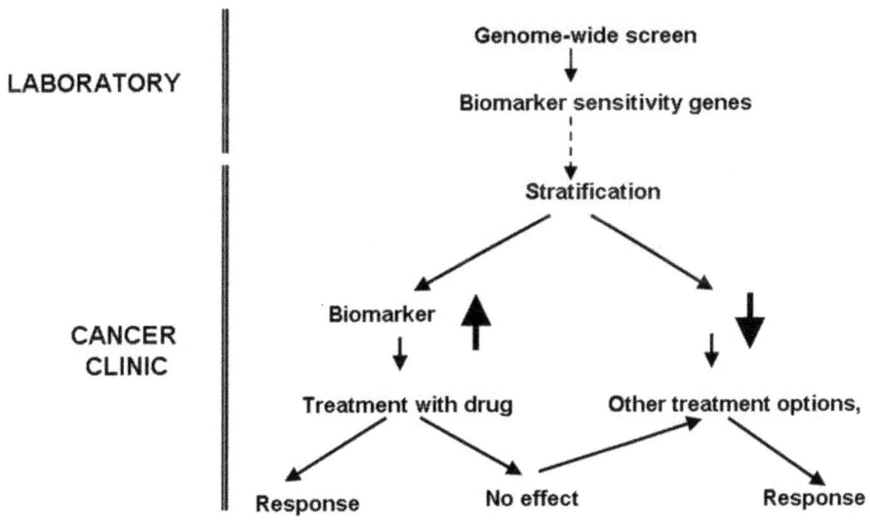

With traditional cytotoxic drugs, the inherent assumption is that efficacy is somehow related to toxicity. Therefore, the primary objective of a phase I trial is to establish the largest dose of a drug that is associated with tolerable toxicity, and this is the dose used in subsequent trials. However, with the development of targeted therapies, this approach might not be optimal or applicable and instead, determining the 'biologically effective dose' might be a more relevant objective of early-phase trials (phase I and phase II). To do this, early-phase clinical trials need to become more advanced, so that observations in patients are complemented by the use of highly sophisticated, laboratory-based technologies—such as genomics, proteomics, and functional imaging—which yield biomarkers of efficacy that relate to the novel mechanisms of action of the candidate. This incorporation of translational research into early-phase clinical trials represents a paradigm shift in drug development, in which Oxford and Harvard have been at the forefront. This new approach will enable the systematic de-prioritization of investigational agents that clearly do not show biological effects early in drug development, on the basis of human pharmacological data rather than relying on data collected via animal models. Therefore, it is anticipated that the incorporation of translational research into early trials will provide critical early data for use in making informed 'go/no-go' decisions. Although this model is described for anticancer drug development, the general principles are applicable to all other disease sites.

Given the growing realisation that animal data does not adequately predict the potential success of a drug, and that human data needs to be collected at the earliest possible stages in the drug development process, the Food and Drug Administration (FDA) and the National Cancer Institute (NCI) in the US have recently introduced the Exploratory Investigational New Drug Applications (eIND) or phase 0 clinical trial. This is a mechanism for obtaining preliminary human data, establishing feasibility, and verifying assay methodology in limited numbers of patients before embarking on a phase I trial. It is hoped that phase 0 clinical trials will further facilitate rational drug selection, help to identify therapeutic failures early in the drug development process, and ultimately shorten the timelines for anticancer drug development. The potential to make earlier and more rational 'go/no-go' decisions coupled with the selection of patients with susceptible disease based on molecular markers increases the probability of demonstrating early drug efficacy and reducing drug development costs.

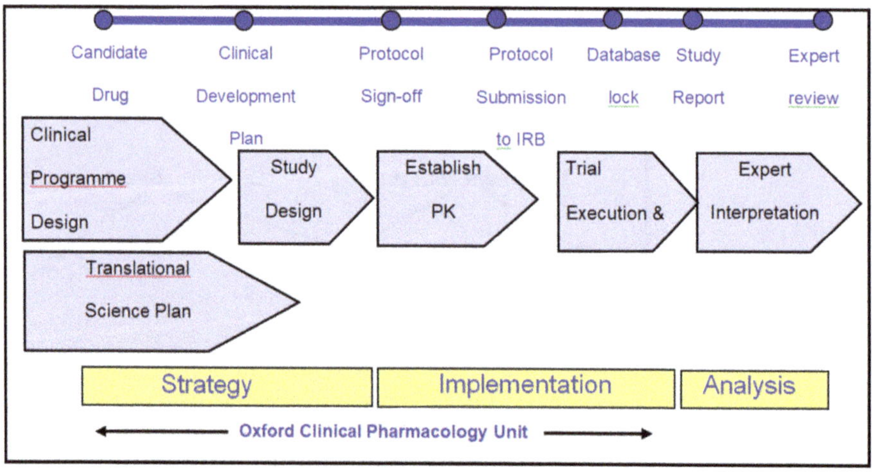

We will work with centres to create a large biorepository of human tumour tissue, permitting us to explore the biology of African cancers. This information will be translated into the clinical context in the form of designs for hypothesis-driven clinical trials, for example, a typical phase 2 trial in which the design has been driven by our predictive biomarker, enriched for African patients who will be recruited into the trial with tumour biopsies screened for biomarker expression, and who will be monitored for their response to the drug treatment. Thereafter, a correlation will be made between biomarker expression and clinical response, allowing the relationship between the biomarker and efficacy to be clarified. Consequently, the phase 3 trial will be enabled to measure the effect of the drug on a tumor type that is much more likely to produce a favorable clinical outcome, because patients will be selected according to the level of biomarker expression

References and further reading

[1] Kerr D 2019 The GHC Win-Win Initiative (Boston, MA: Harvard Medical School) Link to Video https://youtu.be/qpHZ2pIUsQQ

[2] Kerr D, Arnold D, Blay J-Y, Buske C, Carrato A, Gerritsen W and Peeters M 2020 The Oncology Data Network (ODN): A Collaborative European Data-Sharing Platform to Inform Cancer Care *Oncologist* **25** e1-e4

[3] Kerr D J and Pezzella F 2019 *Oxford Textbook of Cancer Biology* (Oxford: Oxford University Press)

[4] Kerr D J, Van De Velde C, Haller D and Baumann M 2016 *Oxford Textbook of Oncology* (Oxford: Oxford University Press)

[5] Johnson R and Kerr D 2015 Publication and dissemination of research *Cancer Research and Clinical trials in Developing Countries* ed D C Stefan (Cham, Switzerland: Springer) pp 201–12

[6] Church D, Kerr R, Domingo E, Rosmarin D, Palles C, Maskell K, Tomlinson I and Kerr D 2014 'Toxgnostics': an unmet need in cancer medicine *Nat. Rev. Cancer* **14** 440–5

[7] Adewole I *et al* 2014 Building capacity for sustainable research programmes for cancer in Africa *Nat. Rev. Clin. Oncol.* **11** 251–9

[8] Kerr D J and Shi Y 2013 Biological markers: tailoring treatment and trials to prognosis *Nat. Rev. Clin. Oncol.* **10** 429–30

[9] La Thangue N B and Kerr D J 2011 Predictive biomarkers: a shift towards personalised cancer medicine *Nat. Rev. Clin. Oncol.* **8** 587–96

[10] Elzawawy A, Khaled H and Omar S *et al* 2013 The role of South and East Mediterranean College of Oncology *Cancer Control* http://cancercontrol.info/cc2013/elzawawy/

[11] The South and East Mediterranean College of Oncology http://semco-oncology.info/

[12] Elzawawy A M 2015 Could African and low- and middle-income countries contribute scientifically to global cancer care? *J. Glob. Oncol.* **1** 49–53

[13] Elzawawy A and Cazap E 2019 ecancer series of global cancer leaders https://ecancer.org/en/video/8112-prof-ahmed-elzawawy-on-global-cancer-control

[14] La Thangue N and Midgley R 2013 Personolized cancer care *How to Get Better Value Cancer Care* ed J A Muir Gray and D J Kerr (Oxford: Offox Press Ltd) pp 100–9

[15] Elzawawy A 2012 Science and affordability of cancer drugs and radiotherapy in the world: win-win scenarios ed R Mohan *Advances in Cancer Management* (Rijeka: InTech) http://intechopen.com/articles/show/title/science-and-affordability-of-cancer-drugs-and-radiotherapy-in-the-world

Chapter 12

The win-win ambassadors

Luca Incrocci

It is known that there is a great need to enhance the effective efforts to fill the huge gaps in value-based clinical oncology care worldwide. The Global Health Catalyst Win-Win Initiative adopts scientific approaches and win-win scenarios that consider all stakeholders. We also emphasize that we are catalysts, consultants, and advisors. We are not competing with, or replacing, any, but we are complementing, empowering, and acting as positive mediators. We are open to all partnerships and collaborations. We are not a funding body. Moreover, to achieve a remarkable increase in clinical oncology services, broad advocacy is needed at all levels worldwide. The required roles of the honorary and distinguished professional Win-Win Ambassadors include serving as high representatives and advocates for the causes of the initiative at different levels and on different global occasions. The distinguished professional ambassadors (who are usually professionals and experts in fields related to cancer) are volunteer experts who can advise and act as catalysts for the establishment and development of clinical oncology—radiotherapy services. We are not marketing certain devices or drugs and we are not agents for any company, but we can offer technical and medical advice about radiotherapy-clinical oncology projects from A to Z, i.e. from the idea until the service is operational and for years afterwards. Our Global Oncology University (Go-U) and ecancerforall (previously ecancer4all) will help. Furthermore, some of the willing Win-Win Ambassadors can help by advising and mentoring the GHC Win-Win young catalysts. The ecancerforall website and the GO-U provide e-platforms to facilitate this. The contribution of one win-win ambassador, HRH Princess Dina Mired was included earlier in this book. In this chapter, we will include the contribution of another win-win ambassador, Professor Luca Incrocci.

My name is Luca Incrocci. I am a radiation oncologist at the Erasmus MC Cancer Institute in Rotterdam, The Netherlands. The department of radiation

doi:10.1088/978-0-7503-3075-6ch12

oncology in Rotterdam is the biggest in the Netherlands and one of the biggest in Europe. We have twelve linacs (of which two are robotic systems), hyperthermia and brachytherapy facilities, and a proton center. We have 33 radiation oncologists, 15 medical physicists, 15 residents in radiation oncology and more than 130 radiation therapy technologists.

Cancer is an emerging public health problem in Africa. The number of cancer patients will double by 2030, due to aging and the growth of the population. This increase is due to societal and economical transitions. What we call Westernization, for example, the use of tobacco, unhealthy diets, and limited exercise all contribute to several chronic diseases and cancer. Cancer receives a low public health priority in Africa because of the limited resources that are mainly used for communicable diseases, such as malaria, HIV/Aids, and tuberculosis. The majority of cancers in Africa are diagnosed at an advanced stage because of the lack of screening and early detection services. Africa also lacks consultants, nurses, pathology workers, health educators, and medical specialists.

What can we do? We can develop health care educational programs, we can increase the number of staff at hospitals and especially at community health centers, and of course, one of the most important things to do is to increase radiotherapy facilities.

In 2011, the general assembly of the United Nations adopted a resolution stating that by 2025, 25% of all non-communicable diseases, including cancer, should be reduced. Radiotherapy can contribute strongly to this reduction. Unfortunately, more than 90% of the population in low- and middle-income countries (LMICs) does not have access to radiotherapy.

Africa has 160 radiotherapy centres, though most of them are in South Africa or Egypt. Only 29 African countries have a radiotherapy facility and their machines, if any, are often more than twenty years old. One misleading assumption is that radiotherapy is not feasible in LMICs and especially in Africa because of the lack of electricity, poor public transport, political instability, and the need for specialized staff. This is not always true. It is true that radiotherapy needs high levels of investment, skills, and resources. It has been calculated that by 2035, there will be a need for more than 3000 radiation oncologists, more than 2000 medical physicists, and more than 8000 radiation oncology technologists worldwide.

In 2007, the Win-Win Initiative was proposed by Dr Ahmed Elzawawy, professor of clinical oncology from Egypt, with the aim of increasing the affordability of better cancer treatment in the world through a scientific approach. All stakeholders can win with this initiative—not only patients and their families, but also manufacturers of radiotherapy machines and medical devices. In April 2016, the Win-Win Initiative joined the Harvard Global Health Catalyst of Harvard Medical School, becoming one of its activities. I am proud to have joined the Harvard Global Health Catalyst and the Win-Win Initiative as an ambassador and I am proud to be one of the volunteers. Erasmus MC can assist with the training of medical physicists, radiation oncologists, and radiation therapists. Erasmus MC can organize workshops in Africa and offer training activities at the Erasmus MC Cancer Institute. We can help in developing online and offline courses, share our treatment protocols, and offer advice through teleconferencing. Let's do this together!

The following is a link to a full video contribution by Professor Luca during the GHC Win-Win Initiative on May 25, 2019, at Harvard Medical School, Boston, MA, USA: https://youtu.be/UwTMsvNldqg.

Chapter 13

Key steps for youth inclusion in global health efforts

Lydia Asana, Marielle Ngamije, Ntami Echeng, Victoria Ainsworth and Andres Diaz

While global health scholarships and practices continue to gain popularity, opportunities abound in terms of practical methods and shared templates for engaging key stakeholders in both current and anticipated needs. One such anticipated need is that of the sustainability of human resources for ongoing innovation, coordination, and impact. This is particularly true for low and middle-income countries and underserved populations within affluent nations. While good intentions and initiatives can be found, it is important to invest not only in the technology and funding needed to sustain programs, but also in engaging, equipping, and entrusting young people with roles and responsibilities that contribute to global health initiatives in mutually beneficial (win-win) ways.

13.1 Introduction

Global Health Catalyst (GHC) programmes have long sought to identify ways in which the diverse interests and experiences of young people can contribute to increasing access to global health care, advocacy, research, and education (C.A.R.E.). The leaders of GHC programs have recognized this need and have consistently engaged young adults as catalysts for global health. These young catalysts have been involved in a number of roles, for example, as event participants, volunteers, mentees, research associates, presenters, and publication contributors. By intentionally engaging, equipping, and entrusting young people with defined roles and responsibilities, GHC programs have established a growing global network of GHC Young Catalysts committed to furthering the global health program goal of increasing global access to health C.A.R.E.

doi:10.1088/978-0-7503-3075-6ch13

13.2 Engage

Key methods of engaging young people in global health programs include identifying relevant groups of young people, such as students in relevant classes, clubs, or programs. Once identified, win-win relationships are formed with these entities and young people are invited to participate in global health projects around the world. They are given the opportunity to serve in short, medium, or long-term programs or single events, with perks, such as support for attending and/or presenting at global health events, including GHC Summits. Examples of activities include providing social media engagement services, researching content for health education programs, or staffing information desks at events. Examples of GHC collaborations include working with medical humanities students under Dr Lindy Davidson at the University of South Florida's Honors College. These students in diverse academic majors have contributed to both national and international global health activities by lending skills in communications, computer science, management, and the sciences. Similarly, establishing a relationship with the student-led African Students Organization at the University of Central Florida has resulted in numerous long-term GHC volunteers and team members. Some who started as undergraduate students are now in medical school, have earned graduate degrees in public health, or are serving as social work professionals. A partnership with a nonprofit organization provided logistical support for annual summits in which students designed flyers, facilitated check-in, and documented sessions. Students and associates of GHC team members have been engaged in research and writing projects.

13.3 Equip

It is important to provide the proper context and tools to enable young people to value opportunities to be engaged and make meaningful contributions. In the case of GHC programmes, team members visit identified groups to provide information on programmes and opportunities. Interested young people then receive additional, detailed information related to the proposed project. Such information includes the cultural context as well as a program overview, goals, and a description of how specific assignments contribute to this goal. Where needed, particularly for long-term engagement, specific skills and program processes are included in young catalyst training and mentoring. Long-serving GHC Young Catalysts have been mentored to present at conferences or co-publish. Many have received support in their personal educational and career goals through mentorship, recommendations, and access to key professionals in their field. By ensuring that young people possess or gain useful context, skills, and access to professional development, we make their experience more rewarding, both for the participants and for the programmes or events they are engaged in.

13.4 Entrust

Once young people are engaged and equipped to contribute to global health efforts, they must be given the opportunity to genuinely do so. Based on the experience, skills, and individual drive of the participant, appropriate levels of responsibility and autonomy should be considered. Opportunities should be created for young people to contribute ideas, content, and program components in order to gain from their innovative minds and methods. In addition, granting opportunities to contribute beyond basic tasks communicates that young people are a valued part of the team.

The organizers of the 2019 GHC Summit included a session dedicated to youth engagement. This session was characterized by presentations by young catalysts on topics including research, medical missions, global disabilities, and advocacy for overlooked health conditions. Experienced professionals interested in the session primarily played an observational role while over forty young catalysts ranging from high schoolers to young professionals from Africa, Asia, Europe, North America, and South America actively participated, facilitated, and later reported on this segment of the global summit. During an interactive segment, young catalysts played a key role in facilitating small group discussions on global healthcare, advocacy, research, and education. For this segment the forty participants formed four small groups for guided discussions. Below are the guided questions posed and a summary of the reported recommendations made by participating young catalysts.

In what ways can young global health catalysts extend and promote the work and impact of the Global Health Catalyst?

- Learn from the successes and failures of existing educational programs
- Establish cross-cultural programs focused on tangible, practical support beyond just data, statistics, and terminology that is better suited to professionals
- Consider the culture, customs, beliefs, and faith practices of target groups and tailor efforts to specific target groups
- Invest in counseling to address stigma and misinformation before embarking on care initiatives
- Incorporate the diversity of cultures and disciplines into collaborative, integrated teams in research, education, care, and advocacy

What strategies can be employed to extend and promote the work and impact of the global health catalyst summit through young adults?

- Create an open-source database of information to support science and research education and careers for young people
- Identify and integrate the things that excite practitioners and young people into the process of engaging young catalysts as early as middle and high school
- Employ a grass-roots approach, entrusting college students with responsibilities that build a sense of ownership in leading community efforts
- Employ a combination of success stories and influencers from within a given community when working in a given community
- Create an infrastructure that supports the return of the diaspora and the inclusion of young catalysts in global outreach programs and policies

What challenges may arise in this effort?

- Lack of buy-in from young people who do not always feel their voices are heard and from communities who may not see young people as a valuable resource
- Logistics of coordinating global efforts, identifying key target populations, matching young people to appropriate tasks, and incorporating diversity of interests and experiences
- Policies and structures that inhibit youth involvement, and limited knowledge to access support in navigating the same
- Retention: the ongoing motivation, development, and recognition of young catalyst contributions is more challenging than initial engagement
- Resources to support young catalysts who need mentorship, training, and funds for transportation, conference fees, and other related costs

As illustrated in the insightful summary outcomes from the 2019 GHC Summit Young Catalysts session, young people are willing and able to participate in global health efforts. When entrusted with tasks, they are able to deliver thoughtful and innovative contributions. In order for these contributions to meet real needs, young people need to be equipped with context and guidance. Armed with this knowledge, compatible youth populations can be engaged through concerted efforts. Global Health Catalyst programs have enjoyed the benefits of engaging, equipping, and entrusting young adults with diverse cultural and educational backgrounds. In keeping with the GHC win-win approach, numerous young people have also been supported through training, mentoring, recommendations, and support. Some are now medical students, some are pursuing advanced research or professional degrees in areas of medical research, others are entering the workforce with graduate public health training, and still others have made educational and career changes in order to more directly influence global health outcomes. The contributors to this chapter exemplify each of these scenarios. Including youth in current global health efforts provides meaningful support to all parties involved, the youth, the programs, and of course, those served worldwide; a win-win-win.

Part III

Scientific resource-saving and better value cancer treatment approaches: the first wing of the Win-Win International Scientific Initiative

Chapter 14

A general overview for scientific resource-saving and better-value cancer treatment approaches

Ahmed Elzawawy

All chapters of this book are directed to all the stakeholders except this part III as it is directed particularly to cancer care professionals, scientists, health industries and health economists. This part contains more specialized medical terms. The objective of this chapter is to present some examples of the published studies and ideas of many authors. We don't claim that all these approaches are exclusive or final solutions. Nevertheless, it shows that there are unlimited approaches for scientific studies and researches that could lead to lower the total costs without diminishing cancer treatment outcome. This could potentially increase opportunities of patient-centered value of cancer care. The win-win doesn't present just one more book or some more declarations or slogans, but, by presenting these examples, we call for more enormous scientific approaches in the real world. As we emphasized several times in the win-win movement—and in this book—that this would serve millions of human's beings with cancer in the world, to boost progress of science implementation, to save the health systems economies from collapse and to flourish health industries. All would win! As we presented in the chapters before, the first wing of the win-win movement implies the explorations of scientific approaches for cost sparing and how to increase affordability of better-value cancer care in the world. Readers can access more relevant examples of our previous publications, working meetings like those during ASCO conferences and ESMO and ESMO Global Policy Committee and ecancer videos on the web http://www.icedoc.org/winwin.htm. After the introduction, the chapter covers total cost of cancer care including personalized cancer care, and also discusses the choosing wisely campaign

14.1 Introduction

In this chapter, we focus on an exploration of examples of published and ongoing scientific research and approaches that could lead to resource sparing and better-value

doi:10.1088/978-0-7503-3075-6ch14

radiotherapy and systemic cancer therapy. Some of the presented examples take breast cancer as a model that could be expanded to other cancers worldwide. Breast cancer is the world's most frequently diagnosed cancer among women. Moreover, nearly all of the diagnostic and treatment modalities are used in breast cancer care [1–3].

The win-win initiative suggests that clinical oncologists should not automatically copy the protocols or guidelines of international societies or groups if they do not fit the local patients and conditions. For example, by definition, cancer treatment guidelines can be very useful as guides, but should not be considered as obligatory pathways for treating every patient in every community of the world. Useful approaches and protocols can be tailored in scientific evidence-based ways in order to consider how to get better-value, patient-centered healthcare according to the real conditions of your patients in different communities. This means that there is room for a wide range of scientific works and publications that are relevant to real-world practice [1, 2].

14.2 The total cost and not solely the prices of drugs or devices per se

As we have emphasized several times in the win-win movement—and in this book—this would serve millions of human beings with cancer in the world, boost the progress of the implementation of science, save health system economies from collapse, and help health industries to flourish. All would win! We consider the resource sparing of the total cost of clinical oncology care and not solely the prices of radiotherapy devices and cancer drugs per se.

In France, the contribution of drug costs to the total cost of cancer care was less than 20% [4].

In the USA, Barlas posed the question 'are hospital prices a bigger problem than drug prices?' and he presented these statistics [5]:

- Overall, hospitals represent 33% of U.S. healthcare costs; physician and clinical spending account for 20%; drugs account for 10%.
- Total U.S. hospital spending in 2017 reached $1.1 trillion, compared with $333 billion for prescription drugs, according to the findings of the Centers for Medicare and Medicaid Services (CMS).
- For the year ending December 31, 2017, hospital costs rose by 4.6%, compared with a 0.4% rise in drug costs, again according to the CMS. For the previous year, hospital costs rose 5.6%, or more than two-and-a-half times the rate of inflation. Drug costs rose by 2.3% in 2016. Hospital spending increases outpaced drug increases again in 2018.

However, in recent years there has been more skyrocketing in the prices of new drugs than ever.

Ideally, value-based pricing of drugs or approval-based pricing using incremental cost-effectiveness (ICER), expressed per quality-adjusted life year (QALY) gained in relation to the average national income, would be a promising method for setting limits on the cost of new treatments [6].

In the UK, the National Institute for Health and Clinical Excellence (NICE) evaluates the clinical and cost effectiveness of oncological interventions, explicitly considering their cost per QALY gained, and provides the UK National Health Service (NHS) with advice about which treatments should be covered. A value-based pricing system of approval for medicines has been adopted in the UK. It is proposed that such a system will recognize innovation, unmet need, and the burden of disease, factors that should favor the funding of cancer medicines [7].

U.S. healthcare payers, health economists, and policymakers are looking for strategies to combat high drug prices and spending. In the United States, spending on prescription drugs grew by an average of 3.6% annually from 2008 to 2017, a rate far more rapid than in other developed nations such as France, where retail drug spending declined during the same period.

To control spending, France sets maximum prices for new products that reflect the added value of the new drug compared with a comparative product. The country also forbids price increases after a new drug's launch and, after five years, lowers prices and obtains additional discounts based on market competition. France also requires manufacturers to pay refunds if spending exceeds a national pharmaceutical spending cap set by Parliament. By retaining approaches used in France, private and public payers in the U.S. could reduce drug spending without restricting access to new drugs. France's pharmaceutical cost-control strategy has two parts. First, the government contracts with manufacturers to purchase new medications at a price that reflects their added therapeutic value. Second, it uses a budget restraint to keep national health insurance (NHI) drug spending in line. [8, 9]. Using regulation versus relying on markets to advance goals is at the center of a long-standing debate in U.S. health policy. Many analysts contend that regulation is inefficient and prevents competition. The example of France shows that regulation does not prevent price competition and can even make use of market prices.

No country's system can be fully replicated in the U.S. or any other country, whether it is rich or less affluent. However, lessons cane be learned by studying how countries such as France achieve lower drug prices. The French system determines maximum drug prices based on added therapeutic value and external reference pricing. It employs negotiation to set prices and limits price increases. It limits total spending to a global budget. Each approach might be implemented in the United States or inspire similar reforms in different countries [9]. We stress that the value of interventions or treatments should be patient-centered and that it also varies in different communities and under different conditions.

From the above, we stress that in the win-win movement, 'scientific studies' means not only medical, clinical, pharmacological, medical physics, health industry innovation, and informatics studies but also economic research, business model studies, and all aspects that contribute to increasing access to better-value cancer care in the world.

14.3 Personalized cancer medicine and better-value outcomes for patients

In 2011, Elzawawy stated that there is sometimes an overlap between the term 'targeted therapy' and the broader meaning of the term 'personalized medicine'. He proposed that the term 'personalized treatment' would move away from the notion of only hitting one target in the tumor with a drug—usually expensive—to the broader concept of considering evidence-based studies of medical factors, biological tumor factors, and human factors such as personal expectations and priorities without compromising the overall outcome. Hence, it would include more aspects of the human host, such as the variability of pharmcogenomics, pharmacodynamics, and pharmacokinetics for different drugs, and other personal variations in human beings and their socioeconomic aspects. [2, 10]

Moreover, we suggest that the term 'precision cancer treatment' should include a prediction of the risks and toxicities of treatment in real daily practice in the real world, which may differ among patients as individuals and for different communities, ethnicities, and pharmacogenomics aspects.

14.4 The 'choosing wisely' campaign

14.4.1 Choosing wisely in medical practice

Overtreatment and unnecessary care and their consequences for patient safety and health system sustainability are issues of increasing concern [11].

In 2002, the American Board of Internal Medicine (ABIM) Foundation published 'Medical professionalism in the new millennium: *a Physician Charter'*, which stated that physicians have a responsibility to promote health equity when some health resources are scarce [12]. In 2010, physician Howard Brody recommended that medical specialty societies, being stewards of a field, ought to publish a list of five things they would like to see changed in their field and publish it for their members [12–14].

In 2012, The ABIM led Choosing Wisely as a United States-based health educational campaign about unnecessary healthcare, unnecessary tests, treatments, and procedures. To conduct the campaign, the ABIM Foundation asked medical specialty societies to make five to ten recommendations and then published this information; the medical specialty societies disseminated it to their members [11].

The Choosing Wisely campaign became an international multispecialty initiative. The campaign has been cited as being part of a broader movement including many comparable campaigns [15]. To date, 25 countries have joined the movement, including Canada (which coordinates the organization) Australia, Brazil, Wales, Germany, Japan, England, Israel, Italy, New Zealand, the Netherlands, Switzerland, and the United States. More than 80 professional societies have participated in this effort, generating a list of more than 550 examples of unnecessary and low-value services. Oncological and other societies have targeted routine tests and treatments that are associated with increasing healthcare costs and patient harm and which do not improve survival or the quality of life [16].

14.4.2 Choosing wisely in clinical oncology

In the United States, escalating healthcare costs represent a central problem for both the federal government and the private sector. The cost of cancer care in the USA is rising exponentially, and cancer care–related spending was projected to reach $173 billion in 2020. A proportion of this expenditure is attributed to unnecessary medical services, which account for an estimated 21% of all healthcare services provided in the United States. This information is particularly useful for policymakers, as it helps them to understand the future burden of the costs of cancer care and to prioritize future resources for cancer research, treatment, and prevention [17].

The American Society of Clinical Oncology (ASCO) is the largest medical professional oncology society in the world committed to conquering cancer through research, education, prevention, and the delivery of high-quality patient care.

The ASCO recognizes the importance of evidence-based cancer care and making wise choices in the diagnosis and management of patients with cancer. After careful deliberation by experienced oncologists, the ASCO highlighted ten categories of tests, procedures, and/or treatments whose common use and clinical value are not supported by the available evidence. These test and treatment options should not be administered unless the physician and patient have carefully considered whether their use is appropriate in an individual case [18, 19]. At the ASCO Choosing Wisely website [19], the reader can view a list of ten items that 'Physicians and Patients Should Question' in oncology: https://www.choosingwisely.org/societies/american-society-of-clinical-oncology/

14.4.3 Recognized limitations, but there are great global needs

There is no doubt that there is a great need all over the world to achieve the aims of Choosing Wisely to reduce the costs of unnecessary medical procedures and treatments. However, the campaign has garnered both praise and criticism, while some of its ideas have spread to other countries. In a study performed in 2015 in the USA, primary healthcare providers found most of the Choosing Wisely recommendations easy to follow, but they felt that some, especially those for symptomatic conditions, would be difficult for patients to accept. Some doctors have said they lack time for the recommended discussions [20]. In the UK, English doctors 'are worried how patients will perceive the initiative' [21]. As stated in the ASCO Choose Wisely website, '*Choosing Wisely's recommendations should not be used to establish coverage decisions or exclusions. But, they are meant to encourage conversation about what is appropriate and necessary treatment. As each patient situation is unique, providers and patients should use the recommendations as guidelines to determine an appropriate treatment plan together*' [19]. Regarding the impact, one of the noted criticisms is that Choosing Wisely does not include an evaluation of its effects on costs, discussions, or medical outcomes [15]. The Choosing Wisely campaign has no intention of scientifically researching its own efficacy, but academic centers and clinics are making plans to independently report on the impact of the campaign [22]. The services targeted by the Choosing Wisely lists have a broad variance in how much impact they can have on patient care and costs [23]. Doctors analyzed many of the services listed as low value by Choosing Wisely and other sources, and found that 25% or 42% of Medicare patients received at least one of these services in an average year, depending on the definition used and there was no significant pattern among different types of physician [24].

The scope of the Choosing Wisely recommendations for cancer care is not well defined. A quality improvement study characterized the scope of these recommendations, focusing on the de-implementation of low-value cancer care, and identified potential gaps for future work [25]. The Choosing Wisely recommendations proposed by some of the most important oncological societies should be considered a starting point and treated with sensitivity by this movement. Nevertheless, the remaining path is still long, especially if a real cultural change in the oncological community must happen before Choosing Wisely becomes a real '*modus operandi*', which means a particular way of doing or implementing something [26].

There are more potential defects in the Choosing Wisely initiative; the greatest, perhaps, is the lack of uniform metrics. It is feasible to state that a test is unnecessary, but what criteria are used to reliably and prospectively define what is necessary? The most important challenge will be the change of attitude in clinical practice for the situations in which the scientific evidence suggests that the proposed intervention has a modest impact, no impact, or could even be harmful. This change is necessary and the challenge should be accepted quickly, so that Choosing Wisely will increasingly come to mean *Choosing Right* [26, 27]. Choosing Wisely has created a principal pathway through which patients and their doctors can discuss when healthcare services may not be needed. Several important steps are still needed to fulfill the promise of Choosing Wisely. It is now time to take those steps [27].

14.5 Financial toxicity tumor board (FTTB)

As explained in different parts of this book, fiscal distress or 'financial toxicity', in which patients experience challenges in paying for treatment, are becoming dominant problems for patients with cancer in the US because of growing care costs and the policies of health insurance underwriters, which aim to reduce their levels of spending.

For that reason, the first Financial Toxicity Tumor Board (FTTB) was launched in September 2019 by the Levine Cancer Institute (LCI) [28]. The LCI is composed of more than 40 hospitals and 900 offices that provide more than 12 million encounters per year and sees more than 18,000 new cases per year in North Carolina, South Carolina, and Georgia (USA).

The FTTB is modeled on the concept of a conventional multidisciplinary tumor board with participation from physicians, nurses, financial counselors, nurse navigators, social workers, and administrators who meet monthly. They are focused on the financial toxicity, financial worry, and fear experienced by patients with cancer. The FTTB is linked to a Patient Assistance Program for oncologic pharmaceutical agents, as this domain constitutes a critical area of financial toxicity for many patients.

As a result of the function of the FTTB, around $60 million of personal expenditure has been avoided for nearly 1800 patients, in addition to more than $1.3 million of copayment[1] assistance that was provided for financially challenged patients.

[1] In the US, a copayment or copay is a fixed amount for a covered service, paid by a patient to the provider of a health service each time a medical service is accessed (https://en.m.wikipedia.org/wiki/copayment).

The FTTB is a proactive example of the management of financial toxicity through the use of a multidisciplinary board. Raghavan *et al* from the LCI [28] stated that FTTBs could substantially ameliorate the growing international problem of financial distress or toxicity.

6. In the win-win movement, we emphasize the great need for tackling the problem of the increasing costs of cancer care worldwide [29]. It is time to move forward wisely and to increase the value of cancer care through clinical research [30]. Therefore, we—in the win-win movement and in this book—consider the Choosing Wisely campaign with appreciation and call for an enhancement of Choosing Wisely to include a broader evidence-based scope, to ensure the pragmatic feasibility of the campaign worldwide. So, we suggest that the Choosing Wisely campaign should adopt the win-win notions—that belong to all—and accordingly advocate for global collaborations and partnerships to conduct unlimited scientific explorations of evidence-based, value-based, and patient-centered innovative approaches that consider patients' physical, social, and personal conditions, their ethnicities, and patient expectations in different communities [1, 31]. The interests of different parties would be considered. Hence, it would be a big global Choosing Wisely Campaign, from which all the cancer care stakeholders in the real world would gain, and in particular, cancer patients.

7. Encouraging probable futuristic approaches: one example is the Genomic-Adjusted Radiation Dose (GARD). Scott and colleagues recently published a proposal to integrate genomics into radiation dosing decisions on August 4, 2021. Hence, the GARD-based framework could be the new model for personalizing radiotherapy prescription doses in clinical practice [32]. Until now, radiotherapy has dropped behind the vast progress made in targeted agents in systemic cancer therapy [33].

In our view, we see that in spite of the fact that that the tests could be expensive and that they would surely need advanced technology, with well-planned interinstitutional and industry cooperation, the tests could be further developed and used widely in the west. With more organized and focused North-South cooperation, these tests could also be applied in the South. As value could be defined as input in relation to output, GARD could lead to better radiotherapy results and also to the avoidance of unnecessary radiotherapy.

8. Final note: as cited here, in this chapter, we have focused on giving examples of scientific medical approaches. However, we emphasize that win-win notions have a broad scope that could include all the scientific studies and proposals that could lead to increased access to better-value cancer care. One example is an article recently published in August 2021, which stated that reducing the cost of healthcare entails a care redesign. The New England Journal of Medicine (NEJM) Catalyst Insights Council members discussed initiatives for decreasing healthcare costs, such as healthcare transitions and home-based care models [35].

A survey of the NEJM Catalyst Insights Council shows a desire for greater price transparency, but slow progress in understanding the costs of care. Care redesign offers an opportunity, but fee-for-service payment remains a problem [35]. The top activities with the greatest potential of containing the total cost of care for healthcare delivery organizations are: (1) care redesign (61%), (2) studies of data that show the cost of care to healthcare delivery organizations (41%), (3) shifting to ambulatory/outpatient settings (40%), (4) studies and data to show the cost of care to patients (35%), (5) more efficient use of clinical work (29%), (6) digital technology such as artificial intelligence and data analytics (22%), (7) novel payer contracts (19%), (8) clinical documentation improvement initiatives (14%) [35].

All the above recommendations and suggestions are important, but I see that according to the win-win scientific notions, without focused scientific studies, explorations, and clinical research in the real world, most of the recommendations will remain plans or wishes. For example, shifting to ambulatory/outpatient settings without comprising the outcomes for patients would require scientific evidence-based studies and innovative ideas (some examples are shown in the next chapters). Moreover, I emphasize that data on costs, information for care providers, and discussions with patients would be inethical and inhuman without an enormous scientific movement that includes the contribution of most—if not all—scientific bodies, institutions, and organizations to provide alternative cost-effective and value-based treatments tailored to patients in different communities and under different conditions. To consider realities, and to pass the phase of recommendations and dreams, win-win scenarios, smart ideas, and every effort should be used that consider the interests of different stakeholders. Hence, all would win in the real world!

Examples of scientific approaches are presented in the next chapters in Part III of this book.

References and further reading

[1] *The Win-Win Initiative* www.icedoc.org/winwin.htm and www.icedoc.net/winwin.htm

[2] Elzawawy A 2012 Science and affordability of cancer drugs and radiotherapy in the world—Win-Win scenarios *Advances in Cancer Management* ed R Mohan (Rijeka: InTech)

[3] Elzawawy A 2007 Breast cancer as a model to improve outcome of cancer care in low- and middle-income countries has now been published in the following paginated issue of *World J. Surg* **39** 693–4

[4] Amalric F 2007 Analyse economique des couts de cancer en France. Impact sur la qualité de vie, prevention, depistage, soin, recherche. Institut National Du Cancer, France

[5] Barlas S 2019 Are hospital prices a bigger problem than drug prices?: Congress doesn't know, doesn't care *P & T* **44** 259–99 https://ncbi.nlm.nih.gov/pmc/articles/PMC6487976/

[6] Sullivan R, Peppercorn J and Sikora K *et al* 2011 Delivering affordable cancer care in high-income countries *Lancet Oncol.* **12** 933–80

[7] NICE News 2011 NICE responds to government plan to introduce value based pricing. NICE News, March 21, 2011

[8] Valérie Paris 2005 'Pharmaceutical regulation in France 1980–2003,' *Int. J. Health Plan. Manag.* **20** 307–28

[9] Rodwin M 2019 What can the United States learn from pharmaceutical spending controls in France? Commonwealth Fund, Nov. 2019 https://doi.org/10.26099/tasq-my53 https://commonwealthfund.org/publications/issue-briefs/2019/nov/what-can-united-states-learn-drug-spending-controls-france

[10] La Thangue N and Midgley R 2013 *Personalized Cancer Care in How to Get Better Value Cancer Care* ed M Gray and D Kerr (Oxford, UK: Offox Press)

[11] Loring B, Ineson S and Sherwood D *et al* 2019 Choosing wisely means choosing equity *NZMJ* **132** 1496 https://nzma.org.nz/journal-articles/choosing-wisely-means-choosing-equity

[12] Cassel C and Guest J 2012 Choosing wisely—helping physicians and patients make smart decisions about their care *JAMA* **307** 1801–2

[13] Brody H 2010 Medicine's ethical responsibility for health care reform—the top five list *New Engl. J. Med.* **362** 283–5

[14] Brody H 2012 From an ethics of rationing to an ethics of waste avoidance *New Engl. J. Med.* **366** 1949–51

[15] Wikipedia 2020 Choosing wisely. December, 2020 https://en.wikipedia.org/wiki/Choosing_Wisely

[16] Choosing Wisely Canada 2012 Choosing wisely international campaigns https://choosingwiselycanada.org/campaign/international/

[17] Mariotto A B, Yabroff K R and Shao Y *et al* 2011 Projections of the cost of cancer care in the United States: 2010–20 *J. Natl. Cancer Inst.* **103** 117–28 (Erratum in *J. Natl. Cancer Inst.* **103** 699)

[18] Schnipper L 2013 *A Top Five List List in Oncology in How to Get Better Value Cancer Care* ed G Muir and D Kerr (Oxford, UK: Offox Press)

[19] American Society of Clinical Oncology (ASCO) 2019 Ten things physicians and patients should question https://choosingwisely.org/societies/american-society-of-clinical-oncology/

[20] Zikmund-Fisher B J, Kullgren J T and Fagerlin A *et al* 2017 Perceived barriers to implementing individual choosing wisely recommendations in two national surveys of primary care providers *J. Gen. Intern. Med.* **32** 210–7

[21] Vogel L 2015 Choosing wisely around the world *CMAJ* **187** E341–2

[22] Wang S 2013 Group urges health-test curbs *Wall Str. J.* February 20, 2013

[23] Morden N E, Colla C H and Sequist *et al* 2014 Choosing wisely—the politics and economics of labeling low-value services *New Engl. J. Med.* **370** 589–92

[24] McWilliams J M, Zaslavsky A M, Jena and Anupam B *et al* 2018 Analysis of physician variation in provision of low-value services. *JAMA Int. Med.* **179** 16–25

[25] Baskin A S, Wang T, Berlin N L and Skolarus T A *et al* 2020 Scope and characteristics of choosing wisely in cancer care recommendations by professional societies *JAMA Oncol.* **6** 1463–5

[26] Saletti P, Sanna P and Gabutti L *et al* 2018 Choosing wisely in oncology: necessity and obstacles *ESMO Open* **2018** e000382

[27] Kerr E A, Kullgren J T and Saini S D 2012 Choosing wisely: how to fulfill the promise in the next 5 years *Health Aff.* **36** 2012–8

[28] Raghavan D, Keith N A and Warden H R *et al* 2021 Levine cancer institute financial toxicity tumor board: a potential solution to an emerging problem *JCO Oncol. Pract.* **17** e1433–9

[29] Elzawawy A 2008 Breast care systemic therapy: the need for more economically sustainable scientific strategies in the world *Breast Care* **2008** 434–8

[30] Lichter A S 2018 From choosing wisely to using wisely: increasing the value of cancer care through clinical research *J. Clin. Oncol.* **36** 1387–8

[31] Elzawawy A 2019 Harvard global health catalyst win-win initiative. where we are and where we go? 2019. A Keynote speech, Global Health Catalyst Summit May 24–26, 2019, Harvard Medical School, Boston, MA, USA https://youtu.be/KqxevKZZyzE

[32] Scott J G, Sedor G, Ellsworth P, Scarborough J A, Ahmed K A, Oliver D E, Eschrich S A, Kattan M W and Torres-Roca J F 2021 Pan-cancer prediction of radiotherapy benefit using genomic-adjusted radiation dose (GARD): a cohort-based pooled analysis *Lancet Oncol.* **22** P1221–9

[33] Kaidar-Person O, Poortmans P and Salgado R 2021 Genomic-adjusted radiation dose to personalise radiotherapy *Lancet Oncol.* **22** P1200–1

[34] Bees J 2021 Reducing the cost of care requires care redesign *NEJM Catalyst Innov. Care Deliv.* **2**

[35] Gupta R 2021 Clinicians want to know the costs of care *NEJM Catalyst Innov. Care Deliv.* **2**

IOP Publishing

Approaching Global Oncology
The win-win model
Ahmed Elzawawy and Wilfred Ngwa

Chapter 15

Examples of scientific explorations for resource-saving better-value cancer drug systemic therapy

Ahmed Elzawawy

In this chapter, we present examples of literature describing scientific studies that could reduce the total cost of systemic cancer treatment (SCT) without compromising outcomes for patients. Some of the cited approaches lead to decreasing the need for chemotherapy hospitalization and eventually the total cost. As we mentioned in the previous chapter, most of the presented examples take breast cancer as a model that could be expanded to other cancers in the world.

Decreasing the need for chemotherapy hospitalization

15.1 Outpatient regimes

In most cancer treatments, the use of intravenous (IV) infusion chemotherapy protocols that require fewer hospitalizations is possible. There are already options for the outpatient regimen and oral therapy. However, there is a need to develop more of these protocols, based on scientific, pharmacological, and clinical information studies and innovative research. The adoption of this policy by cancer societies, its advocacy by such societies, and the awareness of oncologists about the increasing necessity to lessen hospitalizations for chemotherapy are also required.

We can learn from the crisis of COVID-19 pandemic and the shift to more outpatient regimens for cancer chemotherapy. One example is the shift to the combination of oral capecitabine and IV outpatient oxaliplatin in colorectal cancers replacing—as far as possible—protocols that necessitate admission to hospital.

15.2 The oral route for SCT

The oral route for the administration of chemotherapy could lower the cost of patient transportation, the administration of drugs by infusion, hospitalizations, and

doi:10.1088/978-0-7503-3075-6ch15

the subsequent costs of the adverse effects of hospitalization. The potential to receive an oral formulation would be a good option for patients, as it allows more convenient administration, requires less time to be spent at an infusion center, and offers the potential that many patients may not need a port-a-cath or other access device. Hence, it could lower the total cost by reducing the costs of patient transport, drug infusions, and hospitalizations. Moreover, it may improve quality of life, potentially lessen the burden, and be relatively more comfortable for patients and families [1].

15.2.1 Some of the known oral cancer drugs

Several oral cancer drugs have already shown breast cancer responses, such as capecetabine, cyclophoshamide, vinorelbine, etoposide, and oral hormonal therapies such as tamoxifen, anastrazole, letrozole, exemestane, and progesterone.

15.2.2 Examples of new oral cancer drugs

More pharmacological and clinical research to develop oral forms is warranted. Hence, most known cancers could have treatment regimes that are totally or partially administrated via the oral route. The pros and cons of the oral route for the administration of chemotherapy should be carefully studied in each community in scientific and realistic ways [1]. For new drugs, we recommend further pricing revisions for oral drugs and the other forms of non-IV infusion in order for them to be competitive (or not much higher than the total cost of drugs plus the cost of administration, medical staff, and hospitalization).

15.2.3 Oral taxane

In the category of first-line single-agent treatments, an oral taxane, tesetaxel, produced confirmed responses in 45% of 38 patients with HER2-negative, hormone receptor–positive metastatic breast cancer and stable disease in 37%, yielding a clinical benefit rate of 82% [2]. Five hundred and fifty-nine patients have been treated with tesetaxel, including 496 who received it as a monotherapy and 63 in combination with capecitabine. In metastatic breast cancer, tesetaxel has shown significant single-agent activity in two multicenter phase II trials [2, 3].

Unlike paclitaxel and docetaxel, tesetaxel has potent activity against p-glycoprotein-overexpressing tumors; the p-glycoprotein efflux pump mediates gastrointestinal (GI) absorption as well as chemotherapy resistance. Since tesetaxel is not pumped out by p-glycoprotein, it does not need to be given intravenously. The drug also is more bioavailable than other taxanes, and is highly soluble, so it does not require solubilizing agents such as polyethoxylated castor oil and accordingly it removes the need for prophylactic steroids. It has a half-life of about eight days, which allows it to be active for the whole 21-day cycle. The oral drug is given every three weeks and is associated with less alopecia and neuropathy than the levels of alopecia and neuropathy historically reported for parenteral taxanes. Over 1200 people have been treated with tesetaxel in 26 clinical studies. In 19 studies, it was administered as a monotherapy, and it was administered in a combination regimen in the remaining seven studies. Unfortunately, according to a press release issued by

Odonate Therapeutics on March 23, 2021, the clinical package data for tesetaxel is unlikely to support FDA approval. Therefore, clinical development of the oral chemotherapy agent tesetaxel is being discontinued for the treatment of metastatic breast cancer, colorectal cancer, and other solid tumors after the FDA provided feedback on a pre-new drug application [4].

15.3 Ongoing development of other chemotherapy routes

Ready-to-use formulations for subcutaneous (SC) administration significantly reduce pharmacy time, as no medicine preparation time is required.

15.3.1 Subcutaneous trastuzumab and pertuzumab

The FDA has approved a SC trastuzumab formulation for HER2+ breast cancer. Moreover, the randomized, open-label, phase 3 FeDeriCa trial tested the safety profile of SC pertuzumab and trastuzumab plus hyaluronidase in 500 patients with HER2-positive early breast cancer, and showed them to be non-inferior to IV infusions. Overall, the evidence shows that SC administration of monoclonal antibodies offers a faster, more convenient, and less invasive treatment option for HER2-positive breast cancer than IV infusions [5].

The SC administration of rituximab has been used for patients with CD20+ non-Hodgkin's lymphoma (NHL), CD20+ diffuse large B-cell lymphoma or follicular lymphoma [6, 7], and chronic lymphocytic leukemia (CLL) [8].

Patients received rituximab intravenously followed by a single dose of rituximab subcutaneously at one of three fixed doses (1400, 1600, or 1870 mg) in cycle 6. The primary objective was to identify a fixed SC dose that would achieve comparable rituximab serum trough concentrations to those achieved with the standard four-weekly 500 mg m^{-2} rituximab IV dose.

Over 80% of patients preferred SC rituximab over IV rituximab. The most common reasons cited included less time spent in clinic (69%), feeling more comfortable during administration (37%), and less emotional distress (29%) [6]. Satisfaction surveys were also administered as part of the MabEase study, which showed higher scores for 'impact on the activities of daily living', 'convenience', and 'satisfaction' when comparing SC rituximab with IV rituximab [9]. Although the literature supports improved patient satisfaction with the SC formulation, the decision to switch from IV to SC rituximab should be made only after thorough discussion with the patient, as some few patients may experience 'needle phobia' or otherwise prefer IV administration.

15.3.2 Another new exciting example of mode of administration is transdermal estradiol in prostate cancer [10]

Transdermal estradiol therapy produced an effective tumor response. Cardiovascular toxicity and other morbidities were substantially reduced compared with those expected of oral estrogen.

The incidence of gynecomastia was negligible. Transdermal estradiol therapy prevented andropause symptoms, improved quality of life scores, and increased bone density. Transdermal estradiol costs a tenth of the current therapy cost, with the potential for considerable economic savings, compared to conventional hormone therapies.

A new nebulizer device for treating lung cancer with the chemotherapy drug cisplatin could deliver small doses and result in quicker responses without the potential for renal damage which arises with the current IV method of administration [11, 12].

The use of the pulmonary route is a promising way to decrease the severe systemic toxicities associated with chemotherapy. Inhaled chemotherapy has been proved to be feasible and safe in phases I, Ib/IIa, and II of clinical trials. Inhalation allows high drug doses to be administered directly to lung tumors without prior distribution in the organism. Severe systemic toxicities are consequently reduced. However, the lack of improvement in the benefit/risk ratio, compared with conventional chemotherapy, in addition to higher financial costs (due to the requirement for specific hospital facilities and an inhalation procedure that limits environmental contamination) mean that inhalation has been underexploited in lung tumor therapy. Nevertheless, a changing trend has been observed in the past decade with the introduction of new pharmaceutical technologies, such as particle engineering in DPI formulations and nanomedicine.

Pharmacokinetic studies have taken place with the aim of lowering drug dose (and therefore the cost) by changing the infusion regimen.

The phase I/II trials of the prolonged infusion of low-dose gemcitabine are one example. The usual dose of 1000 to 1250 mg m^{-2} used for one patient might be enough for four to five patients and produce comparable results for the responses of solid cancers, such as non-small-cell lung cancer (NSCLC) and breast, pancreatic, and bladder cancers [13, 14].

15.4 Less frequent cycles with comparable efficacy

15.4.1 Zoledronic acid (Zometa) 4 mg every twelve weeks (instead of four weeks) in bone metastases

It may be time to change the dosing schedule of Zoledronic acid to every twelve weeks instead of every four weeks.

Zoledronic acid, a potent bisphosphonate, is commonly administered to patients with bone metastases to reduce the risk of skeletal-related events (SREs). However, there have been concerns regarding its long-term monthly administration.

A randomized study was conducted at 102 clinical trial centers in the United States from March 3, 2006, to July 25, 2013. Patients with bone metastases from breast cancer received 4.0 mg of IV zoledronic acid every four or twelve weeks with placebo for interim infusions for one year. The study randomized 416 women (⩾18 years old) with bone metastases from breast cancer who previously received nine or more doses of zoledronic acid and/or pamidronate during the first ten to fifteen months of therapy.

Another important trial included 1822 patients with three different diseases including prostate cancer, breast cancer, and multiple myeloma who were randomly assigned to receive zoledronic acid every twelve weeks or every four weeks for two years [2]. The primary endpoint was incidence of developing any skeletal-related event (SRE) [15, 16]. The twelve-week regimen of zoledronic acid was non-inferior to the four-week regimen for the proportion of patients experiencing one or more SRE [15, 16].

15.4.2 Nivolumab

Although there is no dispute that these drugs are highly effective for some patients, there are opportunities to reduce prescribing costs through a reduction in unit dosage, frequency, or duration of dosing. In this article, as Ratain and Goldstein [17] stated that time is money, we specifically focus on nivolumab in the context of its recent label change from 240 mg every two weeks to 480 mg every four weeks [17].

15.4.3 Atezolizumab

Goldstein D A and Ratain M J, searched for right dose and frequency for a atezolizumab. It is a PD-L1 inhibitor, approved for use in patients with NSCLC, small cell lung cancer, urothelial carcinoma (UC), and triple-negative breast cancer. As with other checkpoint inhibitors, initial studies used weight-based dosing, prior to switching to a strategy of fixed dosing for all patients. The authors advocated using a standard 840 mg dose, but with a dosing interval greater than the recommended interval of two weeks, i.e. every three or four weeks. Besides, as another alternative, they used therapeutic drug monitoring (TDM) to individualize the frequency of dosing, with the objective of maintaining a therapeutic trough concentration. A minimum blood plasma concentration reached by a drug prior to the administration of a second dose (Cmin) of $\geqslant 6\ \mu g\ ml^{-1}$ was proposed earlier as a conservative target, based on preclinical studies [18]. After the completion of the studies, this TDM strategy would not only reduce the use of scarce healthcare resources, it would also provide increased convenience for patients, requiring fewer visits to the infusion suite. An alternative, and even cheaper, method of dosing individualization could use albumin changes as a surrogate for clearance changes. This approach has been previously investigated for durvalumab [18, 19]. In an era of both personalized medicine and budget constraints, the dosing of atezolizumab provides great opportunity.

15.4.4 Pembrolizumab dosing every eight to twelve weeks

A phase II trial (ClinicalTrials.gov identifier: NCT04032418) studied how well pembrolizumab (Keytruda, Lambrolizumab) given every twelve weeks worked compared to administration every three weeks in treating patients with NSCLC. Immunotherapy using monoclonal antibodies, such as pembrolizumab, may help the body's immune system to attack cancer, and may interfere with the ability of tumor cells to grow and spread. Giving pembrolizumab every twelve weeks may provide similar disease control with fewer treatments for patients with NSCLC, compared to administration every three weeks. Demonstrating that twelve-week dosing is as effective as three-week dosing may also have a significant impact when the costs of these medications are considered [20, 21].

15.5 Shorter courses

15.5.1 Shorter-course trastuzumab could be an option in HER2-positive early breast cancers

Current guidelines recommend one year of anti-HER2 antibody therapy as part of the standard adjuvant treatment for HER2-positive early breast cancer patients based on the duration of treatment used in pivotal registration trials.

It would be interesting to determine whether a shorter course of trastuzumab could potentially achieve similar efficacy with a lower risk of side-effects and reduced costs.

The short-HER trial randomly selected 1254 HER2-positive early breast cancer patients for either nine weeks or one year's treatment with trastuzumab; both groups also received chemotherapy. Both groups had similar disease-free survival and a lower risk of cardiac toxicity resulted for a nine-week course of adjuvant trastuzumab compared to that resulting from treatment for one year [22].

Another study [23] that constituted the largest phase 3 randomised trial to compare six months with twelve months of trastuzumab demonstrated the non-inferiority of reduced-duration trastuzumab, which caused less cardiotoxicity, fewer severe adverse events, and more cost-effectiveness, with an average cost saving of nearly £10 000 (€11 300) per patient. These results support the consideration of reduced-duration trastuzumab for women at a similar risk of recurrence to those included in the trial. Patients were recruited from 152 centres in the UK. We randomly assigned patients with HER2-positive early breast cancer, aged 18 years or older and with a clear indication for chemotherapy, using a computerized minimization process (1:1), to receive either a six-month or a twelve-month course of trastuzumab delivered every three weeks intravenously (a loading dose of 8 mg kg^{-1} followed by maintenance doses of 6 mg kg^{-1}) or subcutaneously (600 mg), given in combination with chemotherapy (concurrently or sequentially) [23].

15.6 Dose optimization of new oncology drugs

Outside oncology, drugs are usually evaluated to optimize the therapeutic index in randomized dose-ranking trials prior to essential phase III trials. It is logical that the dosing of non-cancer drugs considers this notion and does not select the highest dose that patients can tolerate (the maximal tolerated dose (MTD)), particularly if that dose could produce chronic toxicities. In fact, this is aligned with sound pharmacological rules and with global regulatory guidance, such as that of the USA Food and Drug Administration (FDA) [24]. Surprisingly, this rule is not obligatory for groups of new cancer drugs, such as monoclonal antibodies and kinase inhibitors. Many early-phase studies of modern targeted therapies still continue to seek the MTD, and rely on this MTD for later phase trials and potential labeling [25, 26].

Historically, for the chemotherapy of cancer, there was a general belief that more or a higher dose is better. It is surely not the case that this notion is still valid for new targeted cancer drugs, such as monoclonal antibodies and kinase inhibitors?

In 2021, Ratain and Lichter [27] stated that we should seek the optimal dose, i.e. the lowest dose that gives the maximum biologic and clinical effect, since once the target is fully inhibited—or the receptor saturated—there is no reason to give a higher dose. Thus, dosing to toxicity is illogical and conflicts with the principles of clinical pharmacology that are widely accepted outside of oncology.

15.6.1 A plea from Mark Ratain and Allen Lichter to empower the FDA

There is a great need for dose-optimization evidence for all new cancer drugs, including targeted cancer drugs and monoclonal antibodies. Accordingly, in a plea published in The ASCO Post on January 20, 2021, Mark Ratain and Allen Lichter argued that the FDA should require pharmaceuticals companies to optimize the dose as a condition of likely accelerated approval. They also requested that the FDA should demand that all sponsors submit a new drug application (NDA) to provide evidence of dose optimization in accordance with its own guidance document, with the exception of breakthrough drugs, for which it would be permitted to optimize the dosing regimen after approval as a post-marketing condition [27].

Once a targeted oncology drug is labeled and approved by the FDA at a non-optimized highest dose, it is expensive and time-consuming to go back and redo a dose-optimization strategy. It is more sensible to do this work upfront, or alternatively, for the FDA to negotiate an appropriate strategy that would permit rapid approval while also achieving the goal of minimizing adverse events. It is high time for the FDA to reject the obsolete maximally tolerated dose concept for modern targeted oncology drugs. However, there is also an opportunity for the FDA to require that sponsors optimize dosing upfront, either before or soon after approval as a post-marketing condition [26].

Although the FDA has done so for several drugs, the vast majority of oncology drugs over the last decade have been developed and approved at their maximally tolerated dose, leading to off-target adverse events that may be fatal, as in the case of Ibrutinib [28, 29].

Furthermore, Ratain and Lichter gave a striking latest example of a new drug application filed by Amgen. That relates to 'Sotorasib', previously known as AMG-510, for the treatment of patients with KRAS G12C mutated locally advanced or metastatic NSCLC following at least one preceding systemic therapy [27, 30]. A similar drug, 'Adagrasib', is being developed by Mirati Therapeutics [31]. Both drugs are thrilling and promising. KRAS G12C mutant tumors primarily consist of NSCLCs and colorectal cancer [31, 32].

Clearly, Amgen has made a marvelous discovery and preclinical effort. In the Phase 1 trial, Amgen aimed to give the maximally tolerated dose (MTD) of Sotorasib to patients with KRAS G12C mutant tumors (NSCLCs) [32]. The protocol used a Bayesian logistic regression model that aimed to elicit dose-limiting toxicity in 20% to 33% of the patients, regardless of the fact that the drug may be effective without any toxicity, given its mutant target; it has been stated that most probably the starting dose of 180 mg—and not the concept of the MTD of 980 mg—is expected to be safe as well as potentially efficacious [27].

Besides, the Amgen phase I trial recommended the administration of Sotorasib under fasting conditions, without any apparent validation, and showed high variability—a finding commonly observed for drugs whose absorption is augmented by food [33]. Therefore, there is no evidence that the dosing regimen used in the Amgen pivotal trial (960 mg with daily fasting) is optimal. In fact, it is likely that a much lower dose of the drug administered with food may have a superior therapeutic index [27].

Optimization to the lowest dose that produces the maximum biologic and clinical effects could be one of the scientific approaches to reducing the costs of drugs and potential adverse events by developing off-label dosing regimens that use pharmacologically justified dosing. This is aligned with the 'interventional pharmacoeconomics (IVPE)' term coined by Ratain, Goldstein, and Lichter. While pharmacoeconomics is an observational science that usually focuses on the value and affordability of pharmaceutical interventions, the proposed concept of interventional pharmacoeconomics (IVPE) means an attempt to disruptively decrease drug prescription costs through the development of new dosing regimens while maintaining equivalent efficacy [34, 35].

In the Win-Win movement, we appreciate the plea of Ratain and Lichter and we call for advocacy for it, as it could contribute to the optimization of therapeutic index and reduce the costs of new targeted and monoclonal drugs for patients with cancer everywhere in the world.

As shown in different parts of this book, our previous publications, and presentations, the Win-Win movement focuses on scientific approaches that could lead to an increase in the affordability of better-value cancer care, including lowering the total costs of cancer care as one of these approaches [36]. Scientific studies that aim to decrease the high costs of cancer drug prescriptions by initiatives such as this urgently needed initiative, IVPE, constitute important components of approaches to reduce the total costs of cancer care.

In the win-win movement and in this book, we emphasize the huge gap in the affordability of better-value cancer care and the need for a big global campaign and forum. The direction of all-important scientific initiatives is urgently needed. We describe this book using a new term coined by Ahmed Elzawawy as a 'living book', which includes links to videos. The First International Summit on Interventional Pharmacoeconomics, June 29th–July 1st, 2020, Chicago, USA, organized by The Value in Cancer Care Consortium included important presentations by distinguished experts in dose optimization; therefore, we present here a link to the recorded videos of this very relevant first conference, which can be viewed at The ASCO Post website [37].

Moreover, as we cited on different occasions in this book, after publication, links for feedback, proposals, and suggestion will be available to all readers. Hence, our objective is that the publication of this book should be the start of a global stimulus and not an endpoint.

The costs of targeted cancer therapy drugs routinely exceed US $100 000 per patient-year of treatment, endangering patient access and adherence to cancer therapy, and threatening whole health systems [38]. Targeted therapies, such as monoclonal antibodies and oral small molecules, now comprise the bulk of anticancer drug expenditure, while newly developed oral drugs experience sustained price increases of >10% annually. This trend is not expected to change [39].

15.7 Examples of proposals and scientific studies that aim to lower dosage while retaining comparable efficacy

15.7.1 Ibrutinib (Imbruvica) used in patients with chronic lymphocytic leukemia

Reducing the dose from 420 mg to mg 140 daily.

A pilot study (NCT02801578) of lower doses of ibrutinib in patients with chronic lymphocytic leukemia (CLL) was completed and published. During the phase 1 trial of ibrutinib, lower doses (2.5 and 5 mg kg^{-1}) resulted in similar Bruton's tyrosine kinase (BTK) target occupancy assays to those for the highest dose tested (12.5 mg kg^{-1}). These pharmacokinetic/pharmacodynamics (PK/PD) data demonstrate that after the first cycle of ibrutinib at the standard 420 mg d^{-1} dose, the dose can be reduced without losing biological activity. The clinical efficacy of lower doses needs to be systematically evaluated.

Such dose reductions would lower drug cost, lessen untoward toxicity, and facilitate rationale-based combinations [40, 41].

15.7.2 Erlotinib (Tarceva) used in patients with non-small-cell lung cancer and pancreatic tumors

Reducing the dose from 150 mg to 100 mg or 50 mg daily [40].

This is a promising approach. Further studies are needed to reduce the dose to either 100 or 50 mg as optimum without compromising the outcome [40].

15.7.3 Dasatinib used to treat a certain type of chronic myeloid leukemia

Reducing the dose from 100 to 50 mg daily.

Dasatinib (Sprycel) is a tyrosine kinase inhibitor (TKI). TKIs are therapies that block proteins involved in cancer cell growth. Dasatinib is currently used to treat chronic-phase chronic myeloid leukemia (CP-CML) at a dose of 100 mg per day. This dosage can cause myelosuppression and pleural effusions. Low-dose dasatinib continued to demonstrate faster and deeper molecular responses in comparison with standard-dose dasatinib and imatinib. The lack of new safety signals was also noted during this follow-up and it was suggested that dasatinib given at 50 mg per day may be an appropriate option for initial CML-CP treatment [40, 42].

15.7.4 Pembrolizumab used in patients with non-small cell lung cancer, melanoma, bladder, head, and neck cancer: converting from a flat 200 mg dose to a 2 mg kg^{-1} dose of pembrolizumab

Pembrolizumab (formerly lambrolizumab, brand name Keytruda) is a humanized antibody used in cancer immunotherapy. This comprises use in melanoma, lung cancer, head and neck cancer, Hodgkin lymphoma, and stomach cancer. It is given by slow injection into a vein.

Personalized dosing of pembrolizumab from a flat 200 mg dose to 2 mg kg^{-1} dose may have the potential to save approximately $0.825 billion annually in the United States, most likely without impacting outcomes. This option is to be considered for the first-line management of PD-L1-positive advanced lung cancer [43].

Value-based prescribing strategies that do not compromise outcomes for new oral oncology drugs alone could save US $12 billion and more globally per year. This approach does not compromise the outcome and efficacy, and it could save the US $94 000 per patient-year for new oral oncology drugs alone, with a similar opportunity for long-lived parenteral monoclonal antibodies [40]

15.8 Examples of dose reduction using food effects and drug interactions through pharmacokinetic-based studies

- Lapatinib: Converting from 1250 mg with fasting to 500 mg with food
- Abiraterone: converting from 1000 with fasting to 250 mg with food
- Pazopanib: converting from 800 mg with fasting to 600 mg with food
- Certinib (Zykadia): capsules converting from 750 mg with fasting to 450 mg with food
- Venclexta (Venetoclax): capsules converting from 400 mg or 600 mg to 70 mg daily when taken with 300 mg posaconazole

15.8.1 Lapatinib

Converting from 1250 mg with fasting to 500 mg with food

Lapatinib is an oral dual tyrosine kinase inhibitor of both epidermal growth factor receptor and ERBB2; it is approved for advanced ERBB2-positive breast cancer. Pharmacokinetic-based studies include an example that showed that 500 mg lapatinib taken orally with food and a beverage containing CYP3A inhibitors (such as grapefruit juice) and not on an empty stomach as stated, may be as effective as 1250 mg (i.e. the current FDA approved dose) without food. This change could reduce the dose and costs of lapatinib by around 60%. For this expensive drug the habitual dose for one patient is around 1250–1500 mg per day; in addition, there is an opportunity to save the cost of the treatment of diarrhoea due to lapatinib. It has been suggested that the diarrhea is caused by the unabsorbed drug in the gut [44, 45]. Pharmacokinetic studies that pursue ways to enhance the bioavailability of agents could markedly decrease the required doses and associated treatment costs. Strategies include the support of clinical trial processes to pursue evidence to support less costly and optimal therapeutic efficacy outcomes [14, 45].

15.8.2 Abiraterone

A recent study of oral agents approved by the US FDA in the last ten years [46] demonstrated that oral oncology drugs have generally been labeled as requiring fasting, despite the fact that food can create up to a four-fold increase in bioavailability.

The apparent bias for labeling oncology drugs for fasting is exemplified by abiraterone acetate, which was approved for marketing in the United States on April 28, 2011, for the treatment of metastatic prostate cancer. Abiraterone acetate is a prodrug of abiraterone, an inhibitor of CYP17 that decreases the extratesticular formation of androgens.

Most notably, it has a food effect greater than that of any other marketed drug (five- to tenfold, depending on fat content), yet it is labeled to be taken while fasting [47]. Studies have shown that a low abiraterone dose of 250 mg once daily with food was non-inferior to the standard dose of 1000 mg abiraterone in castration-resistant prostate cancer. However, the marked effect of a high-fat meal (a tenfold increase in exposure) implies that absolute bioavailability in the fasting state is no more than 10%. This is most likely to be the result of low absorption under fasting conditions, because 77% of the administered drug is excreted as abiraterone (or its prodrug acetate) in feces. So, Ratain posed a provocative question 'do we really need to flush our few successful products down the toilet?' [48].

Tannock, 2018, stated that the ability to use a highly effective drug at a quarter of the dose, and hence a quarter of the price, could have the enormous consequence of making it available to many men with this common disease who would not otherwise receive it, some in developed countries and many more globally [49]. Unlike some institutions that deny its importance, Tannock stressed the important consequences of the trials in demonstrating the non-inferiority of low-dose abiraterone with food, largely because of the greed of a company in setting an inappropriate price that bears no relationship to the cost of the development and manufacture of abiraterone acetate. Unfortunately, because of the inappropriate pricing of the drug ($8000 to $10 000 per month in the United States for standard treatment), many men will be denied the drug. Even in developed countries, few can afford it in poor and middle-income countries, even though it is manufactured and sold in India for approximately one twentieth of the US price [49]. It also would send a message to the pharmaceutical industry that flawed drug development has financial consequences. After all the above, given the high attrition rate for oncology drugs, we ask you all 'do we really need to waste some of our successful products and the resources of patients and communities?'

Pazopanib has been licensed for advanced soft tissue sarcoma and metastatic renal cell carcinoma (kidney cancer) in a fixed oral daily dose of 800 mg taken while fasting. It is usually given after other treatments have failed. However, ingesting pazopanib with food may improve patient comfort and reduce adverse GI events. Moreover, a food intervention resulting in a better absorption can lead to a lower dose, which could reduce treatment costs. Published studies have shown that an intake of 600 mg pazopanib with food resulted in a bioequivalent exposure and was preferred over a standard pazopanib dose without food. No significant differences were seen in GI toxicities under both intake regimens. Patients seemed to be more positive about their feelings about side-effects and satisfaction with their therapy when pazopanib was taken with food. Forty-one of the patients (68%) preferred the intake with a continental breakfast. (Trial registration: ClinicalTrials.gov [NCT02138526].)

Seven hundred and fifty mg of ceritinib in the fasting state is used for patients with anaplastic lymphoma kinase (ALK)—rearranged metastatic NSCLC. Four hundred and fifty mg of ceritinib with food had a similar exposure and a more favorable GI safety profile than 750 mg of ceritinib in fasting patients with ALK-positive NSCLC. An ASCEND-8 randomized phase 1 trial showed that 450 mg of ceritinib with food had a similar exposure and a more favorable GI safety profile than 750 mg of ceritinib in fasting patients with ALK-positive NSCLC [51].

Venclexta is a prescription medicine used to treat adults with CLL or small lymphocytic lymphoma (SLL). In combination with azacitidine, decitabine, or low-dose cytarabine, it is used to treat adults with newly-diagnosed acute myeloid leukemia (AML).

The effect of posaconazole, a strong cytochrome P450 3A (CYP3A) inhibitor and a commonly used antifungal agent, on the pharmacokinetic properties of venetoclax, a CYP3A substrate, was evaluated in patients with acute myeloid leukemia to determine the dose adjustments needed to manage this potential interaction. Patients with acute myeloid leukemia received 300 mg of posaconazole plus reduced doses of venetoclax (50 or 100 mg) instead of 400 mg or 600 mg to account for the expected increase in venetoclax plasma concentration. Blood samples were collected before dosing and up to 24 h after the venetoclax dose. The results are consistent with the inhibition of the CYP3A-mediated metabolism of venetoclax. Posaconazole can be used for antifungal prophylaxis in patients with acute myeloid leukemia receiving venetoclax after reducing the venetoclax dose by at least 75%. (ClinicalTrials.gov identifier: NCT02203773 [52].)

15.9 Generic equivalents and biosimilars of cancer chemotherapy drugs

Our published view indicates that we stress not taking the proposal of using cheaper generic cancer drugs or biosimilars as a magic wand and as an ideal solution for more cost-effective treatments without assuring the following: (a) their flow of production; (b) their affordability; (c) that generic drugs and biosimilars are of proven good quality; (d) and that they show better value in patient cancer care (the inputs and costs related to a patient-centered outcome) [53, 54].

Therefore, we also stress that generic and biosimilar drugs could be of much more value if there were global regulatory consistency and trust in the good quality and flow of drugs. We suggest the formation of an international body of experts or programs to assure the quality, bioequivalence, and costs of generic cancer drugs, in particular, in LMICs. Hence, better value could be obtained from these drugs. The Win-Win movement advocates what we published previously: that the quality, bioequivalence, and bioavailability of generic drugs should be assured—worldwide and particularly in developing countries—by regulations and by developing a transparent system for international testing [55, 56].

A generic of good quality or an 'original, brand' essential drug would be more cost-effective than generics with lower quality and outcomes, even if the latter have lower prices. Also, first-line treatment using tested, good-quality drugs could reduce the need for second- and third-line treatments, which are usually more expensive. Besides the risk for patients, the results of clinical trials and research in low- and middle-income countries (LMICs) would be doubtful if they were performed using drugs of questionable quality, even if they were used in the control arm. So, we see that the question should not be whether to use a brand or a generic drug in certain indication for certain patients in a certain community, but it should be about what better value we could get under the given conditions [53, 54].

15.10 Repurposing and repositioning drugs

The development of new drugs is not enough for cancer management, in particular when we consider the escalation of high prices. Newer indications of old drugs and innovative indications and uses of older drugs constitute one of the approaches that deserve more research, incentives, and regulations. There are two chapters in this book about this topic.

15.11 Pharmacogenomics studies and value-based treatment

Pharmacogenomics is a branch of genetics that studies individual genetic variations in how drugs work, their efficacy, and their adverse effects. Radiogenomics refers to the same science but for radiotherapy. This science offers a partial explanation for the inter-patient variability in treatment response commonly observed in oncology. Small variations in the patient germ line DNA sequence (genotype), including single nucleotide polymorphisms (SNPs), can alter the expression and functional activity of an encoded protein. Often, genetic variants leading to clinically relevant functional changes occur in noncoding 'intron' regions of the genome or in 'exons' that code for protein expression [57]. These changes may lead to differences in drug distribution, metabolism, activity, and toxicity in different individuals [58].

Pharmacogenomic studies have been suggested to guide adjustments for the effective use of some drugs, such as tamoxifen. Patients can be classified as poor, intermediate, or extensive metabolizers, according to their genetic variation in CYP2D6, a key enzyme in tamoxifen metabolism. However, further prospective studies of CYP2D6 and this topic are warranted, as recent controversies have taken place regarding the significance and value of the adoption of routine clinical CYP2D6 testing [59].

In the win-win global scientific initiative, we adopt the saying: 'Science is an endless search for the truth'. The road leading to facts is endless and enjoyable. In fact, once again, not every exciting scientific finding can be translated into the same expected clinical value in short- and the long-term clinical research and trials.

Probable variations in human host and tumor biology, real local socioeconomic conditions and the priorities of problems, cost-effectiveness, cost utility, as well as available services, including supportive treatment differently affect the overall outcome of cancer treatment.

Specifically, pharmacogenomics and radiogenomics are among the possible reasons why the protocols and treatment guidelines produced by renowned organizations and societies do not yield the same responses and outcomes in different communities and ethnicities; hence, these guidelines should not be copied by different communities without adaptation and without considering different local factors and their value in scientific and realistic ways [1].

Most genetic studies only use white participants. This will lead to greater health inequality. The under-representation of non-European groups is problematic for scientific and ethical reasons. The effects of gene variants that are present only in the unstudied groups remain unknown, which means that important clues about the causes of diseases might be missed. Such undiscovered genes will not be included when testing for genetic diseases. Therefore, a person carrying one of them could wrongly obtain a negative genetic test result and might be told that they are not at increased risk of developing a disease. In recent years, efforts to collect multiethnic data have increased. One example is the UK Biobank, a collection of data from half a million British people which is accessible to any bona fide researcher. It includes some 35 000 DNA samples from people who are either non-European or 'mixed race'. Yet 92% of the research papers on the UK Biobank only used the data from the European-descent samples. Therefore, collecting data does not automatically solve the problem of non-white representation in research [60].

Genetics and pharmacogenomics studies may lead to better customization of treatment in order to achieve better outcomes. This would also avoid the waste of expensive treatments that yield smaller or insignificant responses in different ethnicities and communities with different disease presentations. As shown earlier in this book, value could be defined as input in relation to outcome; hence, better-value cancer care may be achieved by some of these studies.

15.12 Evidence-based medicine could reduce costs and achieve equal or better outcomes

Most programs use minimum criteria to develop their pathways; these typically include assessments of efficacy and toxicity. A few pathway programs go beyond this and delineate treatment options based on maximum survival benefits, effectiveness, quality of life, minimal toxicity, and cost-saving advantages.

One way in which evidence-based medicine (EBM) can help to reduce the costs of cancer care is by optimizing the appropriate use of less expensive drugs. For example, if treatment pathways point to two potential therapies that are largely equivalent in efficacy and toxicity, yet these two drugs vary enormously in cost, pathway programs that consider cost as a factor would ultimately point to the less expensive drug [55, 61].

15.13 More spending on cancer drugs could have lower value

In the first chapter of this book, there are sections about value in terms of patient outcome relative to the input. However, in this chapter, we cite the following points:

In terms of economic value, higher spending does not mean higher economic return.

Cancer drugs have become more effective. However, a high degree of variation with regard to their measure of health and economic value was found in nine industrialized countries. Real-world cancer drug use and expenditure was examined for the period from 2004 to 2014 in the United States, Australia, Canada, France, Germany, Italy, Japan, Sweden, and the United Kingdom. The United States accounted for nearly 56% of cancer drug expenditure in 2014 across all countries evaluated in this study but only received 12.6% of the global total net economic return generated in that year from oncology drug care. At the other end of the scale, Japan achieved close to seven times as much return in terms of health gain per dollar spent on cancer drugs as the United States did [62].

Cancer is the most expensive condition to treat per capita. Growth in US cancer drug expenditures is not primarily driven by consumption (which would mean an increase in the number of treated patients) but by high prices for brand-name drugs, mainly protein kinase inhibitors and monoclonal antibody antineoplastics [62].

15.14 Reduction in the use of expensive supportive care drugs without strong evidence

Physicians should, wherever possible, adhere to pathways that are less likely to prescribe expensive anti-emetics, growth factors, and other supportive care drugs (which are no less costly) in the absence of strong evidence to validate their use [63].

15.15 Value-based reduction in overall therapy

A study in the US showed that out of those chemotherapy patients with ten major cancer diagnoses who were identified as dying in an inpatient setting, 24% received chemotherapy within 14 days of death and 51% received chemotherapy within 30 days of death [1, 64]. Third and fourth lines of treatment rarely change the course of the disease and can cause incapacitating adverse effects. Palliative and supportive care to should be considered along the way in combination with different lines of treatment. However, for the sake of patients' quality of life and to lessen the burden on patients and families, it should only be proposed in certain late stages [65, 66].

The issue of overtreatment raises many controversies. It is a difficult decision [66]. We cannot always predict when death will occur. Doctors may ask themselves, who am I to decide? While we all remember the time-honored saying of Hippocrates: 'first, do no harm', patients in general do not like to hear 'no cancer treatment' [65].

To be clear, this is not a call to routinely abandon chemotherapy in deteriorating patients with progressive, non-responsive late stages. But, let us think together about incentives that could be provided (financial, scientific, career, psychological support, recognition, and other incentives) to oncologists and cancer care professionals in order to avoid overtreatment and to be on the side of more sensible approaches, such as palliative and supportive care that may include evidence-based better-value palliative chemotherapy [65].

Treatment guidelines backed by evidentiary support lead physicians to confidently recommend the most effective therapy as the first-line treatment using standard order sets that define dosage strengths and the number of cycles. For many cancers, especially solid tumors in adults, each successive line of treatment is less efficacious than the preceding line. When patients with late-stage disease face difficult decisions, some will wish to continue a line of treatment no matter what. Others express a desire to improve their quality of life, and many state that they would prefer to die at home rather than in the hospital [66]. Third and fourth lines of treatment rarely change the course of the disease and can cause incapacitating adverse effects. More often than not, if a patient's cancer has not responded to (or has progressed) after the first or second line of treatment, the best course for that patient may be to transition into palliative care. A study analyzing Medstat 2007 data in the US revealed that out of those chemotherapy patients with ten major cancer diagnoses who were identified as dying in an inpatient setting, 24% received chemotherapy within 14 days of death and 51% received chemotherapy within 30 days of death [64].

While we cannot always predict when death will occur, pathways can help guide physicians in making decisions and treatment recommendations pertaining to whether to offer additional cycles of a treatment or move to second, third, and further lines of treatment. They can also provide practical guidance that can be helpful in end-of-life care discussions. This includes demonstrating that transitioning to hospice care can improve both the patient's and the family's quality of life and can reduce the costs borne by the family and underwriters by avoiding unnecessary and ineffective chemotherapy administered within a few weeks of death [61].

15.16 Less toxic pathways

Unfortunately, it has been reported that 58% of potentially fatal adverse events are not listed in the initial USA FDA drug label and 38% are not reported in any published randomized trial [67].

Bach (2020) stated that the voice of the patient is missing in drug-safety reporting [68].

When there are two or more options for treatment with no significant difference in response, but one of them is less toxic, then the decision should be for the less toxic choice. Toxicities may add more suffering for patients, more costs for the treatment of adverse effects, and may affect quality of life. As far as possible, this should be discussed with patients, as they may be biased by information they obtained from internet and other sources [61].

One of the most common reasons that patients require hospitalization during treatment is adverse effects and complications caused by the agents. Less toxic on-pathway regimens can result in fewer or less severe adverse reactions, therefore reducing the number of unplanned hospital visits [61].

15.17 The missed global campaign: the fight against counterfeit medicines

15.17.1 Counterfeit medicine is worth 200 billion USD and causes one million deaths annually in the world

According to the World Health Organization (WHO), the International Criminal Police Organization (Interpol), and the United Nations (UN) Office on Drugs and Crime (UNODC), over one million people die annually from counterfeit medicines. Such medicines have serious impacts on population health, including treatment failure, toxicity, and a contribution to antimicrobial resistance.

Medicine counterfeiting is worth $200 billion annually; medicine counterfeiting is now one of the most lucrative counterfeiting business segments in the world, with very light legal consequences. A $1000 investment yields upward of $400 000. It is a really profitable business. The value–volume ratio for fake medicines is higher than for many illegal drugs.

15.17.2 Medicines for life-threatening conditions account for 60% of counterfeit medicines

Only ten years ago, most the counterfeit medicines were for lifestyle conditions, such as weight loss. However, medicines for the treatment of serious life-threatening conditions such as cancer, HIV/AIDS, tuberculosis, and malaria now account for 60% of all counterfeits [69, 70].

15.17.3 The highest number of reported counterfeit medicines comes from developing countries

About 70% of counterfeit medicines originate from India and China. However, other regional counterfeiting operations are increasing their share. These include operations based in Europe, Africa, and the frontier of South East Asia. Myanmar, Cambodia, and Laos mostly sell to Malaysia and Indonesia. South America, in particular, Colombia and Mexico, mostly sell to the USA and Canada [70–73].

15.17.4 Price is a factor that drives the demand for counterfeit medicines

In most markets, consumers who cannot afford medicines on the conventional health market seek prescriptions from the parallel health system. Such prescriptions come from open drug markets in the case of Africa and South East Asia. Up to 70% of the prescriptions sourced through these channels are estimated to be counterfeit.

15.17.5 Are there proposed solutions?

One of the proposed solutions is to develop devices that can rapidly determine the quality of a medicine. We present here the idea of a new device with a link to more information, as we don't mention the name of the device and company here. The device has a proprietary artificial intelligence (AI) platform which uses a handheld nanoscanner to enable rapid drug quality checking by drug regulators and pharmacies across the world. It checks the chemical quality of a drug versus a pure reference compound using a proprietary AI model and databases. Using the device platform, drug regulators and pharmacies can quickly determine the quality of a drug in less than 30 seconds using a mobile phone. Drugs that fail the screening test are sent to a centralized lab for a confirmatory test. It is currently used in Myanmar and is about to be deployed by a major regulator in West Africa. Since it is 20 times cheaper than existing handheld spectrometers, it is well suited for deployment across resource-poor countries. Drug regulators and pharmacies worldwide may use such devices for the rapid quality assurance of imported and purchased medicines before they are distributed and dispensed. This will make importers and suppliers accountable, since they will no longer be able to supply substandard drugs, as regulators and pharmacies will have a tool that determines a drug's quality. Effective large-scale approaches are required to tackle the growing global problem of counterfeit medicines. Importantly, this includes accurate and scalable tools that facilitate the rapid detection of such medicines to promote accountability and enable global monitoring—especially in low-resource settings. As a low-cost tool that enables this detection, this tool aims to make an important contribution to making medicines safe globally [73].

Unfortunately, it is rare to point to this serious problem of counterfeit medicines in medical articles or conferences. Hence, the question is: how we can expect better-value healthcare and drug therapy while this serious defect persists?

Many serious and realistic win-win scenarios and campaigns involving the relevant international, national, and community authorities are needed to develop many approaches for global access to affordable and reasonable essential medicines. All would win (except the offenders responsible for counterfeit medicines; however, their families would get access to true medicines)!

15.18 Control of the utilization of a drug as a primary strategy

We give here an example from the USA. If this the case in a rich country, then control of utilization should be mandatory in less affluent countries.

In the USA, policymakers have targeted Medicare drug spending from many angles to drive down healthcare costs. Current drug prices propel the healthcare industry's rising medical cost trend, which was projected to rise by 6% in 2020. Medicare is not immune, accounting for 30% of the nation's retail prescription drug spending in 2017. The costs are projected to rise by 4.6% per enrollee over the next decade [74].

In the USA, the primary strategy Medicare uses to limit the utilization of a drug (or another healthcare good or service) is to limit coverage of the payment for it. The program does so by actively determining in which settings the drug is or is not 'reasonable and necessary' through either national or local coverage decisions. When these coverage decisions result in restricted guidelines for the use of the drug, the result is decreased utilization. For instance, in 2007, Medicare narrowed the coverage of erythropoiesis-stimulating agents (ESAs) for cancer treatment. Medicare not only limited the types of patient who could receive ESAs but also the clinical scenarios in which they could be used as reported by Centers for Medicare & Medicaid Services [75]. One of the biggest companies that sells ESAs in the USA reported to their investors in August 2007 that changes in coverage for ESAs by the Centers for Medicare and Medicaid Services (CMS) would reduce the annual sales of the company's ESA from approximately $1 billion to $200 million among Medicare patients [75].

In the win-win, our goal is not at all against the sales of drugs per se, but we support saving the whole system and benefitting all dimensions of cancer care in the world. The strategy of controlling the utilization of drugs by whatever mechanism in each country would assure a more reasonable and justified utilization of drugs (or services). Otherwise, the chaos in their utilization in some less affluent countries opens the door wide for the use of these drugs when they are not necessary, while omitting patients who are in great need. This is also due to the well-known widespread local corruption in many countries, which goes by many names, such as commissions, percentages, or rewards of any kind; these abuse the resources of countries and individuals, patients and families without a cost-effective or measured outcome for patients. This, finally to could lead to increasing difficulties in the markets of those of countries at the forefront of newer products and innovation in cancer diagnosis and treatment [1].

Hence, in the Win-Win Movement, we clearly support transparent, scientific, and value-based measures. However, their implementation and global success need all readers and key players to coordinate in a global campaign.

15.19 Win-Win notions, the pharmaceutical response to interventional pharmacoeconomics studies, the Choosing Wisely initiative, and other scientific initiatives to reduce the cost of cancer drug treatments

The main pioneers of the IVPE studies stated that pharmaceutical companies anticipated strategies with which to confront studies that lead to dose optimization and the reduction of waste, hence, those that potentially lead to decreased costs and increased cost-effectiveness of new cancer drugs [34].

In fact, we pose the question 'do all readers and all stakeholders imagine that leftover cancer drugs in vials that go to waste cost around $3 billion annually in the USA?' This because many top-selling cancer drugs in the United States are only available in single-dose vials, and the vial only comes in one size. This is particularly true for drugs whose dosage is based on a patient's weight or body size and that come in single-dose packages. The sum of $3 billion represents the sales of a leading radiotherapy equipment manufacturer (Varian Medical Systems) for the whole world in the year 2019. This includes all their products, including linear accelerators and informatics. This also constitutes more than 50% of the market for radiotherapy equipment in the world [76, 77].

Surprisingly, the waste of $3 billion in the US could be cut down by providing these drugs in multiple sizes of vial. Another suggestion that needs further study is to follow a system of sharing vials by pooling patients who get the IV drug within 6 h on the same day. The opened vial has to be kept under an IV hood for no longer than 6 h, and then it must be discarded because sterility can no longer be guaranteed. This is as agreed by Medicare and Medicare Services (CMS), but is still not accepted by the Centers for Disease Control and Prevention (CDC) in the US. The increase in the amount of drug sold per treated patient lead to increased profits for manufacturers. It is sad to cite what has been published by many authors, which is that there is an increase in the unjustified profits of oncologists and hospitals in the US and some parts of the world. Even if the profits represent small percentages, they can equate to large amounts of money, given that many of these drugs cost thousands of dollars per vial [35, 76, 78].

Several policy options should also be explored. Regulators could require manufacturers to provide drugs in a reasonable set of size options to ensure the amount of wasted drug is low, say 3%. An alternative to that would allow manufacturers the freedom to select vial sizes but also require them to refund the cost of leftover drugs. This option could be achieved through certified disposal and a virtual return.

Policymakers should also revisit the current FDA guidance on appropriate packaging for intravenous drugs in single-dose vials and encourage the FDA, the CDC, the CMS, and the US Pharmacopeial Convention to reconcile their views on vial contents and vial sharing. It could be also suggested in all countries that the patient funder or the insurance company should pay for the prescribed dose only. If there is a large amount of waste, the manufacturer refunds the hospitals or the physicians. It could also be suggested in all countries that the patient funder or insurance company should pay for the prescribed dose only. If there is a large amount of waste, the manufacturer refunds the hospitals or the physicians. This option could be achieved through certified disposal and a virtual return.

These steps could, in turn, lead to healthcare cost savings for all oral patent-protected oncology products, suggesting that an opportunity for savings of at least 50% may exist for a large number of drugs without forgoing outcomes for patients [40].

Some examples are cited here from the literature [78–80]. One example is that of bortezomib (*Velcade*, Millennium), which is used to treat multiple myeloma. It is only available in the US in a 3.5 mg vial, which is much larger than the average required dose, which Dr Bache and colleagues calculated to be 2.5 mg. That figure is based on the drug's dose of 1.3 mg m^{-2} and the average cancer patient.

Another example is that of pembrolizumab (*Keytruda*, Merck), which was previously sold in 50 mg vials (as a powder that needs to be reconstituted into a liquid). However, in February 2015, the manufacturer introduced a larger, 100 mg vial (as a liquid), and the 50 mg vial became unavailable. 'Merck withdrew the 50 mg vial and replaced it with a 100 mg vial. The increase in revenue from this switch is substantial and it is estimated to add about $1 billion in revenue over the next five years.' Dr Bache and colleagues arrived at this estimate using the example of a 70-kg patient who requires a dose of 140 mg (the drug is dosed at 2 mg kg^{-1}). Three 50 mg vials would previously have been required, leaving only 10 mg unused. But now that the supply is limited to 100 mg vials, 60 mg is wasted.

Dr Bach pointed out that pembrolizumab was approved in Europe last summer and it is being sold in the smaller, 50 mg vials. Bortezomib is sold in 1-mg vials in the United Kingdom: 'One would have to assume that this is due to closer scrutiny of pricing in Europe' [78].

In contrast, it is quite possible to market a drug with negligible waste. One case in point is bendamustine (*Treanda*, Cephalon), which is sold in a variety of vial sizes (25 mg, 45 mg, 100 mg, and 180 mg) that can be combined to reach its dose of 100 mg m^{-2} almost precisely. The authors calculate that only 1% of bendamustine is wasted.

A similar example can be seen in the setting of oral drugs. The 'You&I' program [79] for ibrutinib aimed to remove the 140 mg capsule from the market, limiting dosing flexibility, while pricing newly introduced tablet formulations (140–560 mg) at three times the price of the 140 mg capsule [80].

In a story of limited but encouraging success, the drug makers eventually reversed ibrutinib's 'You&I' program following public outrage [79]. The English High Court backed the National Health Service's (NHS's) off-label use of bevacizumab to reduce costs, despite manufacturer objections [81].

Other strategies used to oppose scientific studies that aim to lower the cost of new cancer drugs, IVPE, and the Choosing Wisely campaign is that according to multiple experts and authors, pharmaceutical companies adopt tactics that include paying physicians to prescribe on-label in opposition to experts who study dose de-escalation [35, 80]. Moreover, there are still legal and regulatory actions that discourage IVPE practices [35].

As we have explained since the start of the Win-Win movement and in different parts of this book is that we are not calling for confrontations or fights between different stakeholders. It has become clear that the majority of cancer patients have no access to cancer care, or at least no access to value-based care that is adapted to patients in their specific communities. This serious burden that affects millions of cancer patients and their families has increased in recent decades and will be further aggravated in upcoming years. The impact of COVID-19 and the post-pandemic situation add another negative crisis. The whole system will suffer more from the risk of collapses or the failure of some sectors. As we already mentioned in this book, an ASCO report sadly stated that nearly 40% of cancer patients in the USA abandon science-based professional oncology care because of their fear of skyrocketing costs and their burden to them and families. Hence, we can imagine how this state of affairs is more tragic in less affluent countries and how it will be aggravated in forthcoming years. There is no doubt about the essential role of industry in creating progress and innovation for cancer diagnosis and treatment. The Win-Win notion implies that all will gain, which includes the manufacturers of cancer drugs and radiotherapy devices. This notion could be expanded to other, non-cancerous diseases [82].

In the win-win movement, we call for an examination of the real incentives of all stakeholders, including industries, oncologists, hospitals, and governments in order to achieve the objective of access to care for millions of cancer patients in the real world. For further details, we ask the reader to view an example of the win-win publications using online access [54]. This also explain why we tackle the situation of access to cancer care, the shortage of cancer drugs, and pharmaco-economic interventions in the US, while our scope is the whole globe. It is clear that most of the key players innovating in the fields of cancer treatments and cancer drugs, old and new, are in the USA, Europe, and Japan. Moreover, the decisions and regulations of the FDA and the guidelines of American organizations for on-label prescriptions are at least viewed—if not followed—in most of the world, despite differences in communities, ethnicities, pathologies, and socioeconomic statuses.

15.19.1 Repairing the compensation system used for oncologists in the USA

As we deal with the real world, the notions of the Win-Win Movement consider the incentives and interests of all stakeholders. It is vital to explore the issue from the oncologists' perspective as well. Medical oncology is a cognitive specialty without many of the associated procedures that provide a financial boost. Many private oncologists in the USA depend on the incentive of the drug prescription reimbursement.

The system must be repaired so that oncologists may be correctly remunerated for their services while avoiding ethical conflicts. To be transparent, patients should have access to information regarding all the kinds of profit that might influence an oncologist's drug choices and thus affect costs and copayments [83]. The first proposal is to pay physicians salaries, as most academic centers do, so that oncologists do not have to rely on chemotherapy sales for income [84]. The second proposal is to adopt clinical pathways in which the fees of practices are paid for disease management and not based on the prices of prescribed chemotherapy [54, 83]. The New York Times published a plan to overhaul cancer care in the US which suggested that the payment system needs to change from fee-for-service towards a system of bundled payments. This is not far from the European idea of 'remuneration for the acts of oncologists', which involves the payment of one fee for all the services of caring for a cancer patient. Hence, the oncologist would be paid for a consultation, advice, a partial diagnosis, or the treatment he/she provided regardless of whether he/she prescribed or not and what he/she prescribed. This would remove the incentive to prescribe more expensive drugs when older generics are equally effective. The oncology community cannot make these changes alone. The government is deeply involved and has to help. Everyone engaged in cancer care needs to help improve it [85, 86]. The third proposal involves 'remuneration for pharmacists' that depends on the number of prescriptions served regardless of the content and number of drugs present in the prescriptions. It may be an audacious idea; however, innovative solutions particularly need to be generated when we are faced with a complicated problem with economic complexities [65].

As mentioned earlier in this chapter, there are many scientific examples of the reduction of costs without sacrificing efficacy, and when, for new oral oncology drugs alone in the US, we could save $94 000 of the $100 000 per patient-year in savings, with a similar opportunity in long-lived parenteral monoclonal antibodies, then we should advocate for more studies in the world in this direction, which should be the leading trend in the real world [18].

In the Win-Win Movement, we see that that with more scientific studies, research, and initiatives like some of the important examples cited in this chapter, the more the affordability of value-based cancer treatment could be improved. Education, training, studies, research, and publications directed to those objectives are essential elements.

As mentioned earlier in this chapter, there are many scientific examples of cost reduction without sacrificing efficacy and when we could save $94 000 of the $100 000 per patient-year in the US in savings for new oral oncology drugs alone, with a similar opportunity for long-lived parenteral monoclonal antibodies, then we should advocate for more studies in the world in this direction, which should be the leading trend in the real world [40, 54].

The oncology community cannot make these changes alone. Governments are deeply involved and have to help. Everyone engaged in cancer care needs to help improve it [85]. Hence, there is a great need for a global win-win campaign, in which all find an international platform for all, while the internal entity, independence, freedom, and credit of each body all are strictly respected.

Note from the author:
As we mentioned in the introduction and in some parts of this book, we present examples of the published studies of many authors and scientists directed to the reduction of costs without compromising the outcome for patients. We emphasize that we do not claim to present the whole wisdom or the final solutions to the challenges of the question of the affordability of cancer care worldwide. However, the objective of this book is to be a call for all readers and key players to contribute in forming a global campaign and movement in which all would gain and win. We do not claim any credit.

This first edition of book is not the end. All readers are invited to send feedback, suggestions, and ideas focused on how to increase the affordability of better-value cancer care to one of the available links : http://icedoc.net/feedback.html and http://icedoc.org/feedback.html. Replies will arrive by e-mail and or via websites, e.g. www.ecancerforall.com, http://www.icedoc.org/Books.htm and http://www.icedoc.net/Books.htm. It is, in the expression I coined, ‘a living book’. Therefore, it is a continuous global forum and a platform in which all are invited to contribute and to lead some of the many approaches and initiatives. We—personally—do not claim any personal credit. The Win-Win Movement and this book belong to all.

Moreover, the feedback will be filtered, summarized, and edited in special chapters or in the main text in a next edition or a next book.

References and further reading

[1] Elzawawy A 2012 Science and affordability of cancer drugs and radiotherapy in the world: win-win scenarios ed R Mohan *Advances in Cancer Management.* (Rijeka: InTech) http://intechopen.com/articles/show/title/science-and-affordability-of-cancer-drugs-and-radiotherapy-in-the-world

[2] Seidman A D, Schwartzberg L S and Gudena V K *et al* 2018 Activity of tesetaxel, an oral taxane, given as a single-agent in patients (Pts) with HER2-, hormone receptor + (HR+) locally advanced or metastatic breast cancer (MBC) in a phase 2 study. *J. Clin. Oncol.* **36** 1042–1042

[3] Miller K D 2021 CONTESSA: oral taxane meets primary endpoint—*Medscape*—Jan 06, 2021

[4] Odonate therapeutics announces discontinuation of development of tesetaxel *News Release* March 22, 2021 https://bit.ly/3u1rMPh

[5] Tan A R, Im S A and Mattar A *et al* 2021 Fixed-dose combination of pertuzumab and trastuzumab for subcutaneous injection plus chemotherapy in HER2-positive early breast cancer (FeDeriCa): a randomised, open-label, multicentre, non-inferiority, phase 3 study *Lancet* **22** 85–97

[6] Rummel M, Kim T and Plenteda C *et al* 2015 Prefmab: Final Analysis Of Patient Satisfaction With Subcutaneous Versus Intravenous Rituximab In Previously Untreated Cd20+ Diffuse Large B-Cell Lymphoma Or Follicular Lymphoma *Value in Health.* **18** A469

[7] Rummel M, Kim T M and Aversa F *et al* 2017 Preference for subcutaneous or intravenous administration of rituximab among patients with untreated CD20+ diffuse large B-cell lymphoma or follicular lymphoma: results from a prospective, randomized, open-label, crossover study (PrefMab) *Ann. Oncol.* **28** 836–42

[8] Assouline S, Buccheri V and Delmer A *et al* 2015 Pharmacokinetics and safety of subcutaneous rituximab plus fludarabine and cyclophosphamide for patients with chronic lymphocytic leukaemia *Br. J. Clin. Pharmacol.* **80** 1001–9

[9] Pieternella L, Irit A and Henriette B *et al* 2017 Efficacy and safety of subcutaneous and intravenous rituximab plus cyclophosphamide, doxorubicin, vincristine, and prednisone in first-line diffuse large B-cell lymphoma: the randomized MabEase study *Haematologica.* **102** 1913–22

[10] Ockrim J L, Lalani E N and Laniado M E *et al* 2003 Transdermal estradiol therapy for advanced prostate cancer-forward to the past? *J. Urol.* **169** 1735–7

[11] Rosière R, Berghmans T and De Vuyst P *et al* 2019 The position of inhaled chemotherapy in the care of patients with lung tumors: clinical feasibility and indications according to recent pharmaceutical progresses *Cancers* **11** 329

[12] University of Strathclyde 2011 Inhaler treatment for lung cancer *ScienceDaily* 11 October

[13] Zwitter M, Kovac V and Smrdel U *et al* 2005 Phase I-II trial of low-dose gemcitabine in prolonged infusion and cisplatin for advanced non-small cell lung cancer *Anticancer Drugs* **16** 1129–34

[14] Elzawawy A M 2015 Could African and low- and middle-income countries contribute scientifically to global cancer care? *J. Glob. Oncol.* **1** 49–53

[15] Hortobagyi G N, Van Poznak C and Harker W G *et al* 2017 Continued treatment effect of zoledronic acid dosing every 12 vs 4 weeks in women with breast cancer metastatic to bone: the OPTIMIZE-2 randomized clinical trial *JAMA Oncol.* **3** 906–12

[16] Himelstein A L, Foster J C and Khatcheressian J L *et al* 2017). Effect of longer-interval vs standard dosing of zoledronic acid on skeletal events in patients with bone metastases: a randomized clinical trial *JAMA* **317** 48–58
[17] Ratain M J and Goldstein D A 2018 Time is money: optimizing the scheduling of nivolumab *J. Clin. Onc.* **36** 3074–6
[18] Goldstein D A and Ratain M J 2019 Alternative dosing regimens for atezolizumab: right dose, wrong frequency *Cancer Chemother. Pharmacol.* **84** 1153–5
[19] Baverel P G, Dubois V F S and Jin C Y *et al* 2018 Population pharmacokinetics of durvalumab in cancer patients and association with longitudinal biomarkers of disease status *Clin. Pharmacol. Ther.* **103** 631–42
[20] ClinicalTrials.gov. Pembrolizumab every 12 weeks versus every 3 weeks in treating patients with non-small lung cancer https://clinicaltrials.gov/ct2/show/NCT04032418
[21] Ratain M J, Goldstein D A and Lichter A S 2019 Interventional pharmacoeconomics—a new discipline for a cost-constrained environment *JAMA Oncol.* **5** 1097
[22] Conte P F, Frassoldati A and Bisagni G *et al* 2021 Nine weeks vs 1 year adjuvant trastuzumab: long term outcomes of the ShortHER randomised trial *Ann. Oncol.* **32** S37–47
[23] Earl H M, Hiller L and Vallier A L *et al* 2019 PERSEPHONE Steering Committee and Trial Investigators. 6 versus 12 months of adjuvant trastuzumab for HER2-positive early breast cancer (PERSEPHONE): 4-year disease-free survival results of a randomised phase 3 non-inferiority trial *Lancet* **393** 2599–612
[24] U.S. Food and Drug Administration (FDA) 1996 U.S. Food and Drug Administration: E4 dose-response information to support drug registration https://fda.gov/regulatory-information/search-fda-guidance-documents/e4-dose-response-information-support-drug-registration
[25] Lichter A S 2018 From Choosing Wisely to Using Wisely: Increasing the Value of Cancer Care Through Clinical Research *J. Clin. Oncol.* **36** 1387–8
[26] Ratain M J 2014 Targeted therapies: redefining the primary objective of phase I oncology trials *Nat. Rev. Clin. Oncol.* **11** 503–4
[27] Ratain M J and Lichter A S 2021 Empowering the FDA to require dose optimization of all new oncology drugs *The ASCO Post* https://ascopost.com/issues/january-25–2021/empowering-the-fda-to-require-dose-optimization-of-all-new-oncology-drugs/?bc_md5=aeb816f3fcdef2642f363a6c644bdba9&utm_source=TAP-EN-012021-INTL&ut%20m_medium=email
[28] Salem J E, Manouchehri A and Bretagne M *et al* 2019 Cardiovascular toxicities associated with ibrutinib *J. Am. Coll. Cardiol.* **74** 1667–78
[29] Ratain M J, Moslehi J J and Lichter A S 2020 Ibrutinib's cardiotoxicity: an opportunity for post-marketing regulation *JAMA Oncol.* **7** 177–8
[30] Amgen 2020 Amgen submits sotorasib new drug application to U.S. FDA for advanced or metastatic non-small cell lung cancer with KRAS G12C mutation https://amgen.com/newsroom/press-releases/2020/12/amgen-submits-sotorasib-new-drug-application-to-u-s--fda-for-advanced-or-metastatic-non-small-cell-lung-cancer-with-kras-g12c-mutation
[31] Jänne P A, Rybkin I I and Spira A I *et al* 2020 KRYSTAL-1: Activity and Safety of Adagrasib (MRTX849) in Advanced/ Metastatic Non–Small-Cell Lung Cancer (NSCLC) Harboring KRAS G12C Mutation *Eur. J. Cancer* **138** S1–2
[32] Hong D S, Fakih M G and Strickler J H *et al* 2020 KRAS G12C inhibition with sotorasib in advanced solid tumors *New Engl. J. Med.* **383** 1207–17
[33] Kang S P and Ratain M J 2010 Inconsistent labeling of food effect for oral agents across therapeutic areas *Clin. Cancer Res.* **16** 4446–51

[34] Ratain M J, Goldstein D A and Lichter A S 2019 Interventional pharmacoeconomics—a new discipline for a cost-constrained environment *JAMA Oncol.* **5** 1097–8
[35] Serritella A V, Strohbehn G W and Goldstein D A *et al* 2020 Interventional pharmacoeconomics *Clin. Pharmacol. Ther.* **108** 487–93 https://ascpt.onlinelibrary.wiley.com/doi/full/10.1002/cpt.1853
[36] The global health catalyst: win-win movement www.icedoc.net/winwin.htm
[37] American Society of Clinical Oncology (ASCO) 2020 The first international summit on interventional pharmacoeconomics, June 29th–July 1st, 2020, Chicago, USA. Video recordings of the sessions of the can be viewed at the ASCO Post https://ascopost.com/Meetings/?m=First+International+Summit+on+Interventional+Pharmacoeconomics
[38] Shih Y C T, Smieliauskas F, Geynisman D M, Kelly R J and Smith T J 2015 Trends in the cost and use of targeted cancer therapies for the privately insured nonelderly: 2001 to 2011 *J. Clin. Oncol.* **33** 2190–6
[39] US Food and Drug Administration (FDA) Hematology/oncology (cancer) approvals and safety notifications https://fda.gov/drugs/resources-information-approved-drugs/oncology-cancer-hematologic-malignancies-approval-notifications
[40] Ratain M J and Lichter A S 2018 Potential for value-based prescribing of oral oncology drugs. *Ann. Oncol.* **29** viii562
[41] Chen L S, Bose P and Cruz N D *et al* 2018 A pilot study of lower doses of ibrutinib in patients with chronic lymphocytic leukemia *Blood.* **132** 2249–59
[42] Naqvi K, Jabbour E and Skinner J *et al* 2019 Long-term follow-up of lower dose dasatinib (50 mg daily) as frontline therapy in newly diagnosed chronic-phase chronic myeloid leukemia *Cancer* **126** 67–75
[43] Goldstein D A, Gordon N and Davidescu M *et al* 2017 A Phamacoeconomic analysis of personalized dosing vs fixed dosing of pembrolizumab in firstline PD-L1-positive non-small cell lung cancer *J. Natl. Cancer Inst.* **109** djx063
[44] Messori A 2007 Effect of food on Lapatinib pharmacokinetics *J. Clin. Oncol.* **25** 5332–3
[45] Ratain M J and Cohen E E 2007 The value meal: how to save $1,700 per month or more on lapatinib *J. Clin. Oncol.* **25** 3397–8
[46] Kang S P and Ratain M J 2010 Inconsistent labeling of food effect for oral agents across therapeutic areas: Differences between oncology and non-oncology products *Clin. Cancer Res.* **16** 4446–51
[47] ZYTIGA—Accessdata.fda.gov https://accessdata.fda.gov/drugsatfda_docs/label/2011/202379lbl.pdf
[48] Ratain M J 2011 Flushing oral oncology drugs down the toilet *J. Clin. Oncol.* **29** 3958–9
[49] Tannock I F 2018 Low-fat abiraterone food effect is of great consequence *J. Clin. Oncol.* **36** 3058–9
[50] Lubberman F J E, Gelderblom H and Hamberg P *et al* 2019 The effect of using pazopanib with food vs. fasted on pharmacokinetics, patient safety, and preference (DIET study) *Clin. Pharmacol. Ther.* **106** 1076–82
[51] Cho B C, Kim D W, Bearz A and Laurie S A *et al* 2017 ASCEND-8: a randomized phase 1 study of Ceritinib, 450 mg or 600 mg, taken with a low-fat meal versus 750 mg in fasted state in patients with anaplastic lymphoma kinase (ALK)-rearranged metastatic non-small cell lung cancer (NSCLC) *J. Thorac. Oncol.* **12** 1357–67
[52] Agarwal S K, DiNardo C and Potluri J *et al* 2017 Management of venetoclax-posaconazole interaction in acute myeloid leukemia patients: evaluation of dose adjustments *J. Clinthera.* **39** 359–67

[53] Elzawawy A and Kerr D 2013 Variation in the availability of cancer drug generics in the United States of America *Ann. Oncol.* **24** 17–22
[54] Elzawawy A 2015 The shortage of essential cancer drugs and generics in the united states of america: global brain storming directions for the world *Int. J. Cancer Clin. Res.* **2** 016
[55] Elzawawy A 2008 Breast care systemic therapy: the need for more economically sustainable scientific strategies in the world *Breast Care* **3** 434–8
[56] Cazap E, Jacobs I, McBride A, Popovian R and Sikora K *et al* 2018 Global acceptance of biosimilars: importance of regulatory consistency, education, and trust *Oncologist.* **23** 1188–98
[57] Guttmacher A E and Collins F S 2003 Welcome to the genomic era *New Engl. J. Med.* **349** 996–8
[58] Connolly R and Stearns V 2009 The role of pharmacogenetics in selection of breast cancer treatment *Curr. Breast Cancer Rep.* **1** 190–7
[59] Lash T L, Lien E A, Sorensen H T and Hamilton-Dutoit S 2009 Genotype-guided tamoxifen therapy: time to pause for reflection? *Lancet Oncol.* **10** 825–33
[60] Kuchenbaecker K, Vassos E and Peterson R 2019 https://theconversation.com/most-genetic-studies-use-only-white-participants-this-will-lead-to-greater-health-inequality-125150 And Accessed also in http://gheg-journal.co.uk/2019/12/genetic-studies-health-inequality/
[61] Kolodziej M A 2011 Does evidence-based medicine really reduce costs? *Oncology* **25** 214–8 https://cancernetwork.com/view/does-evidence-based-medicine-really-reduce-costs
[62] Salas-Vega S and Mossialos E 2016 Cancer drugs provide positive value in nine countries, but the united states lags in health gains per dollar spent *Health Affairs* **35** 813–23
[63] Neubauer M A, Hoverman J R and Kolodziej M *et al* 2010 Cost effectiveness of evidence-based treatment guidelines for the treatment of non-small-cell lung cancer in the community setting *J. Oncol. Pract.* **6** 12–8
[64] Fitch K and Pyenson B 2010 *Cancer Patients Receiving Chemotherapy: Opportunities for Better Management.* (New York: Milliman Inc.)
[65] Elzawawy A 2013 Better value chemotherapy *How to Get Better Value Cancer Care* ed J A Muir Gray and D J Kerr (Oxford, UK: Offox Press Ltd) ch 6
[66] Wennberg J E, Fisher E S and Goodman D C *et al* 2008 *Tracking the Care of Patients with Severe Chronic Illness: The Dartmouth Atlas of Health Care 2008* (Lebanon, NH: The Dartmouth Institute for Health Policy and Clinical Practice Center for Health Policy Research) http://dartmouthatlas.org/downloads/atlases/2008_Chronic_Care_Atlas.pdf
[67] Seruga B, Sterling L, Wang L and Tannock I 2010 Reporting of serious adverse drug reactions of targeted anticancer agents in pivotal phase III clinical trials *J. Clin. Oncol.* **29** 174–85
[68] Bach E 2010 The missing voice of patients in drug-safety reporting *New Engl. J. Med.* **362** 865–9
[69] Counterfeit drugs kill 1 mn people annually: Interpol https://insightcrime.org/news/brief/counterfeit-drugs-kill-1-million-annually-interpol/
[70] Williams L and McKnight 2014 The real impact of counterfeit medications *US Pharm.* **39** 44–6 https://uspharmacist.com/article/counterfeit-meds#:~:text=US%20Pharm.,to%20be%20a%20genuine%20product
[71] Five worrying facts about fake medicines http://pharmafile.com/news/513663/five-worrying-facts-about-fake-medicine

[72] Cartwright R and Baric A 2018 Policy brief: the rise of counterfeit pharmaceuticals in AfricaENACT

[73] RxScanner:Making medicines safe globally http://gheg-journal.co.uk/2019/11/rxscanner-medicines-safe-globally/

[74] Waddil K 2019 How health policy is working to reduce medicare drug spending. health payer intelligence August 13, 2019 https://healthpayerintelligence.com/news/how-health-policy-is-working-to-reduce-medicare-drug-spending

[75] Centers for Medicare & Medicaid Services 2007 Proposed decision memo for erythropoiesis stimulating agents (ESAs) for non-renal disease indications (CAG-00383N)

[76] Medscape 2016 Leftover cancer drugs in vials cost $3 billion annually *Medscape* http://medscape.com/viewarticle/860660?nlid=102735_2201&src=WNL_mdplsnews_160325_mscpedit_honc&uac=96841ST&spon=7&impID=1037730&faf=1

[77] Elzawawy A 2018 GHC summit *The GHC Win-Win initiative* May 25, 2018, Harvard Medical School, Boston, MA https://youtu.be/7R91V4CEH34

[78] Bach P B, Conti R M and Muller R *et al* 2016 Overspending driven by oversized single dose vials of cancer drugs *Brit. Med. J.* **352** i788

[79] Ratain M J, Chen L and Lichter A *et al* 2018 Sales revenues at the potential expense of patient safety: the example of You&iTM https://cancerletter.com/articles/20180413_5/

[80] Singh N, Chang J S and Rachitskaya A V 2017 Open Payments Database: Anti-Vascular Endothelial Growth Factor Agent Payments to Ophthalmologists *Am. J. Ophthalmol.* **173** 91–7

[81] Cohen D 2018 CCGs win right to offer patients Avastin for wet AMD *Brit. Med.* J. **362** k4035

[82] Elzawawy A 2019 ecancer video online July 12, 2019 https://ecancer.org/video/8112/prof-ahmed-elzawawy-onglobal-cancer-control.php

[83] Gatesman M and Smith T 2011 The shortage of essential chemotherapy drugs in the United States *New Engl. J. Med.* **365** 1653–5

[84] Chabner B A 2011 Drug shortages—a critical challenge for the generic-drug market *New Engl. J. Med.* **365** 2147–9

[85] Emanuel E 2013 A plan to fix cancer care *The New York Times* March 23, 2013. https://opinionator.blogs.nytimes.com/2013/03/23/a-plan-to-fix-cancer-care/

[86] Medscape 2013 22 Docs offer plan to fix cancer care *Medscape* https://medscape.com/viewarticle/781476#vp

Chapter 16

Examples of scientific explorations of resource saving for better value in radiotherapy: breast cancer as a model

Ahmed Elzawawy and Wilfred Ngwa

This chapter is a continuation of the previous chapters, but the focus here is on examples that could lead to an increase in the affordability of good-value radiotherapy. Most of the presented examples take breast cancer as a model that could be expanded to other cancers in the world. In the Win-Win Movement, we agree with the American Society for Radiation Oncology (ASTRO)—Choosing Wisely recommendation, in that hypofractionation radiotherapy in breast cancer would be advisable whenever a comparable outcome can be achieved by conventional radiotherapy. We are in favour of increasing the use of evidence-based hypfractionation whenever possible in other localizations, such as the prostate, and for more studies to be undertaken for other indications and in different communities.

16.1 Resource saving in radiotherapy for breast cancer

16.1.1 Postoperative (post-mastectomy and post-lumpectomy) radiotherapy of breast cancer

16.1.1.1 Shorter fractionation for postoperative radiotherapy (hypofractionation)

The UK standardized breast radiotherapy randomized trial START-A for women with early breast cancer (pT1–3a pN0–1 M0), a regimen of 50 Gy in 25 fractions over five weeks was compared with 41·6 Gy or 39 Gy in 13 fractions over five weeks. In START-B, a regimen of 50 Gy in 25 fractions over five weeks was compared with 40.05 Gy in 15 fractions over three weeks. The eligibility criteria included an age over 18 years and no immediate surgical reconstruction. The primary endpoints were local–regional tumour relapse and late normal tissue effects. A ten-year follow-up confirmed that appropriately-dosed hypofractionated radiotherapy is safe and effective for patients with early breast cancer. The results support the continued use

doi:10.1088/978-0-7503-3075-6ch16

of 40.05 Gy in 15 fractions, which has already been adopted by most UK centers as the standard of care for women requiring adjuvant radiotherapy for early invasive breast cancer [1, 2].

FAST-Forward is a multicentre, phase 3, randomized, non-inferiority trial carried out at 97 hospitals (47 radiotherapy centers and 50 referring hospitals) in the UK. Patients aged at least 18 years with invasive carcinoma of the breast (pT1–3, pN0–1, M0) after breast conservation surgery or a mastectomy were eligible. We randomly allocated patients to either 40.05 Gy in 15 fractions (over three weeks), 27 Gy in five fractions (over one week), or 26 Gy in five fractions (over one week) to the whole breast or chest wall. Allocation was not masked because of the nature of the intervention. Twenty-six Gy in five fractions over one week is non-inferior to the standard of 40.05 Gy in 15 fractions over three weeks for local tumor control, and is as safe in terms of normal tissue effects for up to 5 years for patients prescribed adjuvant local radiotherapy after primary surgery for early-stage breast cancer [3].

For now, moderate hypofractionation with 40–42.5 Gy over 15–16 fractions remains the standard of care for the majority of patients with breast cancer who undergo whole-breast radiotherapy without regional nodal irradiation after breast-conserving surgery [4].

Recent studies, however, have demonstrated equivalent tumor control and cosmetic outcomes in specific patient populations with shorter courses of therapy (approximately four weeks). Patients and their physicians should review these options to determine the most appropriate course of therapy. The ASTRO Choosing Wisely campaign recommended considering shorter treatment when initiating whole-breast radiotherapy as part of breast conservation in women with early-stage invasive breast cancer. With comparable tumor control, lower costs, and reduced morbidity, hypofractionation should be strongly considered for the majority of patients with early-stage disease. ASTRO recommended that decisions should be more appropriately individualized based on tumor factors, anatomic considerations, and patient preferences. Dose to the heart, contralateral breast, lung, and other normal tissues should be minimized [5, 6].

With comparable tumor control, lower costs, and reduced morbidity, hypofractionation should be strongly considered for the majority of patients with early-stage disease. ASTRO recommended that decisions be more appropriately individualized based on tumor factors, anatomic considerations, and patient preference. The dose given to the heart, contralateral breast, lung, and other normal tissues should be minimized. A tumor bed boost is recommended for patients aged 50 years or younger with any grade tumor, or in patients aged 51–70 years with high-grade tumors or positive margins. Other recommendations are also included, such as for treatment planning, the technique of whole-breast irradiation (WBI), patient positioning, and other factors [6].

There is a midway solution that could be also reasonable, particularly for low- and middle-income countries (LMICs); the fractionation of 45.0 Gy as 2.50 Gy per fraction in 18 fractions has been used in Port Said, Egypt, for post-mastectomy treatment and in whole-breast radiotherapy (WBRT) after breast conservation surgery [7]. It follows the fractionations practiced successfully for years since the seventies in many French centers [8]. Hence, we reduce the duration and costs by seven sessions of radiotherapy, compared to the conventional radiotherapy of 50.00 Gy in 25 fractions. With this technique alone, we can at least increase the opportunity for radiotherapy for around 30% more patients. Once again, without spending more funds, there is a lot that can be done to increase the affordability of value-based radiotherapy for greater numbers of cancer patients.

We advocate more studies of evidence-based hypfractionation, which should be conducted for other localizations, such as the prostate, and other indications in different communities [9–11].

16.1.2 Accelerated partial breast irradiation

The rationale for accelerated partial breast irradiation (APBI) of small cancers without adverse features predisposing to multicentric recurrence originated from the observation that 80%–90% of breast cancer recurrences after breast conservative surgery and WBI occur in the tumor bed.

The advantage of APBI is that it would resolve the dilemmas regarding chemotherapy and radiotherapy sequencing and could perhaps be more cost-effective [12].

Several techniques, including multicatheter interstitial radionuclide brachytherapy, intracavitary brachytherapy [13], intraoperative radiation therapy, and 3D-conformal external-beam radiation therapy have been proposed. Each of them has its own pros and drawbacks [7].

There are still questions about APBI and its equivalence with WBI, despite its use in some centers the United States and Europe [14]. A total of ten randomized controlled trials involving 15,500 patients with early-stage breast cancer were selected according to the inclusion and exclusion criteria and included in this meta-analysis. The analysis showed that patients receiving APBI had a higher local recurrence rate, but no differences in distant metastasis, breast cancer deaths, contralateral breast cancer, disease-free survival, and overall survival rates [15]. Because the average breast size in some countries, such as Japan, is considerably smaller than in the Western world, the application of APBI to Japanese patients is technically more challenging [16].

The authors' view: Our point of view is that in LMICs, breast cancer cases are usually more advanced [7]. However, APBI could be advised for early breast cancer under certain circumstances, as shown by the example of electronic brachytherapy in a later section of this chapter.

16.1.3 Concurrent boost radiotherapy during the course of whole-breast radiotherapy

One of the ways to shorten the duration of radiotherapy without sacrificing the outcome is to use boost radiotherapy that is given concurrently during the course of WBRT itself, instead of giving it sequentially after WBRT.

The objective is to shorten the duration of radiotherapy without sacrificing the outcome. The boost radiotherapy is given concurrently during the course of WBRT itself, instead of giving it sequentially after WBRT.

There are different ways to deliver concurrent boost radiotherapy (CBRT). In a study by Jalali [17], a concomitant boost (CB) was given to the tumor bed on the non-treatment day of a conventional course, e.g. on Saturdays. Thirty patients with locally advanced breast cancers suitable for breast conservation following neo-adjuvant doxorubicin/epirubicin chemotherapy (CAF/CEF) were recruited for the study. Conventional radiotherapy (RT) to the whole breast was delivered five days a week from Monday to Friday to a dose of 50 Gy, using 6–10 MV photons. In addition, an electron boost to the tumor bed was delivered every Saturday (12.5 Gy/five fractions, a weekly fraction on Saturdays).

It is interesting that there are other studies that delivered the entire course of WBI and CBRT in the same sessions in three weeks. The RT dose to the whole breast was 40.05 Gy at 2.67 Gy per fraction with a CB of 4.5 Gy at 0.3 Gy per fraction. No acute clinical toxicity criteria at grade III or IV and no late soft-tissue toxicity were noted. The cosmetic results observed were good to excellent [19]. These studies demonstrate that giving a CB during whole-breast RT is a viable resource-saving option that does not sacrifice the outcome and the cosmetic results [19].

16.2 Is this a new era of electronic brachytherapy?

In breast cancer treatment, intraoperative radiation therapy (IORT) is a form of APBI in which radiation therapy is delivered, in a single dose, directly to the tumor bed during surgery [20]. IORT allows radiation to be delivered precisely to the area where recurrence is most likely, while reducing compliance issues, radiation exposure to normal tissues, and radiation-induced toxicity [21]. IORT reduces radiation-induced complications associated with WBRT without compromising oncologic or cosmetic outcomes [21–23]. If the final histopathology reveals poor prognostic findings, WBRT can be added. IORT then becomes the boost. IORT given initially does not exclude the potential use of excision and WBRT as a salvage treatment if there is local recurrence in the future.

Two prospective randomized trials, TARGIT-A and ELIOT, suggested that IORT is a safe alternative to WBRT for selected low-risk patients [22–29]. IORT to the tumor was delivered to all 947 tumors during the initial surgical breast-conserving procedure [29]. IORT consisted of 20 Gy delivered to the balloon surface. The system delivers 50-kV x-ray radiation using a balloon applicator. Balloon sizes were chosen that best filled the excision cavity (75% 3–4 cm, 23% 4–5 cm, 2% 5–6 cm). Following IORT balloon placement, the skin-to-balloon distance was measured using ultrasound. The minimum allowable distance for treatment was 8 mm [26, 27].

The teletherapy radiation component of breast conservation treatment requires expensive equipment and a high degree of medical expertise, leading to a lack of availability in rural areas. Many women with early breast cancer who are excellent candidates for breast conservation find that they live too far from a radiation therapy center to make the treatment practical, or they discover that 30–35 treatments are simply too inconvenient and/or too costly [28, 29]. This may lead to unnecessary mastectomies and, in some cases, bilateral mastectomies.

This happens too frequently when excision plus IORT could have been a simple, outpatient, one-day, less expensive, breast-conserving solution for a select subset of low-risk women with early-stage breast cancer. Additionally, biologic subtyping data may allow suitability guidelines for IORT to be refined. The excellent results achieved in patients who received WBRT after IORT support a further exploration of IORT as a planned boost to WBRT in higher-risk patients [28–31].

To summarize the case of electronic brachytherapy, we presented the following at the Global Health Catalyst GHC Summit—Win-Win and in a lecture of the GHC Global Radiation Oncology course [30]:

- Electronic brachytherapy x-ray (eBx) uses a miniaturised x-ray tube instead of radioactive sources
- Used at high dose rates (HDRs) in gynaecological cervix and endometrium, IORT breast, skin, and spinal treatments
- It is clinically tested and reliable

Advantages:

- It avoids isotope administration, transport, handling, and disposal of radioactive isotopes plus subsequent costs
- It avoids additional room shielding with subsequent costs
- There are no radiation risks in the case of system failure
- Electronic brachytherapy eliminates some of the accidents related to radionuclide brachytherapy, such as loss of sources, radiation leakage in the 'off' state, transportation accidents, and radioactive waste
- Outpatient treatment times are the same as those of a fresh (7 Ci) Ir^{192} source
- The source does not decay over time and therefore maintains a constant dose profile
- Minimal stray radiation to normal tissue and organs.
- Minimal shielding required for the operating staff. Medical staff can remain in the room with the patient, as determined by the facility's radiation safety officer
- The device is portable and no bunker is required
- Enables IORT

- Patient-driven advantages:
- Increased access for the patient. Treatment is done in the same surgical operation session, with no need for further visits to hospital.

- Physician-driven advantages:
- Improved dosimetry
- Applicator insertion and treatment set-up similar
- As we stated above: no isotope handling and minimal shielding are required
- It has significant competitive advantages over HDR iridium, due to its more optimal dose targeting that dramatically reduces the dose given to the bladder and rectum

In the Win-Win initiative, we stress that we are not promoting one technology or the products of a certain company, but we cite the example of electronic brachytherapy as an idea that is scientifically interesting. However, as for any interesting new technology, it could be more developed with more ideas and applications.

One of the limiting factors that impedes the use of electronic brachytherapy for interstitial applications is the source dimensions. However, it is highly anticipated that the design of a miniaturized x-ray tube that is closer to the dimensions of an Ir-192 wire is not too far away, and the new era of electronic brachytherapy has just begun [31].

From the authors to the reader: we raise the following question for the reader: in the near future, could electronic brachytherapy be considered as a way to increase the affordability of cost-effective brachytherapy for a greater number of patients by using one transportable machine in a van (car) to serve several units and different cities? Is it time for a new era of electronic brachytherapy—one without radioactive isotopes—in the third decade of the 21st century?

As we mentioned in different parts of this book, the links for feedback are: http://icedoc.net/feedback.html and http://icedoc.org/feedback.html

16.3 Palliative radiotherapy of painful bone metastasis

16.3.1 Single versus multiple fractions

Radiotherapy remains the main modality of management for symptomatic bone metastases. In such cases, the goal of radiotherapy is to provide pain relief and optimize the quality of life (QoL) with minimal displacement, discomfort, hospitalization, and morbidity for patients and also to minimize the cost and time commitment. The performance status and the degree of systemic disease must be considered prior to treatment [32, 33].

The ASTRO Choosing Wisely recommendation for palliative bone metastases is that studies suggest equivalent pain relief can be obtained by the use of 30 Gy in ten fractions, 20 Gy in five fractions, or a single 8 Gy fraction. A single treatment is more convenient, but may be associated with a slightly higher rate of retreatment at the same site [5].

Approximately 25 randomized clinical trials and three meta-analyses have demonstrated the equivalence of single- and multiple-fraction radiotherapy for bone relief from uncomplicated bone metastases. The other advantages of single-fraction radiotherapy include decreased cost and a lower risk of acute effects [34]. A single fraction is preferred when cost utility is considered, a higher rate of retreatment is associated with single-fraction radiotherapy [35]. However, most authors recommend multiple fractionations for the primary treatment of complicated bone metastases for which there is no surgical option, or for postoperative treatment. The goals of postoperative radiation therapy are to decrease pain, promote healing, and minimize the risk of progression [33].

It is worth noting that the treatment of asymptomatic bone metastases may be deferred unless the patient is at risk of a serious adverse outcome, such as spinal cord compression or impending pathological fracture [32].

16.3.2 Half-body radiotherapy

Single-dose hemibody irradiation (HBI) is effective and safe for pain relief in 70%–80% of patients with multiple-site painful metastases. Generally, the dose for lower HBI is 8 Gy in one fraction; for upper HBI, it is 7 Gy in one fraction, with a reduction of the lung dose to 6 Gy in one fraction by partial shielding. Studies also report a decrease in opioid use and the need for localized external-beam radiotherapy. Patients should be pre-medicated with intravenous fluid, antiemetics, corticosteroids, and analgesics to avoid a pain flare-up. Sequential treatment with both upper and lower HBI requires a six-week gap for the recovery of myelosuppression [33, 36]. Middle half-body 3D-conformal radiotherapy (3D-CRT) has been used for widespread bone metastases. The target included the pelvic bones, the lumbar-sacral vertebrae and the upper third of the femurs. The radiotherapy was delivered in 3 Gy fractions, bid, $\geqslant$ 6 h apart, on two consecutive days (total dose: 12 Gy) using the three-dimensional conformal RT (3D-CRT) box technique. Studies have shown that HBI delivered using the 3D-CRT technique is safe and effective [37].

16.3.3 Reduction in the costs of some procedures used to follow up the radiotherapy of bone metastases

The International Bone Metastases Consensus Working Party recommended that the follow-up and evaluation of response should be clinical as far as possible. Therefore, biochemical and imaging studies are not routinely required in the follow-up process. This represents a cost saving [38].

16.4 General measures

16.4.1 General strategic planning of radiotherapy facilities in developing countries

In 1999, a global strategy for radiotherapy was proposed in a consultation for the World Health Organization. It considered different local parameters, including the gross national product (GNP) per capita, which categorized countries in the world into four groups (or levels). Accordingly, a three-tier series of radiotherapy services was proposed, with an internet-based intercommunication strategy [39]. An integrated three-tier radiotherapy service implies the consideration of three levels (primary, secondary, and tertiary) of radiotherapy centre in developing countries, coordinated through a teleradiotherapy network. Such a network could be cost-effective, help to bridge the gap, and give all patients access to state-of-the-art technology in radiotherapy [40].

To explore a feasible cost-effective solution, Datta *et al* [41] suggested ‘optimized teleradiotherapy networks (TRTNets)’ through resource sharing could be a cost-effective and financially viable option to create RT infrastructure and facilitate capacity building toward realizing the 2030 Agenda for Sustainable Development goals in most LMICs. Low-income countries and some LMICs that are not expected to show a positive return on investment (ROI) should be considered for external financial assistance.

16.4.2 Practical modifications of the system of work in radiotherapy departments

There are several points and suggestions that deserve study in order to increase the number of patients treated, for example:

- An increase in the hours of work and shifts, particularly for cobalt machines in developing countries [7].
- An increase in the working days from five to six or seven days per week.
- An increase in the number of fractions from five to six fractions per week. In a study of accelerated (six) fractions per week versus conventional (five) fractions per week for radiotherapy in squamous cell carcinoma of the head and neck in a randomized international multicenter trial with 908 patients conducted by the International Atomic Energy Agency-Accelerated Fractionation (IAEA-ACC) study group, local control was better in the group selected for six fractions per week. In fact, this finding deserves more studies for other tumors particularly the locally advanced lesions [42].
- The reduction of machine downtime in many developing country institutions, which is mainly due to maintenance problems and the lack of a culture of local regular preventive maintenance [43]. In our view, we emphasizes the importance of programs that should developed in order to ensure that most of the problems of machine downtime can be fixed as soon as possible by local teams, either alone, or using prompt telecommunication with the manufacturer's maintenance staff [7].

16.5 Professional education and training

We emphasize that the most mandatory element for resource sparing, cost-effective treatment, i.e. better-value treatment tailored for patients in different communities, is well-trained and regularly updated medical, technical, and maintenance staff. This is a higher priority than sophisticated machines and techniques.

Therefore, customized and regularly updated training is recommended for the local medical, technical, and maintenance staff [7, 30, 39, 43]. We consider this aspect in the educational and training program planning of the Global Oncology University. We indicated that the curricula of clinical oncology provided for LMICs should not be less than those provided for HICs, but they should provide—as far as possible—different valid care options, hints, and pointers to scientific undertakings to solve problems and for research to tailor treatments to get better outcomes for their patients. This is in addition to in-depth knowledge of the readymade resources and guidelines for treatment produced by Western societies and organizations, even though those may not scientifically give the best results for their local patients in real life. Moreover, these curricula address the topic of how to establish and to develop clinical oncology services [30]. These issues deserve more global consideration for effective wide realization if we seriously want to see a breakthrough in the rate of increasing access to clinical oncology services in the world.

16.6 Conclusions

In a recent study conducted in the USA, around one quarter of 135 breast cancer patients undergoing mastectomy with strong indications for radiotherapy did not receive their postoperative radiotherapy. Surprisingly, one of the reasons that they did not receive radiotherapy was their socioeconomic conditions [44]. Hence, even in the US, there are disparities in access to radiotherapy, but surely, its magnitude it is not comparable with the huge shortage in LMICs.

In this chapter, we have just cited examples of what can be done in scientific ways without spending any more or buying machines. By a rough estimation, these actions could double the number of patients treated and hence improve the affordability of radiotherapy, particularly in middle-income countries, without seeking more funds and without compromising the outcome. On the contrary, as shown here, some of the presented options would bring more comfort to patients and hospital visits.

This would not lead to fewer purchases of radiotherapy equipment, but it would increase the opportunities to purchase, because the gap is estimated to be at least 10 000 units in this decade. Contrary to belief, radiotherapy is cost-effective and not that expensive. It is salient to note that the cost of one military jet would represent the entire cost of radiotherapy for a country in some of parts of the world [39]. The approaches cited in this chapter are just encouraging scientific examples, but a lot of scientific, value-based system improvement actions could be taken to make radiotherapy more cost-effective, even though we affirm that contrary to belief, radiotherapy is cost-effective and not that expensive if we that a radiotherapy device can serve for many years.

Hopefully, the successful and effective global campaign that the Win-Win Movement advocates could be one of the stimuli that remarkably increases radiotherapy facilities in the real world.

As we have stated on many occasions, more studies and research are needed in order to evolve evidence-based, cost-sparing, better-value cancer treatment in LMICs, according to what could fit patients in each community e.g. the Africa–Oxford–Harvard Clinical trials and the Cancer Research Consortium, AFROX-H (cited in this book). Clinical investigators from developing countries are the key to appropriately addressing those challenges via the rational utilization of radiotherapy and cancer drugs—both new and old drugs and techniques [7, 30, 43, 45].

In this book, there are relevant chapters by distinguished experts that give more details on different aspects that could lead to increased access to radiotherapy of considerable value in the world.

Once again, there is a need for an international forum in which all willing organizations, local bodies, stakeholders, and manufacturers come to coordinate together—within a win-win atmosphere—to achieve the feasible objective of increasing the availability and affordability of better-value clinical oncology care for millions of underserved cancer patients.

Once again, we do not claim that anyone or a single group could provide all solutions. What we presented here are examples of what could contribute—with the contribution of many other examples and stakeholders—to a remarkable increase in access to radiation oncology services in the world. We do not claim personal credit. We ask all readers and interested bodies to send feedback, suggestions, and ideas focused on how to increase the affordability of better-value cancer care to one of the available links: http://icedoc.net/feedback.html and http://icedoc.org/feedback.html. The replies will be provided by e-mail or by website, e.g. www.ecancerforall.com, http://www.icedoc.org/Books.htm and http://www.icedoc.net/Books.htm. This is a continuous global forum and platform—belonging to all—to which all are invited to contribute and to lead.

References and further reading

[1] The START Trialists' Group 2008 The UK Standardisation of Breast Radiotherapy (START) Trial B of radiotherapy hypofractionation for treatment of early breast cancer: a randomised trial *Lancet* **29** 1098–107

[2] Haviland J S, Owen J R and Dewar J A *et al* 2013 The UK Standardisation of Breast Radiotherapy (START) trials of radiotherapy hypofractionation for treatment of early breast cancer: 10-year follow-up results of two randomised controlled trials *Lancet Oncol.* **14** 1086–94

[3] Brunt A, Haviland J S and Wheatley D A *et al* 2020 Hypofractionated breast radiotherapy for 1 week versus 3 weeks (FAST-Forward): 5-year efficacy and late normal tissue effects results from a multicenter, non-inferiority, randomised, phase 3 trial *Lancet* **395** 1613–26

[4] Krug D, Baumann R and Combs S E *et al* 2021 Moderate hypofractionation remains the standard of care for whole-breast radiotherapy in breast cancer: considerations regarding FAST and FAST-forward *Strahlenther Onkol.* **197** 269–80

[5] Choosing Wisely. American Society for Radiation Oncology ASTRO https://choosingwisely.org/societies/american-society-for-radiation-oncology/

[6] Smith B, Bellon J and Blitzblau R *et al* 2018 Radiation therapy for the whole breast: Executive summary of an American Society for Radiation Oncology (ASTRO) evidence-based guideline *Pract. Radiat. Oncol.* **8** 145–52

[7] Elzawawy A 2012 Science and affordability of cancer drugs and radiotherapy in the world: win-win scenarios ed R Mohan *Advances in Cancer Management* (Rijeka: InTech) http://intechopen.com/articles/show/title/science-and-affordability-of-cancer-drugs-and-radiotherapy-in-the-world

[8] Sarrazin D, Le M and Arriagada R *et al* 1989 Ten year results of randomized trial comparing a conservative treatment to mastectomy in early breast cancer *Radiother. Oncol.* **14** 177

[9] Datta N R, Datta S and Samiei M 2020 Strategies to maximize available resources with minimum cost escalation for improving radiation therapy accessibility in the post-corona-virus disease 2019 era: an analysis for Asia *Adv. Radiat. Oncol.* **6** 100565

[10] Irabor O C, Swanson W and Shaukat F *et al* 2020 Can the adoption of hypofractionation guidelines expand global radiotherapy access? An analysis for breast and prostate radiotherapy *JCO Glob. Oncol.* **6** 667–78

[11] Swanson W, Kamwa F and Samba R *et al* 2021 Hypofractionated radiotherapy in African Cancer Centers *Front. Oncol.* **10** 618641

[12] Sarin R 2005 Partial-breast treatment for early breast cancer: emergence of a new paradigm *Nat. Clin. Pract. Oncol.* **2** 40–7

[13] Rodriguez-Ibarria N, Pinar M B and Garcia L *et al* 2020 Accelerated partial breast irradiation with interstitial multicatheter brachytherapy after breast-conserving surgery for low-risk early breast cancer *Breast* **52** 45–9

[14] Cole C, Bliss J and Poortmans P 2019 Accelerated partial breast irradiation: more questions than answers? *Lancet* **394** 2127–9

[16] Xiang X, Ding Z, Feng L and Li N 2021 A meta-analysis of the efficacy and safety of accelerated partial breast irradiation versus whole-breast irradiation for early-stage breast cancer *Radiat. Oncol.* **16** 24

[16] Mitsumori M and Hiraoka M 2008 Current status of accelerated partial breast irradiation *Breast Cancer* **15** 101–7

[17] Jalali R, Singh S and Budrukkar A 2007 Techniques of tumour bed boost irradiation in breast conserving therapy: current evidence and suggested guidelines *Acta Oncol.* **46** 879–92

[18] Chadha M, Woode R and Sillanpaa J *et al* 2007 Three-week Accelerated Radiation Therapy (ART) schedule with a concomitant in-field boost as treatment for early stage breast cancer *Int. J. Radiat. Oncol. Biol. Phys.* **69** S137

[19] Munshi A 2009 Resource-sparing and cost-effective strategies in current management of breast cancer *J Can Res Ther* **5** 116–20

[20] Harris E E R and Small W Jr 2017 Intraoperative radiotherapy for breast cancer *Front Oncol.* **7** 317

[21] Polgar C, Fodor J, Major T, Sulyok Z and Kasler M 2013 Breast-conserving therapy with partial or whole breast irradiation: ten-year results of the Budapest randomized trial *Radiother. Oncol.* **108** 197–202

[22] Vaidya J S, Joseph D J and Tobias J S *et al* 2010 Targeted intraoperative radiotherapy versus whole breast radiotherapy for breast cancer (TARGIT-A trial): an international, prospective, randomized, non-inferiority phase 3 trial *Lancet* **376** 91–102

[23] Corica T, Nowak A and Saunders C *et al* 2016 Cosmesis and breast related quality of life outcomes after intraoperative radiation therapy for early breast cancer: a substudy of the TARGIT-A Trial *Int. J. Radiat. Oncol.* **96** 55–64

[24] Vaidya J, Wenz F and Bulsara M *et al* 2014 Risk-adapted targeted intraoperative radiotherapy versus whole-breast radiotherapy for breast cancer: 5-year results for local control and overall survival from the TARGIT-A randomised trial *Lancet* **383** 603–13

[25] Veronesi U, Orecchia R and Maisonneuve P *et al* 2013 Intraoperative radiotherapy versus external radiotherapy for early breast cancer (ELIOT): a randomised controlled equivalence trial *Lancet Oncol.* **14** 1269–77

[26] Silverstein M J, Fastner G and Maluta S *et al* 2014 Intraoperative radiation therapy: a critical analysis of the ELIOT and TARGIT trials. Part 1–ELIOT *Ann. Surg. Oncol.* **21** 3787–92

[27] Silverstein M J, Epstein M and Kim B *et al* 2018 Intraoperative radiation therapy (IORT): A series of 1000 tumors *Ann Surg Oncol.* **25** 2987–93

[28] Athas W F, Adams-Cameron M, Hunt W C, Amir-Fazli A and Key C R 2000 Travel distance to radiation therapy and receipt of radiotherapy following breast-conserving surgery *J. Natl. Cancer Inst.* **92** 269–71

[29] Ballard-Barbash R, Potosky A L, Harlan L C, Nayfield S G and Kessler L G 1996 Factors associated with surgical and radiation therapy for early stage breast cancer in older women *J. Natl. Cancer Inst.* **88** 716–26

[30] Elzawawy A An introduction to affordability of better value clinical oncology.lecture: online course of global radiation oncology (CaReER 18–19), Harvard Global Health Catalyst. Global Oncology University GO-U http://icedoc.org/Docs/Elzawawy_8%20Sept.2018_GO_U.pdf http://icedoc.net/Docs/Elzawawy_8%20Sept.2018_GO_U.pdf

[31] Ramachandran P 2017 New era of electronic brachytherapy *World J. Radiol.* **9** 148–54

[32] Janjan N, Lutz S and Bedwinek J *et al* 2009 Therapeutic guidelines for the treatment of bone metastasis : a report from the American College of Radiology Appropriateness Criteria Expert Panel on Radiation Oncology *J. Palliat. Med.* **12** 417–23

[33] Fairchild A and Stephen L 2011 Palliative radiotherapy for bone mestasestas *Decisions Making in Radiotherapy* ed J J Lu and L W Brady (Berlin: Springer) pp 25–42

[34] Chow E, Harris K and Fan G *et al* 2007 Palliative radiotherapy trials for bone metastases: a systemic review *J. Clin. Oncol.* **25** 1423–36

[35] Van den Hout W B, Van der Linden Y M and Steenland E *et al* 2003 Single-versus multiple-fraction radiotherapy in patients with painful bone metastases: cost-utility analysis based on a randomized trial *J. Natl. Cancer Inst.* **95** 222–9

[36] Berg R, Yilmaz M and Høyer M *et al* 2009 Half body irradiation of patients with multiple bone metastases: a phase II trial *Acta Oncol.* **48** 556–61

[37] Macchia G, Ferro M and Cilla S *et al* 2018 Efficacy and safety of 3D-conformal half body irradiation in patients with multiple bone metastases *Clin. Exp. Metastasis* **35** 747–52

[38] Chow E, Wu J and Hoskin P *et al* 2002 International consensus on palliative radiotherapy endpoints for future clinical trials in bone metastases *Radiother. Oncol.* **64** 275–80

[39] Porter A, Aref A and Chodounsky Z *et al* 1999 A global strategy for radiotherapy: A WHO consultation *Clin. Oncol. (R. Coll. Radiol.)* **9** 368–70

[40] Datta N R and Rajasekar D 2004 Improvement of radiotherapy facilities in developing countries: a three-tier system with a teleradiotherapy network *Lancet Oncol.* **5** 695–8

[41] Datta N R, Rogers S and Bodis S 2019 Challenges and opportunities to realize 'The 2030 agenda for sustainable development' by the united nations: implications for radiation therapy infrastructure in low- and middle-income countries *Int. J. Radiat. Oncol. Biol. Phys.* **105** 918–33

[42] Overgaard J, Mohanti B and Bhasker S *et al* 2006 Accelerated versus conventional fractionated radiotherapy in squamous cell carcinoma of head and neck. A randomized international multicentere trial with 908 patients conducted by the IAEA-ACC study group *Int. J. Radiat. Oncol. Biol. Phys.* **66** S13

[43] Bhadrasain V 2005 Radiation therapy for the developing countries *J. Can. Res. Ther.* **1** 7–8

[44] Jagsi R, Abrahamse P and Morrow M *et al* 2010 Patterns and correlates of adjuvant radiotherapy receipt after lumpectomy and after mastectomy for breast cancer *J. Clin. Oncol.* **28** 2396–403

[45] Elzawawy A M 2015 Could African and low- and middle-income countries contribute scientifically to global cancer care? *J. Glob. Oncol.* **1** 49–53

Chapter 17

Challenges for radiotherapy accessibility in the post-COVID-19 era in low- and middle-income countries: strategies to maximize available resources with minimum cost escalation

Niloy R Datta[1], Sneha Datta[2], Massoud Samiei[3]

[1]*Director-Professor, Department of Radiotherapy, Mahatma Gandhi Institute of Medical Sciences, Sevagram, India*
[2]*Animal Production and Health Laboratory, Joint FAO/IAEA Divison of Nuclear Techniques in Food and Agriculture, Department of Nuclear Sciences and Applications, International Atomic Energy Agency (IAEA), Vienna, Austria*
[3]*Senior Consultant, Nuclear Energy, International Atomic Energy Agency (IAEA), Vienna, Austria*

This chapter covers strategies for the maximal utilization of radiotherapy (RT) infrastructure and explores the possibility of creating radiotherapy infrastructure in low- and middle-income countries (LMICs) that do not have any radiotherapy facilities.

17.1 Introduction

According to the World Health Organization (WHO), cancer is the second leading cause of death globally with an estimated 9.6 million deaths in 2018, 70% of which occurred in LMICs [1]. The WHO estimates that the number is likely to double by 2040, and that the LMICs will account for 67% of all cancers. Apart from the higher risk of mortality, cancer also significantly affects the economy. Its impact was estimated to be US$ 1.16 trillion in 2010, and is expected to reach US$ 2.9 trillion by 2030 for LMICs alone [2, 3]. LMICs have been further burdened by the current Coronavirus disease 2019 (COVID-19) pandemic. According to the World Bank, the pandemic could shrink the global economy by around 4.9% and is exacting a massive toll, especially on poor and vulnerable populations [4]. This could significantly hamper efforts to provide optimal cancer therapy, especially in LMICs.

RT, an essential component of cancer management, is estimated to be required for 60.5% of all cancer patients [5]. The lack of adequate RT infrastructure and human resources in LMICs has been well recognized [6–9]. Currently, the mean RT

doi:10.1088/978-0-7503-3075-6ch17

accessibility in LMICs is estimated to be just 33%, primarily due to the lack of adequate RT infrastructure and trained human resources [10]. COVID-19 has forced governments to divert most of their available resources toward healthcare related to the pandemic. Thus, it might be difficult for many countries, especially LMICs, to allocate adequate funds for very capital-intensive ventures, such as RT infrastructure. This could have an unfavorable impact on the targets listed in the United Nations (UN) 'Sustainable Developmental Goals (SDG)', which was proposed to be achieved by 2030, wherein one of the goals is reducing premature mortality from noncommunicable diseases (including cancer) by one third [10, 11].

It is therefore essential to evolve pragmatic strategies that can maximize the utilization of the available RT infrastructure with minimum cost escalation. This is especially important for LMICs who are already challenged by the projected rising cancer incidence in the coming decades and who have grossly inadequate RT accessibility for their cancer patients. The following sections critically analyze these options for LMICs and aim to improve RT accessibility using available resources.

17.2 Magnitude of the problem

The World Bank classified 135 countries as LMICs in 2019, based on their gross national income (GNI) per capita [12, 13]. The classification includes: low-income (n=29 with GNI/capita ⩽ US$ 1035), low-mid income (n=50 with GNI/capita US$ 1036–4045) and upper-mid income groups (n=56 with GNI/capita US$ 4046–12,535). The cancer incidences for 'all cancers excluding non-melanoma cancer' for each country in 2020 among the LMIC group were extracted from the Global Cancer Observatory [14]. Details of the existing RT infrastructure for the same countries were obtained from the DIrectory of RAdiotherapy Centres (DIRAC) of the International Atomic Energy Agency (IAEA), as of November 15, 2020 [15].

According to the IAEA recommendations, the demand for megavoltage teleradiotherapy (TRT) units for each country was quantified by assuming an optimum RT utilization rate of 55% with an assumed reirradiation rate of 10% [5]. Thus, 60.5% of all cancers would require RT. Furthermore, a single TRT unit would treat 500 new patients annually using routine techniques within the normal 8 h working day of a department [5, 8]. These figures could vary; therefore, it is highly desirable that each RT centre should estimate values depending on their RT utilization rates, the proportion of patients reporting for reirradiation, and the number of patients treated per TRT unit/per year. However, for the purpose of this exercise, the values recommended by the IAEA have been used [5, 8]. As the details of the personnel (radiation oncologists, medical physicists, and RT technologists) were not available in the current DIRAC database, the human resources for RT could not be evaluated. It is assumed that adequate human resources are available in each center to work with their existing TRT units.

The cancer incidence was obtained from the Global Cancer Incidence, Mortality and Prevalence (GLOBOCAN) database for 125 LMICs, while the TRT details were listed in 88 of the 135 LMICs (figure 17.1). Thus, the cancer incidence in these 88 countries was reported as 10.98 million, of which 6.64 million would need RT. According to DIRAC, 5350 TRT units and 1201 brachytherapy units were available in these countries, resulting in a mean % RT accessibility of 47.7% (±SD: 34.1, range: 2.3–151.6). It is estimated that a total of 13 289 TRT units would be required

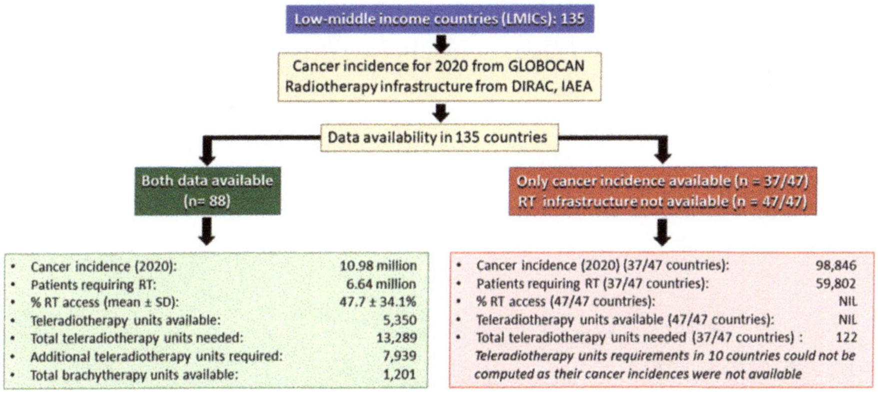

Figure 17.1. Status of radiotherapy (RT) accessibility in LMICs based on available data for cancer incidence (2020) obtained from GLOBOCAN and RT infrastructure data obtained from the DIRAC database (IAEA). Of the 135 LMICs, both data sets were available for 88 countries. It is estimated that 60.5% of all cancer patients will require RT and 500 patients can be treated by a single teletherapy unit annually using standard fractionation. Forty-seven LMICs are presumed to have no RT facilities, as no data was available in the DIRAC database. The RT requirement could thus only be estimated for 37 of the 47 LMICs where only the cancer incidence was available. (Status as of November 15, 2020.)

to provide 100% RT access for these patients. Thus, an additional 7939 TRT units would be required in these 88 countries, ranging from −5 to +3818 for each country (table 17.1, third column). At present, only eight of the 88 LMICs have adequate TRT units, equating to ⩾100% RT accessibility.

Cancer incidence data were available for 37 of the remaining 47 LMICs. Of the 98 846 estimated cancer patients in these countries, RT is likely to be required for 59 082 patients. This would require 122 TRT units, while additional units would be required for the remaining ten countries, based on their cancer incidence. As the details of TRT units were not listed in the DIRAC database, it may be prudent to assume that none of these 47 LMICs (34.8%) currently has any RT facilities.

17.3 Pragmatic strategies for maximizing the utilization of radiotherapy infrastructure with minimal cost escalation

The various strategies for maximizing the utilization of existing RT infrastructure, as discussed below, are feasible only for the 88 countries that currently have TRT units with adequate personnel. It is assumed that 500 patients/TRT unit/year can be treated within the normal eight working hours of a department. The various approaches that could be used to increase patient throughput with minimal cost escalation have been recently discussed for Asia [16]. Using the same framework and parameters, one could adapt them for the 88 LMICs globally. Minor modifications may be required at the individual country level, depending on the type of cancer, local management practices, available human resources, and RT infrastructure. These various strategies include:

i. *Hypofractionated radiotherapy (HFRT) within the eight working hours of a department:* the usual RT fractionation involves the delivery of 1.8 to 2 Gy/fraction for most patients. Patients undergoing radical, postoperative, or

Table 17.1. Changes in the % radiotherapy access and additional teleradiotherapy unit requirements for LMICs resulting from the adoption of various strategies to maximize the utilization of existing radiotherapy infrastructure. (Status as of November 15, 2020.)

Countries	With SFRT and eight working hours		With HFRT and eight working hours		+25% working hours and SFRT		+25% working hours and HFRT		+50% working hours and SFRT		+50% working hours and HFRT	
	% RT access	Additional TRT units	% RT access	Additional TRT units	% RT access	Additional TRT units	% RT access	Additional TRT units	% RT access	Additional TRT units	% RT access	Additional TRT units
Afghanistan	NA	NA	NA	NA	NA	NA	NA	NA	NA	NA	NA	NA
Albania	48.0	5	57.6	4	60.0	3	69.6	2	72.0	2	81.6	1
Algeria	54.0	32	64.8	20	67.4	18	78.2	10	80.9	9	91.7	3
American Samoa	NA	NA	NA	NA	NA	NA	NA	NA	NA	NA	NA	NA
Angola	14.4	18	17.2	14	18.0	14	20.8	11	21.5	11	24.4	9
Argentina	78.6	35	94.3	8	98.2	2	113.9	−16	117.8	−19	133.6	−32
Armenia	27.2	8	32.7	6	34.1	6	39.5	5	40.9	4	46.3	3
Azerbaijan	67.1	5	80.5	2	83.9	2	97.3	0	100.7	0	114.1	−1
Bangladesh	18.0	159	21.6	127	22.5	120	26.1	99	27.0	94	30.7	79
Belarus	69.4	16	83.3	7	86.8	5	100.6	0	104.1	−1	118.0	−5
Belize	NA	NA	NA	NA	NA	NA	NA	NA	NA	NA	NA	NA
Benin	NA	NA	NA	NA	NA	NA	NA	NA	NA	NA	NA	NA
Bhutan	NA	NA	NA	NA	NA	NA	NA	NA	NA	NA	NA	NA
Bolivia	41.9	11	50.3	8	52.4	7	60.8	5	62.9	5	71.2	3
Bosnia and Herzegovina	56.0	8	67.1	5	69.9	4	81.1	2	83.9	2	95.1	1
Botswana	39.7	2	47.7	1	49.7	1	57.6	1	59.6	1	67.5	0
Brazil	51.4	350	61.7	230	64.3	206	74.5	126	77.1	110	87.4	53
Bulgaria	74.8	11	89.7	4	93.5	2	108.4	−2	112.2	−3	127.1	−7
Burkina Faso	NA	NA	NA	NA	NA	NA	NA	NA	NA	NA	NA	NA
Burundi	NA	NA	NA	NA	NA	NA	NA	NA	NA	NA	NA	NA

Cabo Verde	NA	NA	NA	NA	NA	NA	NA	NA	NA	NA	NA	NA
Cambodia	10.1	18	12.1	14	12.6	14	14.7	12	15.2	11	17.2	10
Cameroon	4.9	19	5.9	16	6.2	15	7.1	13	7.4	13	8.4	11
Central African Republic	NA	NA	NA	NA	NA	NA	NA	NA	NA	NA	NA	NA
Chad	NA	NA	NA	NA	NA	NA	NA	NA	NA	NA	NA	NA
China	30.1	3818	36.1	2908	37.6	2726	43.6	2123	45.1	1998	51.2	1569
Colombia	69.0	41	82.8	19	86.3	14	100.1	0	103.5	−3	117.3	−13
Comoros	NA	NA	NA	NA	NA	NA	NA	NA	NA	NA	NA	NA
Congo, DR	NA	NA	NA	NA	NA	NA	NA	NA	NA	NA	NA	NA
Congo, Rep.	NA	NA	NA	NA	NA	NA	NA	NA	NA	NA	NA	NA
Costa Rica	29.8	12	35.7	9	37.2	8	43.2	7	44.7	6	50.6	5
Cote d'Ivoire	10.8	17	13.0	13	13.5	13	15.7	11	16.2	10	18.4	9
Cuba	31.2	40	37.4	30	39.0	28	45.2	22	46.8	20	53.0	16
Djibouti	NA	NA	NA	NA	NA	NA	NA	NA	NA	NA	NA	NA
Dominica	NA	NA	NA	NA	NA	NA	NA	NA	NA	NA	NA	NA
Dominican Republic	91.3	2	109.5	−2	114.1	−3	132.3	−5	136.9	−6	155.2	−7
Ecuador	60.7	14	72.8	8	75.9	7	88.0	3	91.1	2	103.2	−1
Egypt	72.1	46	86.5	19	90.1	13	104.5	−5	108.1	−9	122.5	−22
El Salvador	69.1	4	82.9	2	86.3	1	100.1	0	103.6	0	117.4	−1
Equatorial Guinea	NA	NA	NA	NA	NA	NA	NA	NA	NA	NA	NA	NA
Eritrea	NA	NA	NA	NA	NA	NA	NA	NA	NA	NA	NA	NA
Eswatini	NA	NA	NA	NA	NA	NA	NA	NA	NA	NA	NA	NA
Ethiopia	2.3	85	2.7	71	2.9	68	3.3	58	3.4	56	3.9	49
Fiji	NA	NA	NA	NA	NA	NA	NA	NA	NA	NA	NA	NA
Gabon	93.5	0	112.2	0	116.9	0	135.6	−1	140.2	−1	158.9	−1

(Continued)

Table 17.1. (*Continued*)

Countries	With SFRT and eight working hours		With HFRT and eight working hours		+25% working hours and SFRT		+25% working hours and HFRT		+50% working hours and SFRT		+50% working hours and HFRT	
	% RT access	Additional TRT units	% RT access	Additional TRT units	% RT access	Additional TRT units	% RT access	Additional TRT units	% RT access	Additional TRT units	% RT access	Additional TRT units
Gambia	NA	NA	NA	NA	NA	NA	NA	NA	NA	NA	NA	NA
Georgia	139.9	−5	167.9	−6	174.9	−7	202.9	−8	209.9	−8	237.9	−9
Ghana	17.1	24	20.5	19	21.4	18	24.8	15	25.6	15	29.1	12
Grenada	NA	NA	NA	NA	NA	NA	NA	NA	NA	NA	NA	NA
Guatemala	23.7	16	28.4	13	29.6	12	34.3	10	35.5	9	40.3	7
Guinea	NA	NA	NA	NA	NA	NA	NA	NA	NA	NA	NA	NA
Guinea-Bissau	NA	NA	NA	NA	NA	NA	NA	NA	NA	NA	NA	NA
Guyana	106.1	0	127.3	0	132.6	0	153.8	0	159.1	0	180.4	0
Haiti	NA	NA	NA	NA	NA	NA	NA	NA	NA	NA	NA	NA
Honduras	54.3	6	65.2	4	67.9	3	78.7	2	81.5	2	92.3	1
India	44.0	827	52.8	581	55.0	532	63.8	369	66.0	335	74.7	219
Indonesia	14.3	382	17.2	308	17.9	293	20.8	244	21.5	233	24.4	198
Iran	85.0	21	102.0	−2	106.2	−7	123.2	−23	127.5	−26	144.5	−37
Iraq	57.8	14	69.3	8	72.2	7	83.8	4	86.7	3	98.2	0
Jamaica	54.0	4	64.8	3	67.5	2	78.3	1	81.0	1	91.8	0
Jordan	92.5	1	111.0	−1	115.7	−2	134.2	−3	138.8	−4	157.3	−5
Kazakhstan	105.1	−2	126.1	−9	131.4	−11	152.4	−15	157.7	−16	178.7	−20
Kenya	19.1	51	22.9	40	23.9	38	27.7	31	28.7	30	32.5	25
Kiribati	NA	NA	NA	NA	NA	NA	NA	NA	NA	NA	NA	NA
Korea, DPR	4.3	67	5.2	55	5.4	53	6.2	45	6.4	44	7.3	38
Kosovo	NA	NA	NA	NA	NA	NA	NA	NA	NA	NA	NA	NA
Kyrgyz Rep.	11.9	7	14.3	6	14.9	6	17.3	5	17.9	5	20.2	4
Lao, PDR	20.1	8	24.2	6	25.2	6	29.2	5	30.2	5	34.3	4
Lebanon	106.0	−1	127.2	−5	132.5	−6	153.8	−8	159.1	−9	180.3	−10

Lesotho	NA	NA	NA	NA	NA	NA	NA	NA	NA	NA	NA	NA
Liberia	NA	NA	NA	NA	NA	NA	NA	NA	NA	NA	NA	NA
Libya	73.2	2	87.8	1	91.4	1	106.1	0	109.7	−1	124.4	−1
Madagascar	8.5	21	10.2	18	10.7	17	12.4	14	12.8	14	14.5	12
Malawi	NA	NA	NA	NA	NA	NA	NA	NA	NA	NA	NA	NA
Malaysia	102.3	−1	122.7	−11	127.8	−13	148.3	−19	153.4	−20	173.8	−25
Maldives	NA	NA	NA	NA	NA	NA	NA	NA	NA	NA	NA	NA
Mali	5.9	16	7.1	13	7.4	12	8.6	11	8.9	10	10.1	9
Marshall Islands	NA	NA	NA	NA	NA	NA	NA	NA	NA	NA	NA	NA
Mauritania	56.3	2	67.6	1	70.4	1	81.7	0	84.5	0	95.7	0
Mexico	66.4	83	79.7	42	83.0	33	96.3	6	99.6	1	112.9	−19
Micronesia	NA	NA	NA	NA	NA	NA	NA	NA	NA	NA	NA	NA
Moldova	15.8	16	19.0	13	19.8	12	22.9	10	23.7	10	26.9	8
Mongolia	68.6	2	82.3	1	85.7	1	99.4	0	102.8	0	116.5	−1
Montenegro	102.3	0	122.8	−1	127.9	−1	148.4	−1	153.5	−1	174.0	−1
Morocco	61.9	26	74.2	15	77.3	12	89.7	5	92.8	3	105.2	−2
Mozambique	3.0	32	3.6	27	3.8	25	4.4	22	4.5	21	5.1	18
Myanmar	24.8	67	29.8	52	31.0	49	36.0	39	37.2	37	42.2	30
Namibia	70.7	1	84.9	0	88.4	0	102.6	0	106.1	0	120.2	0
Nepal	24.0	25	28.8	20	30.0	19	34.8	15	36.0	14	40.8	12
Nicaragua	29.2	7	35.0	6	36.5	5	42.3	4	43.8	4	49.6	3
Niger	NA	NA	NA	NA	NA	NA	NA	NA	NA	NA	NA	NA
Nigeria	4.7	142	5.7	117	5.9	112	6.8	95	7.1	92	8.0	80
North Macedonia	41.1	6	49.3	4	51.3	4	59.6	3	61.6	2	69.8	2
Pakistan	26.4	164	31.7	127	33.0	120	38.3	95	39.6	90	44.9	72
Papua New Guinea	6.5	14	7.8	12	8.1	11	9.4	10	9.8	9	11.1	8
Paraguay	62.6	5	75.2	3	78.3	2	90.8	1	93.9	1	106.5	−1

(Continued)

Table 17.1. (*Continued*)

Countries	With SFRT and eight working hours		With HFRT and eight working hours		+25% working hours and SFRT		+25% working hours and HFRT		+50% working hours and SFRT		+50% working hours and HFRT	
	% RT access	Additional TRT units	% RT access	Additional TRT units	% RT access	Additional TRT units	% RT access	Additional TRT units	% RT access	Additional TRT units	% RT access	Additional TRT units
Peru	64.3	30	77.2	16	80.4	13	93.3	4	96.5	2	109.4	−5
Philippines	28.2	130	33.9	100	35.3	94	40.9	74	42.3	69	48.0	55
Russian Federation	68.6	210	82.3	98	85.8	76	99.5	2	102.9	−13	116.6	−65
Rwanda	14.3	12	17.2	10	17.9	9	20.8	8	21.5	7	24.4	6
Samoa	NA	NA	NA	NA	NA	NA	NA	NA	NA	NA	NA	NA
Sao Tome and Principe	NA	NA	NA	NA	NA	NA	NA	NA	NA	NA	NA	NA
Senegal	22.0	11	26.4	8	27.5	8	31.9	6	33.0	6	37.4	5
Serbia	52.9	28	63.4	18	66.1	16	76.6	9	79.3	8	89.9	3
Sierra Leone	NA	NA	NA	NA	NA	NA	NA	NA	NA	NA	NA	NA
Solomon Islands	NA	NA	NA	NA	NA	NA	NA	NA	NA	NA	NA	NA
Somalia	NA	NA	NA	NA	NA	NA	NA	NA	NA	NA	NA	NA
South Africa	75.7	33	90.8	10	94.6	6	109.7	−9	113.5	−12	128.6	−23
South Sudan	NA	NA	NA	NA	NA	NA	NA	NA	NA	NA	NA	NA
Sri Lanka	63.9	11	76.7	6	79.9	5	92.7	1	95.9	1	108.7	−2
St. Lucia	NA	NA	NA	NA	NA	NA	NA	NA	NA	NA	NA	NA
St. Vincent and the Grenadines	NA	NA	NA	NA	NA	NA	NA	NA	NA	NA	NA	NA
Sudan	30.2	23	36.2	18	37.7	17	43.7	13	45.2	12	51.3	10
Suriname	151.6	−1	182.0	−1	189.6	−1	219.9	−1	227.5	−1	257.8	−1

Syrian Arab Republic	23.3	23	27.9	18	29.1	17	33.8	14	34.9	13	39.6	11
Tajikistan	13.9	6	16.6	5	17.3	5	20.1	4	20.8	4	23.5	3
Tanzania	9.2	50	11.0	40	11.5	39	13.3	33	13.8	31	15.6	27
Thailand	48.3	112	58.0	76	60.4	69	70.1	45	72.5	40	82.2	23
Timor-Leste	NA	NA	NA	NA	NA	NA	NA	NA	NA	NA	NA	NA
Togo	NA	NA	NA	NA	NA	NA	NA	NA	NA	NA	NA	NA
Tonga	NA	NA	NA	NA	NA	NA	NA	NA	NA	NA	NA	NA
Tunisia	113.8	−3	136.6	−6	142.3	−7	165.1	−9	170.8	−10	193.5	−11
Turkey	98.5	4	118.2	−41	123.1	−50	142.8	−80	147.7	−86	167.4	−107
Turkmenistan	93.4	0	112.1	−1	116.7	−1	135.4	−2	140.1	−2	158.8	−3
Tuvalu	NA	NA	NA	NA	NA	NA	NA	NA	NA	NA	NA	NA
Uganda	2.4	42	2.8	34	2.9	33	3.4	28	3.5	27	4.0	24
Ukraine	44.1	115	52.9	81	55.1	74	64.0	51	66.2	47	75.0	30
Uzbekistan	21.4	26	25.7	20	26.8	19	31.1	16	32.1	15	36.4	12
Vanuatu	NA	NA	NA	NA	NA	NA	NA	NA	NA	NA	NA	NA
Venezuela, RB	58.8	33	70.5	20	73.5	17	85.2	8	88.2	6	99.9	0
Vietnam	17.5	174	21.0	139	21.9	132	25.4	109	26.3	104	29.8	87
West Bank and Gaza	NA	NA	NA	NA	NA	NA	NA	NA	NA	NA	NA	NA
Yemen, Rep.	5.9	16	7.0	13	7.3	13	8.5	11	8.8	10	10.0	9
Zambia	19.2	13	23.0	10	24.0	10	27.8	8	28.8	7	32.6	6
Zimbabwe	31.2	15	37.5	12	39.0	11	45.3	8	46.8	8	53.1	6
All LMICs	**47.7%[a]**	**7939**	**57.2%[a]**	**5724**	**59.6%[a]**	**5281**	**69.2%[a]**	**3815**	**71.5%[a]**	**3509**	**81.1%[a]**	**2467**

NA: not available as either data for cancer incidence in GLOBOCAN or for teleradiotherapy units in DIARC (IAEA), or both were unavailable. RT: radiotherapy; TRT: teleradiotherapy units; SFRT: standard fractionated radiotherapy; HFRT: hypofractionated radiotherapy; [a]: mean values for LMICs with existing RT infrastructure.

preoperative RT are usually treated with standard fractionation RT (SFRT) schedules of 70 Gy/35 fractions/seven weeks, 60 Gy/30 fractions/six weeks and 50 Gy/25 fractions/five weeks. However, patients on palliative RT are usually treated with a higher dose/fraction, depending on their disease and the site of irradiation. A mild to moderate HFRT could be adopted, whereby the treatment durations for radical, postoperative, and preoperative patients and the two-week palliative RT schedule are reduced by one week each, while keeping the respective total RT doses the same. Correspondingly, this would result in doses per fraction of 2.33, 2.40, 2.5, and 3 Gy for these treatments. As detailed in an earlier publication [16], as a result of these measures, an additional 100 patients could be treated. Thus, at least 600 patients/TRT unit/year could be accommodated with the use of HFRT within the usual eight working hours of a department. This would improve the mean %RT accessibility to 57.2% (±SD: 40.9, range: 2.7–182) from 47.7% with SFRT. The additional number of required TRT units would also drop to 5724 with HFRT from 7939 with SFRT with a normal eight-hour working day (table 17.1, figures 17.2 and 17.3).

ii. *With 25% more working hours and SFRT:* an additional 125 patients/year/TRT unit could be accommodated by increasing the working hours by 25% (2 h for an 8-hour working time of a department). Thus, the estimated number of patients that could be treated by each TRT unit/year could increase to 625. This would improve the mean % RT accessibility to 59.6% (±SD: 42.6, range: 2.9–189.6) and the requirement for additional TRT units would drop to 5281 (table 17.1, figures 17.2 and 17.3).

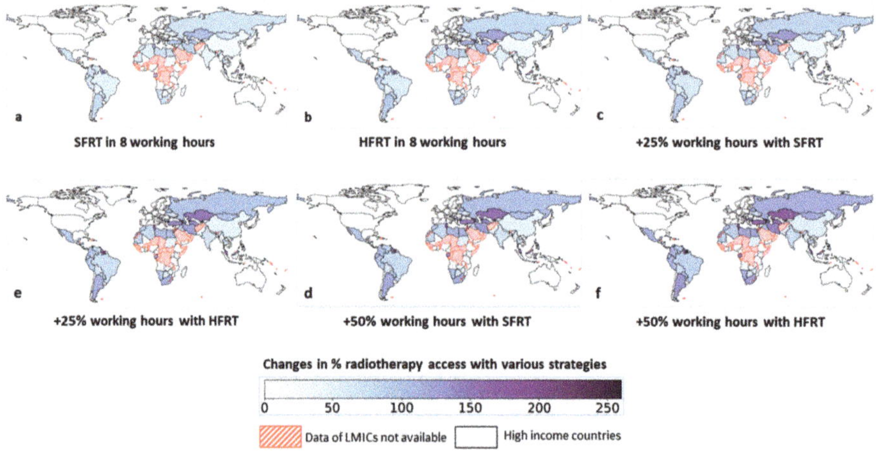

Figure 17.2. Changes in % radiotherapy (RT) access using various strategies in LMICs (a) with standard fractionated radiotherapy (SFRT) in routine working hours of 8 h day^{-1} (b) with hypofractionated radiotherapy (HFRT) within routine hours (c) with 25% additional working hours (+2 h) and SFRT (d) with 25% additional working hours (+2 h) and HFRT (e) with 50% additional working hours (+ 4 h) and SFRT (f) with 50% additional working hours (+4 h) and HFRT. A gradual gain in %RT access is observed from (a) to (f). Details of individual countries are given in table 17.1 (Status as of November 15, 2020). Reprinted from [16], copyright (2020) with permission from Elsevier.

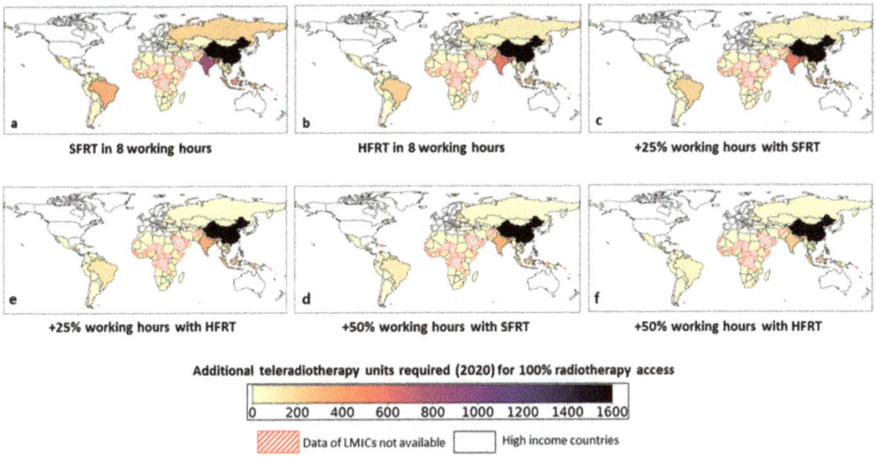

Figure 17.3. Additional teleradiotherapy (TRT) units required as per the status in 2020 for 100% radiotherapy (RT) access in LMICs (a) with standard fractionated radiotherapy (SFRT) for routine working hours of 8 h day^{-1} (b) with hypofractionated radiotherapy (HFRT) within routine hours (c) with 25% more working hours (+2 h) and SFRT (d) with 25% more working hours (+2 h) and HFRT (e) with 50% more working hours (+ 4 h) and SFRT (f) with 50% more working hours (+4 h) and HFRT. A gradual decline in the number of additional TRTs is observed from (a) to (f). Details of individual countries are given in table 17.1 (Status as of November 15, 2020). Reprinted from [16], copyright (2020) with permission from Elsevier.

iii. *With 25% more working hours and HFRT:* a combination of strategies (i) and (ii) could treat an additional 225 patients/TRT unit/year, thereby allowing 725 patients to be treated annually by a TRT unit. This would improve the mean %RT accessibility to 69.2% (±SD: 49.4, range: 3.3–219.9) and the requirement for additional TRT unit drop down to 3815 (table 17.1, figures 17.2 and 17.3).

iv. *With 50% more working hours and SFRT:* a 50% increase in working hours (by four hours) with SFRT could increase the annual number of patients treated by a single TRT unit by 250, thus bringing the total number to 750 patients/TRT unit/year. This would further improve the mean %RT accessibility to 71.5% (±SD: 51.1, range: 3.4–227.5) and the requirement for additional TRT units could drop to 3509 (table 17.1, figures 17.2 and 17.3).

v. *With 50% more working hours and HFRT:* a 50% increase in working hours with HFRT could enable an additional 350 patients to be treated in a single TRT unit. Consequently, 850 patients could be treated per TRT unit annually, thereby achieving a mean %RT accessibility of 81.1% (±SD: 57.9, range: 3.9–257.8). The requirement for additional TRT units would drop to 2467 (table 17.1, figures 17.2 and 17.3).

As these strategies are adopted, a gradual improvement in the %RT accessibility is evident with the same RT infrastructure. Thus, with SFRT and a normal eight-hour working period, only eight of the 88 LMICs are expected to have 100% RT accessibility today. With HFRT and 50% longer working hours, this could improve to 32 out of 88 LMICs (figure 17.4). Consequently, the number of countries which would not need any additional TRTs would increase from ten (with SFRT and 8 h in the working day) to 37 (with HFRT and 50% longer working hours) (figure 17.5).

As the benchmark of treating 500 patients annually in a single TRT unit is based on conventional and relatively simple RT techniques, countries with >100% RT access could practice specialized RT procedures, such as intensity-modulated RT, image-guided RT, stereotactic RT procedures, and others which demand additional

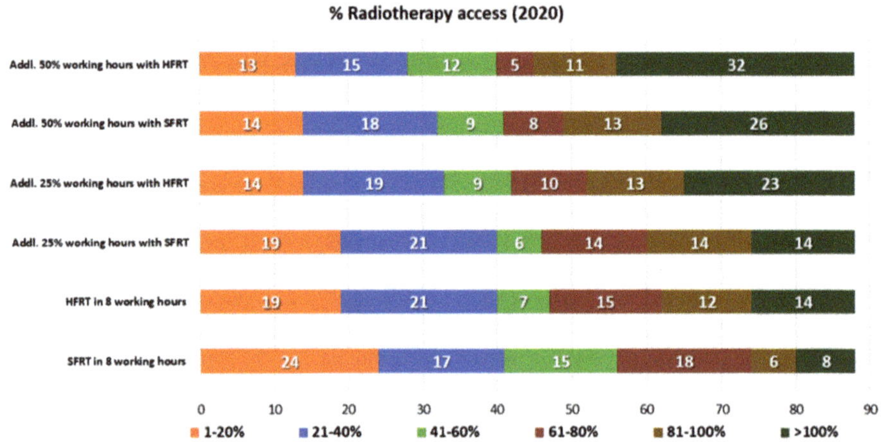

Figure 17.4. Changes in the % radiotherapy access in categories of 1%–20%, 21%–40%, 41%–60%, 61%–80%, 81%–100%, and >100% in 88 LMICs resulting from various strategies used to maximize the utilization of existing radiotherapy infrastructure. (Status as of November 15, 2020.) Reprinted from [16], copyright (2020) with permission from Elsevier.

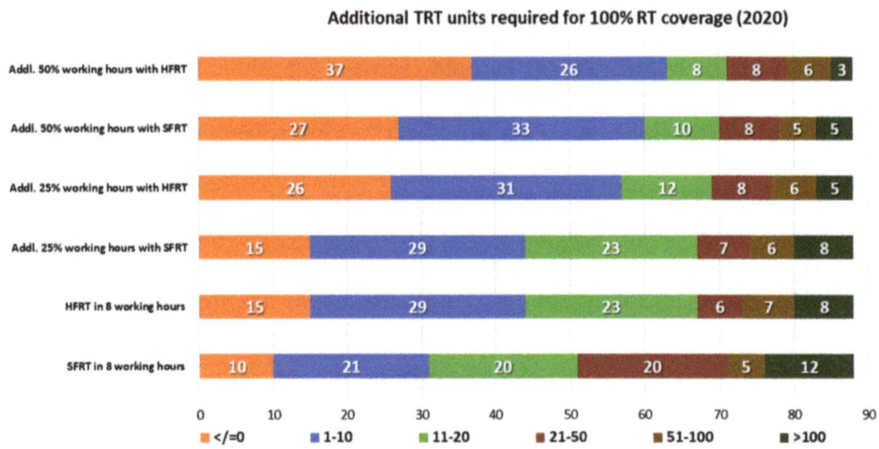

Figure 17.5. Changes in the additional teleradiotherapy units (TRT) required in categories of ⩽0, 1–10, 11–20, 21–50, 51–100, and >100 in 88 LMICs resulting from various strategies used to maximize the utilization of existing RT infrastructure. (Status as of November 15, 2020.) Reprinted from [16], copyright (2020) with permission from Elsevier.

machine time for treatment delivery and stringent quality assurance procedures. Of course, these decisions have to be taken at the level of individual center, depending on the types of case, their suitability, and the available human resources.

It may be noted that additional working hours would also require additional staff. If existing staff are ready to work additional hours, this would be financially rewarding for them. Otherwise, the additional working hours could help to provide new employment opportunities. This could create a win-win situation for patients (who would have reduced waiting times) and existing staff (in terms of additional income) and would also help to create employment opportunities for freshly trained RT personnel, many of whom could have difficulty in getting suitable positions due to a likely slowdown in investments for establishing new RT infrastructure.

17.4 Setting up radiotherapy infrastructure in countries lacking radiotherapy

The strategies discussed above for the maximal utilization of RT infrastructure would be solely applicable to the 88 LMICs that already have TRT units in their cancer center(s). However, one also needs to explore the possibility of creating RT infrastructure in the 47 LMICs that do not have any RT facilities. This requires strong political will and support from various governmental and nongovernmental resources. It may be important to note that it is now quite evident that one could expect a positive return on investment after creating RT infrastructure [10, 17]. The benefits from investments in cancer care would not only keep patients alive and alleviate their suffering, but could also increase direct workforce participation and broader societal contributions. In the long term, after effective treatment, these patients could make a substantial contribution in terms of both direct productivity and indirect societal gains. A recent WHO report estimates that investments in cancer care in LMICs during the 2020–2030 period could save over 7.3 million lives, which through their productivity and societal contributions will add a full social value of US$ 1.315 trillion [1]. The WHO analysis should encourage the above 47 countries to seriously consider setting up RT infrastructure for long-term economic gain.

17.5 Pooling of available resources through the teleradiotherapy network

The present COVID-19 pandemic has made us all more accustomed to working using virtual digital platforms. This could also play an important role in not only further maximizing the individual resources related to RT but also in sharing them between various centers. Telemedicine has been recognized as part of a sustainable healthcare solution in several medical specialties, particularly in LMICs, although its application in radiation oncology is limited and needs to be widened [18].

At present, information transfer in RT relies on standard interfaces such as Health Level 7 (HL7) and DICOM-RT. These could be used to exchange data between different RT centers on a wider geographical scale with the use of current information and communications technology (ICT). This has been applied in many developed countries and found to be cost-effective [19, 20]. The widespread availability of telecommunications technologies provides an opportunity to build a three-tier teleradiotherapy network (TRTNet) by creating primary (PRTC), secondary (SRTC), and tertiary RT centers (TRTC), thereby facilitating RT accessibility and also capacity building [16, 21–23] (figure 17.6).

Briefly, the PRTC could consist of a single TRT unit located in an existing medical center equipped with a computed tomography (CT) scanner and other basic pathological, medical, and surgical facilities. The PRTC would primarily be involved in RT treatment delivery. Treatment planning and brachytherapy applications could be carried out at the SRTC, which would be equipped with two TRT units, a CT simulator, a treatment planning system and a brachytherapy (preferably high-dose-rate) unit. The SRTC would perform treatment planning for patients referred from the PRTC, in addition to those directly attending the SRTC. The RT treatment plans could be transmitted back to the PRTC through the ICT network for teletherapy delivery. All treatments are expected to be delivered using either conventional two-dimensional or three-dimensional conformal techniques. SRTCs should be established in existing hospitals that have pathology departments, adequate medical and surgical facilities, and personnel trained in oncology. These should coordinate the activities of their associated PRTCs and provide technical support for quality assurance (QA). The tertiary RT centers could have state-of-the-art RT facilities and would be responsible for coordinating teaching and training for all the subsidiary centers within the network. If needed, patients could be referred to higher centers for specialized treatments. The tertiary centers would also be the focal points for framing national and regional guidelines to provide uniformity and quality in cancer care.

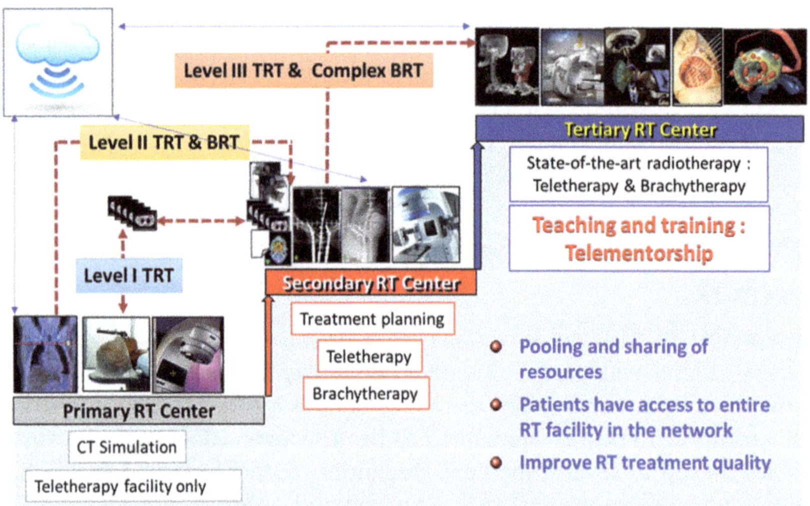

Figure 17.6. A schematic representation of a three-tier teleradiotherapy network integrating primary, secondary, and tertiary radiotherapy centers to pool and share resources, enabling patients to access the entire radiotherapy infrastructure within the network. (Reproduced [16], copyright (2020) with permission from Elsevier.)

A three-tier teleradiotherapy network would allow the pooling and sharing of resources, giving access to the entire range of radiotherapy facilities and improving the quality of radiotherapy [10, 21, 24, 25]. Furthermore, this would also be cost-effective and would prove to be economically viable and particularly feasible in countries with limited human resources. Moreover, this network could be used for patient consultations and the joint evaluation of radiotherapy treatment plans and other details related to patient treatment within the network. Moreover, the same network could be used for teaching and training between these centers by allowing online and structured training programs between the participating centers in a wider network, thus helping capacity building. The three-tier TRTNet could finally be integrated into a teleoncology network that would include telepathology, tele-radiology, telediagnostics, teleconsultation, and telefollow-up and which would also potentially be a key platform for capacity building for all those involved in cancer care.

17.6 Conclusions

The disruptions caused by the present COVID-19 pandemic have affected almost all of us in every sphere of activity worldwide. The resultant economic slowdown is expected to have a ripple effect, leading to the curtailment of many programs that will be treated as nonessential or relegated to a lower priority. While every country, irrespective of its income status, is struggling to emerge from this health and economic crisis, it also forces one to embrace new strategies to mitigate the impact of this pandemic in various fields by adopting alternative cost-effective pathways.

The IAEA has called the growing incidence of cancer in LMICs a 'silent crisis'[26]. The current situation will have a sustained dampening effect on the allocation of resources and therefore make it difficult the fulfill the SDG targets proposed by the United Nations [11]. Thus, alternative means, as discussed above, could maximize the available resource utilization. Since the creation of new RT infrastructure is a capital cost-intensive venture, it may not be accorded preference over other healthcare issues related to the COVID-19 pandemic. Under such conditions, the proposed strategies could be adopted by various RT centers in 88 LMICs to address their limited RT accessibility using their available facilities. These strategies could not only help to considerably improve the % RT accessibility, but would also reduce the need for additional TRT units. However, for the 47 LMICs with no RT infrastructure (which constitute almost one third of the LMICs), a collaborative approach needs to be undertaken by individual countries along with various national and international agencies. Given the provision of optimal cancer treatment, long-term economic gains can be envisaged. This should also motivate and encourage policymakers to adopt cost-effective pragmatic strategies to address the 'silent crisis' in LMICs in the post-COVID-19 era. Furthermore, these strategies could provide solutions to help countries to move toward meeting the targets of the UN 2030 Agenda. In particular, SDG 3, related to health and wellbeing for all, seeks, *inter alia*, to reduce the premature mortality from noncommunicable diseases (including cancer) by one third by 2030 [11]. Achieving this goal would be challenging even under normal circumstances and requires unified and determined action from all stakeholders at a national level to explore realistic and practical solutions for the maximal utilization of their existing infrastructure and human resources.

Note from the Editors:
The authors of this chapter are highly distinguished experts in the field of this topic. They have a known history of publishing in this field. Parts of the chapter are inspired by their recent article, which offered an analysis for Asia [16]:

Datta NR, Datta S, Samiei M (2020). Strategies to Maximize Available Resources With Minimum Cost Escalation for Improving Radiation Therapy Accessibility in the Post-Coronavirus Disease 2019 Era: An Analysis for Asia. *Adv. Radiat. Oncol.* 2021 Jan-Feb; 6(1):100565. doi: 10.1016/j.adro.2020.09.005. Epub 2020 Sep 24. PMID: 32995668;PMCID: PMC7513874.

However, in this chapter, the authors provide a wider view of strategies to maximize available resources with minimum cost escalation in LMICs in the world.

—Ahmed Elzawawy and Wilfred Ngwa

References

[1] World Health Organization 2020 World Cancer Report https://who.int/publications/i/item/who-report-on-cancer-setting-priorities-investing-wisely-and-providing-care-for-all

[2] Stewart B W and Wild C P World Cancer Report. 2014 https://publications.iarc.fr/Non-Series-Publications/World-Cancer-Reports/World-Cancer-Report-2014

[3] Knaul F M A-O H, Mèndez O, Alsan M, Seinfeld J, Marx A, Atun R and Akaza H 2014 *The Global Economic Burden of Cancer.* (Lyon, France: Int. Agency for Reserach on Cancer) http://publications.iarc.fr/Non-Series-Publications/World-Cancer-Reports/World-Cancer-Report-2014

[4] Int. Monetary Fund 2020 World Economic Outlook, April 2020: The Great Lockdown https://imf.org/en/Publications/WEO/Issues/2020/04/14/weo-april-2020#Introduction

[5] Rosenblatt E and Zubizarreta E 2017 *Radiotherapy in Cancer Care: Facing the Global Challenge.* (Vienna: IAEA) https://www-pub.iaea.org/books/iaeabooks/10627/Radiotherapy-in-Cancer-Care-Facing-the-Global-Challenge

[6] Datta N R, Samiei M and Bodis S 2014 Radiation therapy infrastructure and human resources in low- and middle-income countries: present status and projections for 2020 *Int. J. Radiat. Oncol. Biol. Phys.* **89** 448–57

[7] Zubizarreta E H, Fidarova E, Healy B and Rosenblatt E 2015 Need for radiotherapy in low and middle income countries—the silent crisis continues *Clin. Oncol. (R. Coll. Radiol.)* **27** 107–14

[8] Abdel-Wahab M, Fidarova E and Polo A 2017 Global access to radiotherapy in low- and middle-income countries *Clin. Oncol. (R. Coll. Radiol.)* **29** 99–104

[9] Samiei M Challenges of making radiotherapy services accessible in developing countries in cancer control 2013, global health dynamics in association with Int. Network for Cancer Treatment and Research (INCTR) http://globalhealthdynamics.co.uk/cc2013/wpcontent/uploads/2013/04/83–96-Samiei-varian-tpage-incld-T-page_2012.pdf

[10] Datta N R, Rogers S and Bodis S 2019 Challenges and opportunities to realize 'The 2030 Agenda for Sustainable Development' by the United Nations: implications for radiation

therapy infrastructure in low- and middle-income countries *Int. J. Radiat. Oncol. Biol. Phys.* **105** 918–33

[11] United Nations Transforming our world: the 2030 agenda for sustainable development A/RES/70/1 https://sustainabledevelopment.un.org/content/documents/21252030%20Agenda%20for%20Sustainable%20Development%20web.pdf

[12] The World Bank World Bank classification https://datahelpdesk.worldbank.org/knowledgebase/articles/906519-world-bank-country-and-lending-groups

[13] The World Bank World Bank for GNI/capita https://databank.worldbank.org/reports.aspx?source=2&series=NY.GNP.PCAP.CD&country=#

[14] Int. Agency for Research on Cancer Cancer Tomorrow http://gco.iarc.fr/tomorrow/graphic-isotype?type=0&population=900&mode=population&sex=0&cancer=39&age_group=value&apc_male=0&apc_female=0

[15] Int. Atomic Energy Agency DIRAC (DIrectory of RAdiotherapy Centres) https://dirac.iaea.org/Data/CountriesLight

[16] Datta N R, Datta S and Samiei M 2020 Strategies to maximize available resources with minimum cost escalation for improving radiotherapy accessibility in the post COVID-19 era: an analysis for Asia *Adv. Radiat. Oncol.* **6** 100565

[17] Datta N R, Samiei M and Bodis S 2015 Are state-sponsored new radiation therapy facilities economically viable in low- and middle-income countries? *Int. J. Radiat. Oncol. Biol. Phys.* **93** 229–40

[18] Ngwa W, Sajo E and Ngoma T *et al* 2015 Potential for information and communication technologies to catalyze global collaborations in radiation oncology *Int. J. Radiat. Oncol. Biol. Phys.* **91** 444–7

[19] Norum J, Bruland O S and Spanne O *et al* 2005 Telemedicine in radiotherapy: a study exploring remote treatment planning, supervision and economics *J. Telemed. Telecare* **11** 245–50

[20] Ngwa W N T and Zietman A *et al* 2016 Closing the cancer divide through Ubuntu: information and communication technology powered models for global radiation oncology *Int. J. Radiat. Oncol. Biol. Phys.* **94** 440–9

[21] Datta N R, Heuser M and Bodis S 2016 A roadmap and cost implications of establishing comprehensive cancer care using a teleradiotherapy network in a group of sub-Saharan African countries with no access to radiation therapy *Int. J. Radiat. Oncol. Biol. Phys.* **95** 1334–43

[22] Datta N R, Heuser M and Samiei M *et al* 2015 Teleradiotherapy network: applications and feasibility for providing cost-effective comprehensive radiotherapy care in low- and middle-income group countries for cancer patients *Telemed. J. E. Health* **21** 523–32

[23] Datta N R and Rajasekar D 2004 Improvement of radiotherapy facilities in developing countries: a three-tier system with a teleradiotherapy network *Lancet Oncol.* **5** 695–8

[24] Datta N R, Khan S, Marder D, Zwahlen D and Bodis S 2016 Radiotherapy infrastructure and human resources in Switzerland: Present status and projected computations for 2020 *Strahlenther Onkol* **192** 599–608

[25] Hazin R and Qaddoumi I 2010 Teleoncology: current and future applications for improving cancer care globally *Lancet Oncol.* **11** 204–10

[26] International Atomic Energy Agency 2006 PACT: building partnerships to stop the global cancer epidemic (Vienna: IAEA)

Chapter 18

Innovation: low-cost radiotherapy machines and novel ring-based compensator intensity-modulated radiation therapy

Eric Ford, Bishwambhar Sengupta and Kyuhak Oh

This work was presented at the Win-Win session of the The Global Health Catalyst Summit at the Dana-Farber Cancer Institute, Boston, MA, USA. Professor Eric Ford presented an innovative device to facilitate the implementation and reduce the cost of one of the advanced forms of radiotherapy delivery, namely intensity-modulated radiation therapy (IMRT). The following is a link to a video of the session: https://youtu.be/kyTTMtU2SKI.

18.1 Introduction

Radiation therapy is a key tool in the management of cancer. It is recommended for use in 75% to 90% of patients for the cancers that present most commonly in low- and middle-income countries (LMICs) [1] and it is known to be highly cost-effective for healthcare systems [2]. Some key features driving this benefit are the fact that it is non-invasive, allows for organ preservation, and has a low risk of morbidities. To fully realize this potential, however, radiation therapy capabilities must include the most advanced form of delivery, IMRT. The benefit of IMRT can be appreciated in figure 18.1, in which the IMRT plan is better able to limit the radiation dose to the parotid gland (yellow arrow, right). This results in improved salivary function (reduced xerostomia, dry mouth) which results in improved nutritional status for the patient during and after treatment. Although the benefits of radiation therapy and IMRT in particular are well-appreciated, access in LMICs is extremely limited [3]. The reasons for this include its upfront capital cost, staff availability and expertise, and the reliability of equipment [2].

With this in mind, we have undertaken a project supported by the US National Cancer Institutes (NCI, UG3 CA211310-01) to design and develop a technology for IMRT delivery that will provide high-precision therapy in a way that is lower-cost,

doi:10.1088/978-0-7503-3075-6ch18

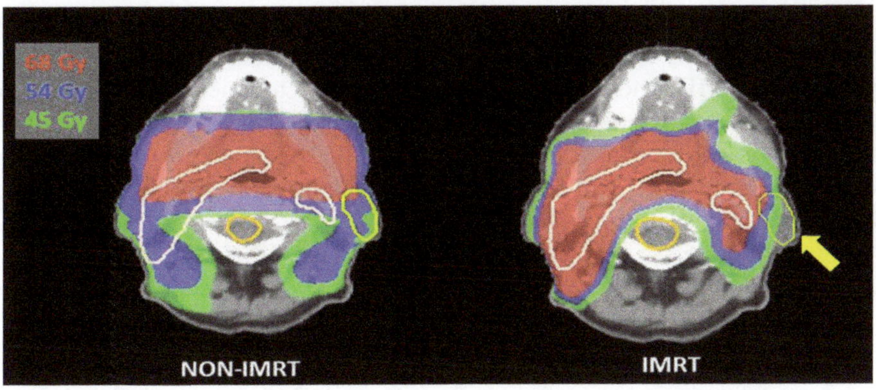

Figure 18.1. A radiation treatment plan using intensity-modulated radiation therapy IMRT (right) vs. one without IMRT (left). IMRT provides for enhanced sparing of the parotid gland (yellow arrow).

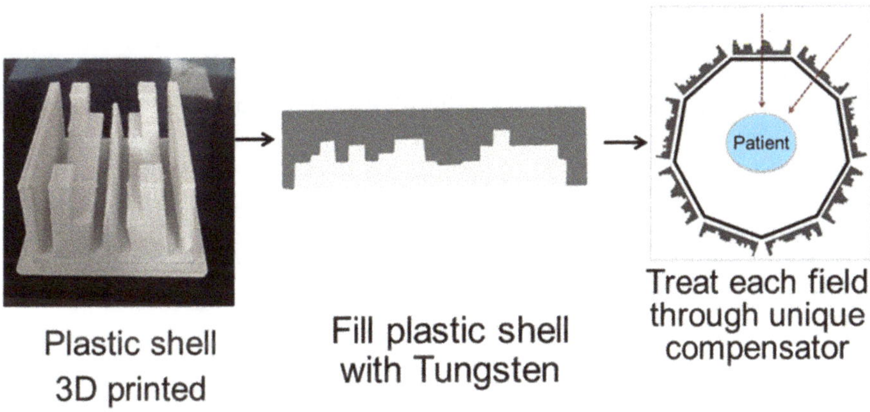

Figure 18.2. IMRT using compensators. In the system developed here, the compensator is 3D printed in plastic and then filled with metal on demand. Each treatment has a set of compensators which are unique to that patient. The materials are recyclable, which reduces cost and waste.

more efficient, simpler, and less demanding in terms of staff requirements. This is achieved by employing a physical metal compensator in the radiation beam, which sculpts the radiation dose (figure 18.2). While compensator-based IMRT is not novel [4], the key innovation here is the delivery system and the ring arrangement, which allows for automatic delivery and safety interlocks. This provides for treatment times at least ten times shorter than in previous iterations of this technology. Treatment planning studies are underway and indicate that even with the older technology of Cobalt-60 teletherapy beams, treatment times are actually shorter than those of a modern system using a linear accelerator, e.g. 7.6 ± 2.0 min vs. 3.9 ± 0.9 min [5]. In addition, the quality of the plan for the radiation treatment is not compromised. The treatment provides a similar radiation dose coverage of the target volumes, along with similar or even improved sparing of organs at risk, compared to current technology.

Further design and validation work is underway with partner sites in India. This work has also recently been coupled with the Rapid Planning Assistant (RPA) being developed at the MD Anderson Cancer Center by Dr Laurence Court and his group [6]. This will provide for automatic treatment planning, which must happen first in preparation for treatment. Together, these technologies should provide for increased access to a vital therapy, reduce costs, and provide benefit to both cancer patients and the healthcare system as whole.

An overview video is available at: https://youtu.be/_0Zq1rXg7lY [7].

References

[1] Delaney G, Jacob S, Featherstone C and Barton M. 2005 The role of radiotherapy in cancer treatment: estimating optimal utilization from a review of evidence-based clinical guidelines *Cancer* **104** 1129–37

[2] Atun R, Jaffray D A, Barton M B, Bray F, Baumann M and Vikram B *et al* 2015 Expanding global access to radiotherapy *Lancet Oncol* **16** 1153–86

[3] Abdel-Wahab M, Bourque J M, Pynda Y, Izewska J, Van der Merwe D and Zubizarreta E *et al* 2013 Status of radiotherapy resources in Africa: an International Atomic Energy Agency analysis *Lancet Oncol.* **14** e168–75

[4] Chang S X, Cullip T J, Deschesne K M, Miller E P and Rosenman J G 2004 Compensators: an alternative IMRT delivery technique *J. Appl. Clin. Med. Phys* **5** 15–36

[5] Van Schelt J, Smith D L, Fong N, Toomeh D, Sponseller P A and Brown D W *et al* 2018 A ring-based compensator IMRT system optimized for low- and middle-income countries: design and treatment planning study *Med. Phys* **45** 3275–86

[6] Kisling K, Zhang L, Simonds H, Fakie N, Yang J and McCarroll R *et al* 2019 Fully automatic treatment planning for external-beam radiation therapy of locally advanced cervical cancer: a tool for low-resource clinics *J. Global Oncol.* **5** 1–9

[7] Ford E 2019 Compensator-based IMRT

Chapter 19

Innovation: lowering the cost of image guidance in radiation therapy using low-dose megavoltage imaging-cone beam CT for accurate radiation therapy delivery

Ross Berbeco

This chapter covers a low-dose approach for accurate radiation therapy delivery presented during the Global Health Catalyst Summit (see https://youtu.be/kyTTMtU2SKI). Professor Ross Berbeco presented an innovative approach for implementing image-guided radiotherapy with reduced purchase and service costs, reduced downtime, and reduced infrastructure requirements.

Image guidance in radiation therapy can save lives and reduce toxicity. It has been demonstrated that improved treatment accuracy and precision through image guidance can improve patient outcomes [1]. High-quality (meaning effective and safe) radiation therapy depends on the accurate delivery of conformal radiation doses to patients. Knowledge of the patient's anatomy at the time of treatment is essential.

Image guidance is not consistently used or readily available in many cancer centers. Obstacles include up front capital costs, ongoing personnel and maintenance costs, education and training, and patient throughput concerns. Even an initial sizable investment in state-of-the-art equipment can be insufficient if the other aspects are not addressed. A center that has an image-guided program that is not adequately supported may end up providing less safe and/or less effective treatments as well as running the risk of extended facility downtime while waiting for service, for example.

An approach that could overcome the challenges listed would require a volumetric imaging technology that is low-cost and low-maintenance. One possible solution is to use the megavoltage (MV) therapy beam for imaging, rather than attaching a kV source and imager to the linear accelerator (LINAC) gantry. The advantages of using MV, rather than kV, imaging include reduced purchase and service costs, reduced downtime, and reduced infrastructure requirements. The additional clinical benefits of using MV imaging include improved penetration of thick anatomy, reduced beam hardening and metal artifacts, and improved Hounsfield units (HU) accuracy for adaptive radiation therapy applications.

However, there are technical challenges to be overcome to achieve high-quality, low-dose MV imaging. The inherent physics of MV photon absorption within the anatomy and within the detector are not as favorable as for kV photons. Poor efficiency in MV imaging leads to low photon counts in the detector, requiring unacceptable radiation dose levels to achieve usable, low-noise images. The interactions of higher-energy photons with the patient anatomy tend to be less dependent on the atomic number (Z) of the anatomy than those of lower-energy photons due to the smaller number of photoelectric interactions. This leads to reduced contrast, particularly for bony anatomy and implanted radiopaque fiducials.

One approach that has been explored is the use of a lower-energy treatment beam (2.5 MV) combined with a high-efficiency detector. The rationale is that the 'softer' x-ray beam should provide better anatomical contrast and improved detector absorption, which would be amplified further by the improved inherent efficiency of the detector. However, maintaining a photon energy spectrum that is higher than those of typical diagnostic x-ray sources (~150 kVp), will retain the advantages of MV imaging.

A possible method for improving detector efficiency for MV imaging is to increase the effective scintillator thickness for greater photon collection. Some strategies for this include: (1) stacking of identical layers, (2) using novel, low-cost, high-efficiency scintillation materials, and (3) stacking combinations of low-efficiency, high resolution scintillator layers with high-efficiency, low-resolution layers.

A multilayer imager (MLI) prototype has been built by combining four identical imager layers, each one equivalent to a standard, commercial single-layer imager [2]. Megavoltage imaging-cone beam computed tomography (MV-CBCT) data was acquired using the MLI at radiation dose levels equivalent to those of the kV-CBCT protocols [3]. Figure 19.1 shows a comparison between CBCT reconstructions acquired with the standard clinical kV on-board imaging (OBI) system, the standard clinical AS1200 MV imager, and the combined four layers of the MLI. The radiation dose levels were nominally equivalent for each imaging modality. The MLI significantly decreases noise, increasing the image quality and detectability of low-contrast materials, compared to MV-CBCT with the standard single-layer detector. It was further found that MV-CBCT with the MLI provided much greater HU accuracy than that of kV-CBCT, indicating that it is better suited for radiotherapy dose planning. This has important implications for cancer centers with limited resources or inconsistent access to CT simulators.

The impact of scintillator composition and thickness on MV-CBCT quality has been studied in analytical modeling studies [4, 5] and experimental measurements [6]. In general, increased photon detection efficiency leads to a decrease in noise, improving contrast and feature detection. Experiments with a novel scintillating

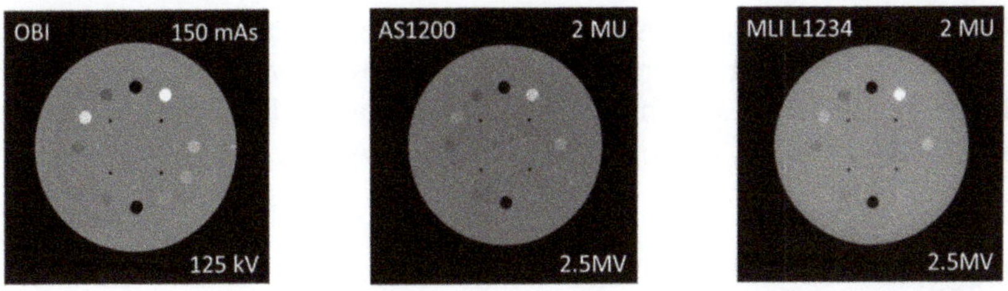

Figure 19.1. Improvements in image quality are shown for the four-layer multilayer imager (MLI). Reconstructed material insert slices are shown for (left) the standard kV on-board imager (OBI) and a 125 kVp source, (middle) the standard single-layer MV detector (AS1200) and (right) the four-layer MLI with all layers combined and 2.5 MV beam delivery. All images were acquired at nominally the same dose. Reprinted from [3], copyright (2020) American Association of Physicists in Medicine.

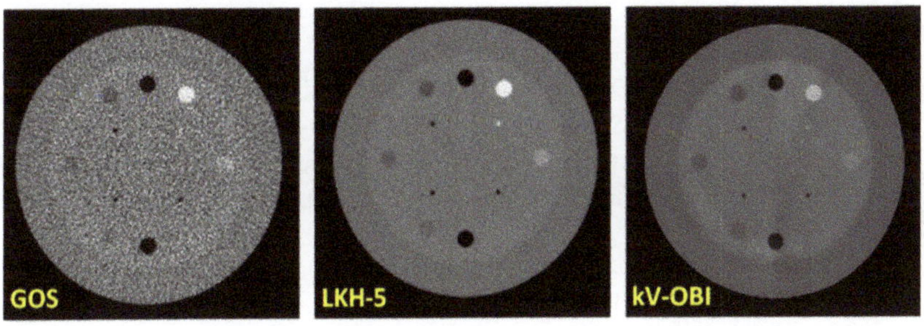

Figure 19.2. The improved noise performance of a novel scintillating glass (LKH-5) enables MV-CBCT image quality to approach that of kV-CBCT, at the same imaging dose (2.7 cGy). (left) The low detection efficiency of a standard commercial single-layer MV detector employing a thin GOS scintillator leads to high-noise MV-CBCT acquisitions, obscuring low-contrast features. (middle) Increased detector efficiency leads to a major reduction in noise relative to the standard GOS MV detector, revealing the low-contrast features. (right) kV-CBCT acquisition with a commercial OBI system is shown for comparison at the same imaging dose level. Reprinted from [6], copyright (2018) American Association of Physicists in Medicine.

glass (LKH-5) demonstrated MV-CBCT image quality approaching that of kV-CBCT imaging, for the same imaging dose (figure 19.2). It was also found that the reduced spatial resolution from thicker scintillators has a negligible effect on feature detection for radiotherapy applications. The improvements in noise performance far outweigh the reduction in resolution, providing a clear direction for further advances.

Overall, these flat-panel detector developments demonstrate that low-dose, high-quality MV-CBCT is achievable with slight modifications of currently available technology. Access to this technology will enable high-accuracy image-guided radiotherapy in low-resource environments, with reduced downtime and other costs associated with auxiliary kV x-ray imaging systems. Further advances, such as adaptive radiotherapy, which may be enabled by this new imaging have the potential to make MV-CBCT an important feature in every resource environment. Manufacturers will welcome the reduced technical overhead, cancer centers will value the reduced capital and maintenance costs, and patients and clinicians will appreciate the low-dose, high-quality imaging and therapy – win, win, win.

Author's note: The ideas presented in this chapter are based on a lecture entitled 'Low-dose MV-CBCT for accurate radiation therapy delivery' that was presented at the Global Health Catalyst Summit, Win-Win session, May 24, 2019 at the Dana-Farber Cancer Institute, Boston, MA, USA [7]. A video is available at: https://youtu.be/kyTTMtU2SKI.

Acknowledgements

The research reported in this chapter was supported, in part, by grants from Varian Medical Systems, Inc. and the National Cancer Institute of the National Institutes of Health under award number R01CA188446. The content is solely the responsibility of the authors and does not necessarily represent the official views of the National Institutes of Health.

References

[1] Bujold A, Craig T, Jaffray D and Dawson L A 2012 Image-guided radiotherapy: has it influenced patient outcomes? *Semin. Radiat. Oncol.* **22** 50–61

[2] Rottmann J, Morf D, Fueglistaller R, Zentai G, Star-Lack J and Berbeco R 2016 A novel EPID design for enhanced contrast and detective quantum efficiency *Phys. Med. Biol.* **61** 6297–306

[3] Myronakis M *et al* 2020 Low-dose megavoltage cone-beam computed tomography using a novel multi-layer imager (MLI) *Med. Phys.* **47** 1827–35

[4] Hu Y H *et al* 2018 Leveraging multi-layer imager detector design to improve low-dose performance for megavoltage cone-beam computed tomography *Phys. Med. Biol.* **63** 035022

[5] Hu Y-H *et al* 2018 Physics considerations in MV-CBCT multi-layer imager design *Phys. Med. Biol.* **63** 125016

[6] Hu Y H *et al* 2019 Characterizing a novel scintillating glass for application to megavoltage cone-beam computed tomography *Med. Phys.* **46** 1323–30

[7] Berbeco R 2019 Low-dose MV-CBCT for accurate radiation therapy delivery *Global Health Catalyst Summit, May 24–26, 2019*

IOP Publishing

Approaching Global Oncology
The win-win model
Ahmed Elzawawy and Wilfred Ngwa

Chapter 20

Smart radiotherapy biomaterials for combining radiotherapy and immunotherapy

Michele Moreau, Sayeda Yasmin-Karim, Victoria Ainsworth, Romy Mueller, Bashkim Ziberi and Wilfred Ngwa

One of the major areas of global cancer health disparity is access to radiotherapy, employed in the treatment of over 50% of cancer patients. Innovative approaches with the potential to significantly reduce the disparities in access to radiotherapy include the use of evidence-based hypofractionated radiotherapy (HFRT) and smart radiotherapy biomaterials (SRBs), which are being developed. SRBs can be employed in place of the inert radiotherapy biomaterials (fiducials and beacons) currently used. Animal studies have established that SRBs can boost both local and metastatic tumor kill when used in conjunction with HFRT. SRBs are particularly attractive, because they represent an evidence-based low-cost approach that makes immunotherapy more accessible using a smart drug delivery approach. This chapter highlights SRB technology, whose clinical translation has the potential to significantly increase access to radiotherapy and immunotherapy for both high-income country (HIC) and low- and middle-income country (LMIC) populations.

20.1 Introduction

Radiotherapy is employed in the treatment of over 50% of cancer patients, either alone, or in combination with other treatments [1]. However, pervasive disparities exist in access to radiotherapy, especially in Africa and for African American populations in the USA [2, 3]. The recent World Health Organization Cancer Report [4, 5] describes the growing global burden of cancer and disparities as alarming; over 70% of 18.1 million cases and 60% of 9.6 million deaths per year occur in LMICs. In LMICs such as those in Africa, where survival rates are amongst the lowest, the cancer burden is projected to reach an alarming 1.4 million new cases and 1 million deaths per year by 2030. The primary drivers of these disparities in incidence and deaths may underlie the higher cancer-related morbidity and mortality

doi:10.1088/978-0-7503-3075-6ch20

rates also seen among African American/immigrant populations in the USA. Innovative approaches that reduce these disparities in access to radiotherapy are crucial in addressing the growing global burden of cancer deaths and associated disparities [1].

Innovative approaches with the potential to significantly reduce disparities in access to radiotherapy include the use of evidence-based HFRT and SRBs [6, 7], which are being developed with support of the National Cancer Institute in a project titled 'Biomaterial Drones for Image-Guided Drug Delivery during radiotherapy'. SRBs may be employed in place of the inert radiotherapy biomaterials (fiducials and beacons) currently used. Preliminary studies have established that SRBs can boost both local and metastatic tumor kill when used in conjunction with HFRT [6, 8]. The major benefits of HFRT, which involves the delivery of larger doses of radiation per treatment fraction in order to complete the full course of treatment over a shorter period of time, include: [7, 9] (1) more patients may have access to treatment, since each patient can come into the clinic less often for radiotherapy, compared to conventional treatment; (2) increased patient convenience; (3) expected cost savings, given the smaller number of fractions. Hence, the use of HFRT with SRBs has great potential to increase access to radiotherapy, and successful outcomes would set the stage for USA–Africa multicentre clinical trials following the delays due to COVID-19 [10].

Figure 20.1 illustrates the mechanism [6] by which SRBs can boost the immune-mediated abscopal effect, whereby radiotherapy at one site may lead to the regression of cancer at different sites that were not treated.

This therapeutic strategy of using SRBs with one fraction of RT has been shown to consistently boost abscopal response rates across several tumor types. In particular, studies have demonstrated that these increased responses are

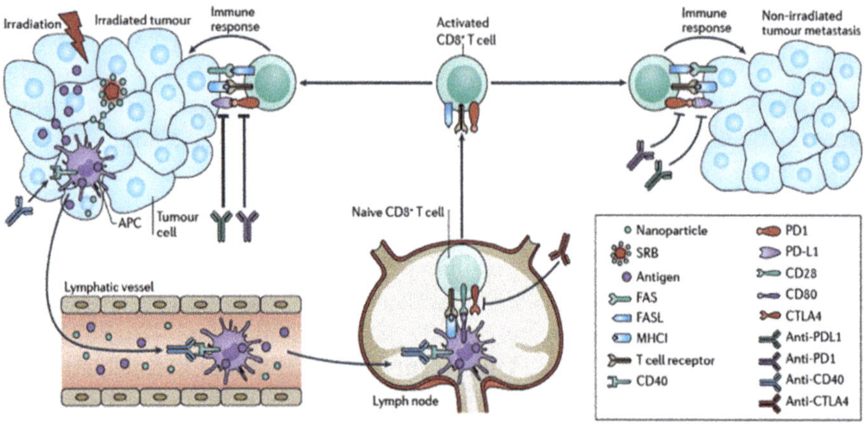

Figure 20.1. Illustration of a new approach using immunogenic SRBs incorporating anti-CD40 payloads to prime the abscopal effect. Sustained slow release of anti-CD40 directly into the tumor microenvironment is designed to boost the abscopal effect, leading to the regression of locally treated tumors and metastases. FASL, FAS ligand; MHCI = major histocompatibility complex class I. SRBs can also provide image guidance with both MRI and CT imaging contrasts. Reprinted from [6] with permission from Springer Nature.

consistent with increased infiltration of antigen-presenting cells (APCs) into the treated tumors and ultimate CD8+ T-cell infiltration into treated and untreated tumors. The use of one fraction of RT has also been shown to be more effective as a strategy for mitigating the immunosuppressive properties of RT on infiltrating APCs and T cells.

In clinical practice, fiducials are currently inserted into a target lesion to act as internal landmarks that enable real-time lesion tracking. Current commercially available fiducial markers come in various shapes and sizes and can be made of gold, titanium, carbon, platinum, or polymer. Fiducial markers serve as reference points for image-guided radiotherapy (IGRT). The visualization of fiducials allows high doses of radiation to be delivered with increased accuracy, limiting exposure of the surrounding healthy tissue.

Most patients in LMICs are diagnosed with metastatic disease. HFRT has already been shown to be an effective approach to reducing treatment times and costs for cancers such as breast and prostate cancers. Additional innovations are needed for patients with metastatic disease, whose prognosis is often poor. In immunotherapy, immune-checkpoint therapy has not, so far, been successful in patients or accessible to many patients due to dose-limiting toxicities, limited eligibility, and costs. Given the poor response to conventional chemotherapy, there is also a need to develop new effective treatment options. SRBs offer a safe approach being developed for use with HFRT to boost the abscopal effect, which causes regression of both local and distant metastatic tumors.

Studies using SRBs show:

1. A robust abscopal effect that causes the regression of both treated (local) and untreated (metastatic) tumors and the prevention of metastasis [6, 11–14]
2. A major statistically significant increase in survival in different tumor models [4–6]
3. Increased infiltration of APCs and T cells, corroborating the abscopal mechanism of action. [4–6]

The use of SRBs for the *in situ* delivery of immunoadjuvants reduces doses substantially, hence causing minimal toxicities shown to be safe in animal studies [15]. The constituents of SRBs include PLGA (a Food and Drug Administration (FDA) approved polymer and nanoparticles). Our results in animals using SRBs with and without one fraction of radiotherapy have resulted in no safety concerns; the surviving animals remain healthy for over 200 days until they are sacrificed [16–18]. The work is now in clinical translation, and multicenter clinical trials are planned to begin in 2021.

20.1.1 Implementation in LMICs

HFRT presents an excellent opportunity for investment in LMICs where radiation therapy occupies a substantial proportion of health expenditure. Work by the Global Task Force for Radiotherapy estimated that the nominal cost of scaling up radiotherapy for demand between 2015–35 is US$26·6 billion in low-income countries, $62·6 billion in lower-middle-income countries, and $94·8 billion in upper-middle-income countries, which amounts to $184·0 billion across all LMICs [1]. The implementation of the SRB approach with HFRT is an exciting opportunity to minimize this cost and increase RT access for cancer management through the adoption of a single fraction or a few fractions of radiotherapy as the new prescription standard. A number of studies in the developed world have already shown the potential to minimize the cost per patient in the delivery of both breast and prostate RT [19–22]. A recent study has demonstrated major savings for American and African healthcare systems [23]. The potential impact of expanding global radiotherapy access has become pertinent, considering that lower fraction schemes and doses also offer equivalent local control, a superior toxicity profile, and noninferior late effects compared to a conventional prescription. The SRB and HFRT approaches also realize other goals of high-quality care, including patient centeredness, timeliness, efficiency, and equity [24, 25].

Innovations such as SRBs, which lead to the efficacy and safety of moderate hypofractionation scheme delivery will make RT affordable to millions. At the moment, studies have reported a low incidence of side-effects for extreme fractionation (less than five fractions) [26] and single fractionation has been demonstrated in small clinical studies for localized prostate cancer using high dose rate (HDR) brachytherapy. Single-fraction prostate external beam radiotherapy can be planned with stereotactic approach while respecting HDR brachytherapy constraints and can possibly be planned and delivered in a single day [27]. Single-fraction RT delivered pre- and intra-operatively have also shown some feasibility for selected breast cancer patients [27–30]. SRBs can serve as next-generation fiducial markers, brachytherapy spacers, and balloon applicators, designed to respond to stimulus and perform additional desirable functions such as the controlled delivery of immunoadjuvants directly into the tumor subvolume, while minimizing normal tissue toxicities [31]. SRBs are cheap and can be used with a single fraction [32].

Figure 20.2 highlights the survival advantage when SRBs are used to deliver immunotherapy anti-CD40. Nanoparticles from the SRBs can provide image guidance, but also amplify damage to tumor cells to further enhance therapeutic efficacy. The rate of release of SRBs may be customized as a function of different parameters, including polymer weight, the pH value of the tumor microenvironment, or the irradiation dose, depending on the type of sensitivity of the smart polymer used to develop the SRB. The approach can also be used for radio-immunotherapy dose-painting, which allows for sustained boosting of the tumor subvolume, including those that are hypoxic and resistant to treatment. SRB polymer components can make the tumor more immunogenic using immunotherapy released by the SRB to prime a robust abscopal response, causing regression of both locally treated and distant untreated tumors. Clinical trials for this approach are currently at the FDA stage; they are expected to begin in 2021 and to involve leading cancer centres in the USA and Africa.

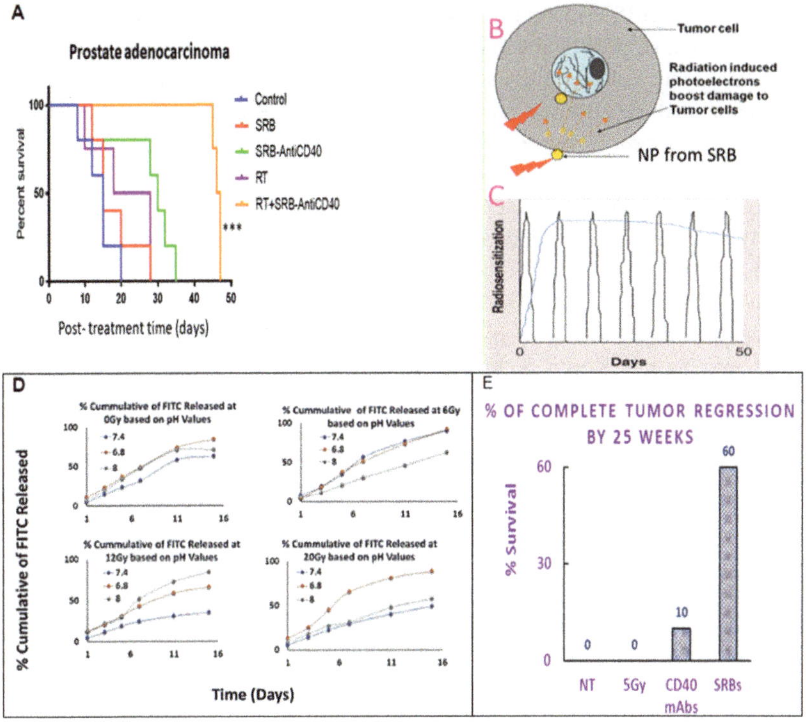

Figure 20.2. (a) Kaplan Meier survival assay for in-animal studies showing an increased duration of survival when treated with SRBs delivering the immunotherapy anti-CD40. (b) Nanoparticles (NPs) in SRBs can enhance the damage caused to tumor cells via the photoelectric effect. (c) Sustained delivery of the immunotherapy/NPs is a significant advantage, as opposed to repeated injections over time. (d) The release profile can be modulated as a function of pH or radiotherapy dose. (e) The use of SRBs can cause complete regression of local and metastatic tumors. Reprinted from [24], copyright (2020) by The American Society of Clinical Oncology.

References

[1] Atun R *et al* 2015 Expanding global access to radiotherapy *Lancet Oncol.* **16** 1153–86

[2] McClelland S *et al* 2017 The pervasive crisis of diminishing radiation therapy access for vulnerable populations in the United States, part 1: African-American patients *Adv. Radiat. Oncol.* **2** 523–31

[3] Ngwa W *et al* 2016 Closing the cancer divide through ubuntu: information and communication technology-powered models for global radiation oncology *Int. J. Radiat. Oncol. Biol. Phys.* **94** 440–9

[4] World Health Organization 2020 *WHO Report on Cancer: Setting Priorities, Investing Wisely and Providing Care for All*

[5] Stewart B W and Wild C P 2014 *World cancer report 2014* WHO https://publications.iarc.fr/Non-Series-Publications/World-Cancer-Reports/World-Cancer-Report-2014

[6] Ngwa W *et al* 2018 Using immunotherapy to boost the abscopal effect *Nat. Rev. Cancer* **18** 313–22

[7] Irabor O C *et al* 2020 Can the adoption of hypofractionation guidelines expand global radiotherapy access? An analysis for breast and prostate radiotherapy *J. Glob. Oncol* **6** 667–78

[8] Moreau M *et al* 2018 Priming the abscopal effect using multifunctional smart radiotherapy biomaterials loaded with immunoadjuvants *Front. Oncol.* **8** 56
[9] Haque W, Verma V, Butler E B and Teh B S 2018 Trends and disparities in the utilization of hypofractionated neoadjuvant radiation therapy for rectal cancer in the United States *J. Gastrointest. Oncol.* **9** 601–9
[10] Ngwa W *et al* 2017 Potential role of the quality assurance review center platform in global radiation oncology *Int. J. Radiat. Oncol.* **99** 956–62
[11] Ngwa W *et al* 2018 Using immunotherapy to boost the abscopal effect *Nat. Rev. Cancer* **18** 313–22
[12] Yasmin-Karim S *et al* 2018 Radiation and local anti-CD40 generate an effective *in situ* vaccine in preclinical models of pancreatic cancer *Front. Immunol.* **9** 2030
[13] Moreau M, Yasmin-Karim S, Kumar R, Irabor O C and Ngwa W 2018 Priming the abscopal effect using multifunctional smart radiotherapy biomaterials loaded with immunoadjuvants *Front. Oncol.* **8** 56
[14] Yasmin-Karim S, Moreau M and Ngwa W 2018 Radiotherapy with no margins *AAPM2018* https://w3.aapm.org/meetings/2018AM/programInfo/programAbs.php?sid=7524&aid=41424
[15] Wood J, Yasmin-Karim S, Mueller R, Viswanathan A N and Ngwa W 2020 Single radiotherapy fraction with local anti-CD40 therapy generates effective abscopal responses in mouse models of cervical cancer *Cancers* **12** 1026
[16] Li D K and Wang W 2020 Characteristics and clinical trial results of agonistic anti-CD40 antibodies in the treatment of malignancies (Review) *Oncol. Lett.* **20** 176
[17] Ngwa W *et al* 2017 Smart radiation therapy biomaterials *Int. J. Radiat. Oncol. Biol. Phys.* **97** 624–37
[18] Krucińska I *et al* 2017 Biological properties of low-toxicity PLGA and PLGA/PHB fibrous nanocomposite implants for osseous tissue regeneration. Part I: evaluation of potential biotoxicity *Molecules* **22** 2092
[19] Knorr D A, Dahan R and Ravetch J V 2018 Toxicity of an Fc-engineered anti-CD40 antibody is abrogated by intratumoral injection and results in durable antitumor immunity *Proc. Natl. Acad. Sci. USA* **115** 11048–53
[20] Hunter D, Mauldon E and Anderson N 2018 Cost-containment in hypofractionated radiation therapy: a literature review *J. Med. Radiat. Sci.* **65** 148–57
[21] Lievens Y 2010 Hypofractionated breast radiotherapy: financial and economic consequences *The breast* **19** 192–7
[22] Mortimer J W *et al* 2016 Use of hypofractionated post-mastectomy radiotherapy reduces health costs by over $2000 per patient: an Australian perspective *J. Med. Imaging Radiat. Oncol.* **60** 146–53
[23] Voong K R *et al* 2017 Long-term economic value of hypofractionated prostate radiation: Secondary analysis of a randomized trial *Adv. Radiat. Oncol.* **2** 249–58
[24] Irabor O C *et al* 2020 Can the adoption of hypofractionation guidelines expand global radiotherapy access? An analysis for breast and prostate radiotherapy *JCO Glob. Oncol.* **6** 667–78
[25] Gupta A, Ohri N and Haffty B G 2018 Hypofractionated whole breast irradiation is cost-effective-but is that enough to change practice? *Transl. Cancer Res.* **7** S469–72
[26] Porter M E 2010 What is value in health care? *N. Engl. J. Med.* **363** 2477–81
[27] Widmark A *et al* 2016 Extreme hypofractionation versus conventionally fractionated radiotherapy for intermediate risk prostate cancer: early toxicity results from the scandinavian randomized phase III Trial 'HYPO-RT-PC *Int. J. Radiat. Oncol.* **96** 938–9

[28] Henderson D, Tree A and van As N 2017 Single fraction external beam radiotherapy for localised prostate cancer: a planning study *Clin. Oncol.* **29** e87

[29] Blitzblau R C *et al* 2015 A phase 1 trial of preoperative partial breast radiation therapy: Patient selection, target delineation, and dose delivery *Pract. Radiat. Oncol.* **5** e513–20

[30] Horton J K *et al* 2015 Preoperative single-fraction partial breast radiation therapy: a novel phase 1, dose-escalation protocol with radiation response biomarkers *Int. J. Radiat. Oncol.* **92** 846–55

[31] Charaghvandi R K *et al* 2017 Treatment constraints for single dose external beam preoperative partial breast irradiation in early-stage breast cancer *Clin. Transl. Radiat. Oncol.* **6** 7–14

[32] Ngwa W *et al* 2017 Smart radiation therapy biomaterials *Int. J. Radiat. Oncol.* **97** 624–37

Chapter 21

Improving access to radiotherapy in LMICs through a collaborative initiative to reduce technology downtime

Taofeeq A Ige, Alexander Jenkins, Manjit Dosanjh, Donna O'Brien, David Pistenmaa and C Norman Coleman

This chapter covers approaches that aim to increase access to radiotherapy care in Africa by reducing machine downtime. It includes a survey design covering this issue across Africa.

Survey respondents listed alphabetically by country
Saad Khoudri, Ismail Zergoug, **Algeria**
Higidio Miezi Eduardo, **Angola**
Surbhi Grover, Remigio Makufa, Memory Nasingo, **Botswana**
Anne Marthe Maison Mayeh, Samba Richard Ndi, Apolinaire Ngnah, **Cameroon**
Tofangui Alain Ouattara, **Cote D'Ivoire**
Khaled El-Shahat, Ehab Attalla, Nashaat Deiab, **Egypt**
Eskadmas Yinesu Belay, **Ethiopia**
Rolland Kayende, **Gabon**
George Felix Acquah, Eric Addison, Emmanuel Amankwaa-Frempong, Hubert Foy, Francis Hasford, **Ghana**
Ejidio Ngigi, **Kenya**
Fadwa Badi, Fairoze El Tashani, Ihab Elburi, **Libya**
Tovo Harivony, Jean Norbert Randriamarolahy, **Madagascar**
Aphousalle Kone, Siaka Maiga, Drissa Samake, **Mali**
Moussa Cheibetta, Ahmedou Tolba, **Mauritania**
Seeven Mootoosamy, **Mauritius**
Salwa El-Boutayeb, **Morocco**
Ainadine Momade, **Mozambique**
Melanie Grobler, Wilfred Midzi, **Namibia**
Simeon Chinedu Aruah, Hassan Ibrahim, Kenneth Nwankwo, **Nigeria**

doi:10.1088/978-0-7503-3075-6ch21

Joel Kra, Pacifique Mugenzi, **Rwanda**
Magatte Diagne, **Senegal**
Graeme Lazarus, Ayron Rule, Chris Trauernicht, **South Africa**
Fawzia Elbashir, Nadir Abd Ellatif Ali, **Sudan**
Hellen Makwani, Shaid Yusufu, **Tanzania**
Leila Farhat, Mounir Besbes, **Tunisia**
Kavuma Awusi, **Uganda**
Mutule Mulape Kanduza, Barbara Mule, Nasangu Augustine Mwale, **Zambia**
Godfrey Azangwe, Lawrence Mhatiwa, Edwin Mhukayesango, **Zimbabwe**

Respondents from outside of Africa
Rebecca Wong, Stephen Breen, Gordon Chan, Daniel Letourneau, Ivan Yeung, **Canada**
Jamal Khadar, **Jordan**
Jacques Bernier, Shelley Bulling, Oscar Matzinger, **Switzerland**
Ajay Aggarwal, Richard Hugtenburg, Michael Pearson, Winston Swaby, Natalie Thorp, Frank van den Heuvel, **UK**
Harmar Brereton, Marvin Glass, Eric Klein, Daniel Petereit, Chris Peters, Scot Remick, Stephen Ryan, David Wazer, **USA**
Deepa Angal-Kalinin, Graeme Burt, David Cheneler, Trevor Hartnett, Peter McIntosh, Boris Militsyn, Suzanne Sheehy, Innovative Technologies towards building Affordable and equitable global Radiotherapy (ITAR) Project, Lancaster University, **UK**

21.1 Introduction

Effectively solving complex cancer care problems in resource-constrained settings requires an understanding of the issues and the formation of trusted partnerships with those who experience them.

In recognition of the extreme shortfall of radiotherapy (RT) capacity in low- and middle-income countries (LMICs), especially in Sub-Saharan Africa, the International Cancer Expert Corps (ICEC) sponsored and the European Organization for Nuclear Research (CERN) hosted a workshop at CERN in November 2016 to define the design characteristics of an affordable, robust, and high-quality novel medical linear accelerator (LINAC) as part of a sophisticated RT system that will function more reliably in challenging environments and also require fewer specialists to plan radiation treatments, to deliver the treatments, and to service and repair the RT system [1]. In this and subsequent workshops supported by the UK Science and Technology Facilities Council (STFC), which had extensive participation by representatives from LMIC countries, the LMIC representatives enumerated time after time that frequent equipment failures, maintenance and service shortcomings, a lack of well-trained key personnel, as well as country-specific healthcare challenges severely impacted their ability to treat cancer patients using LINACs.

It was determined that the current LINAC prototype design process requires finer detailed information from a broad representation of LMICs regarding the obstacles to providing treatment with LINACs. Fortunately, through this experience, true partnerships have now been formed with several of the LMIC representatives who were able to attend the workshops at CERN, in the UK, and in Botswana. In turn, they were able to develop a collaboration among leaders of RT facilities in all 28 African countries that offer LINAC-based RT. This chapter presents the rationale for team building to derive baseline data and the questionnaire created with the input of facilities in these 28 African countries for comparison with data from Jordan and selected high-income countries (HICs).

21.2 The problem being addressed

Globally, cancer is the second most prevalent cause of death among non-communicable diseases (NCDs) [2]. It is estimated that the annual global cancer incidence will rise from 17 million cases in 2018 to as many as 27.5 million cases in 2040 [3]. About 65 to 70% of this increase will occur in LMICs, where cancer is a major cause of morbidity and mortality [4]. As expected, the negative economic impact is greater and is especially problematic for these countries as a result of premature deaths and the loss of years of productivity [5–7]. Because RT has a role in the cure or palliation of over 50% of patients with cancer, Abdel-Wahab *et al*, Barton *et al*, Zubizarreta *et al*, and Atun *et al* [8–11] argue that RT is a critical and cost-effective component of a comprehensive cancer control plan. The importance of making RT available is emphasized further in the 2015 Global Taskforce on Radiotherapy for Cancer Control (GTFRCC) report, which highlighted the health, societal, and economic benefits of increasing the capacity for RT treatment by 25% before 2025 [11]. Since many LMICs have inadequate or no RT centres, it is projected that to meet the RT demand in LMICs over the next two to three decades, there will be a need for around 5000 additional RT machines in Africa [11]. While many LMICs provide RT using cobalt-60 machines, LINACs can provide better state-of-the-art treatment without the environmental and potential terrorist risks that arise due to the radioactive sources in cobalt-60 machines [12]. The 66th United Nations General Assembly and the UN Sustainable Development Goals (SDG) have emphasized addressing the burden of NCDs, among which, cancer ranks as the second highest [13].

Unfortunately, there is a severe shortfall in RT capacity in LMICs, especially in sub-Saharan Africa [14]. Based on the IAEA recommendation of one RT machine per 200 000 in the population, the shortfall for each country in Africa that has cobalt-60 and/or LINAC technology for patient treatment is shown in table 21.1, which is derived from data provided by the International Atomic Energy Agency [14]. The table does not include the 27 countries that have neither a cobalt-60 machine nor a LINAC.

21.3 Methodology

The ICEC sponsored and CERN hosted a workshop in 2016, which was the first key action step in defining the design characteristics of an affordable and high-quality novel medical LINAC as part of a sophisticated RT system that will function more reliably in challenging environments and also require fewer specialists to plan radiation treatments, deliver the treatments, and service and repair the RT system [1]. A multidisciplinary team of international experts

Table 21.1. Radiation therapy treatment capacity in Africa compared to selected HICs and a middle-income country (countries are listed from most RT units per person and the best access to the fewest RT units per person for the poorest access) [14].

Country	Pop. in millions	People per machine	RT units in use	RT units needed[1]	RT Capacity (%)
USA	331	8700	3827	1655	231.2
Switzerland	8.6	119,000	72	43	167.4
Canada	37.6	132,400	284	197	144.2
UK	67.9	195,000	348	340	102.4
Jordan	9.9	762,000	12	50	26.0
African countries with LINACs					
Mauritius	1.27	423,000	3	6	50.0
Tunisia	11.7	509,000	23	58	39.7
S. Africa	59	608,000	97	295	32.9
Egypt	102	857,000	119	510	23.3
Morocco	36.9	880,000	42	184	22.8
Gabon	2.2	1.1M	2	11	18.2
Libya	6.9	1.15M	6	34	17.6
Algeria	43.8	1.18M	37	219	16.9
Namibia	2.5	1.25M	2	12	16.7
Zimbabwe	14.8	2.1M	7	74	9.5
Botswana	2.3	2.3M	1	11	9.1
Mauritania	4.6	2.3M	2	23	8.7
Kenya	53.8	4.89M	11	269	4.1
Rwanda	10.5	5.25M	2	52	3.8
Senegal	16.3	5.43M	3	81	3.7
Sudan	43.9	5.49M	8	219	3.7
Zambia	17.9	6M	3	89	3.4
Ghana	31.0	7.75M	4	155	2.6
Angola	32.9	11M	3	164	1.8
Tanzania	59.7	11.9M	5	298	1.7
Cote d'Ivoire	26.4	13.2M	2	132	1.5
Madagascar	27.7	13.85	2	138	1.4
Mali	20.2	20.2M	1	101	1.0
Nigeria	206	29.4M	7	1027	0.7
Cameroon	26.5	26.5M	1	132	0.8
Mozambique	31.2	31.2M	1	156	0.6
Uganda	45.7	45.7M	1	228	0.4
Ethiopia	115	115M	1	575	0.2

[1] (IAEA standard is one RT machine per 200 000 in the population)

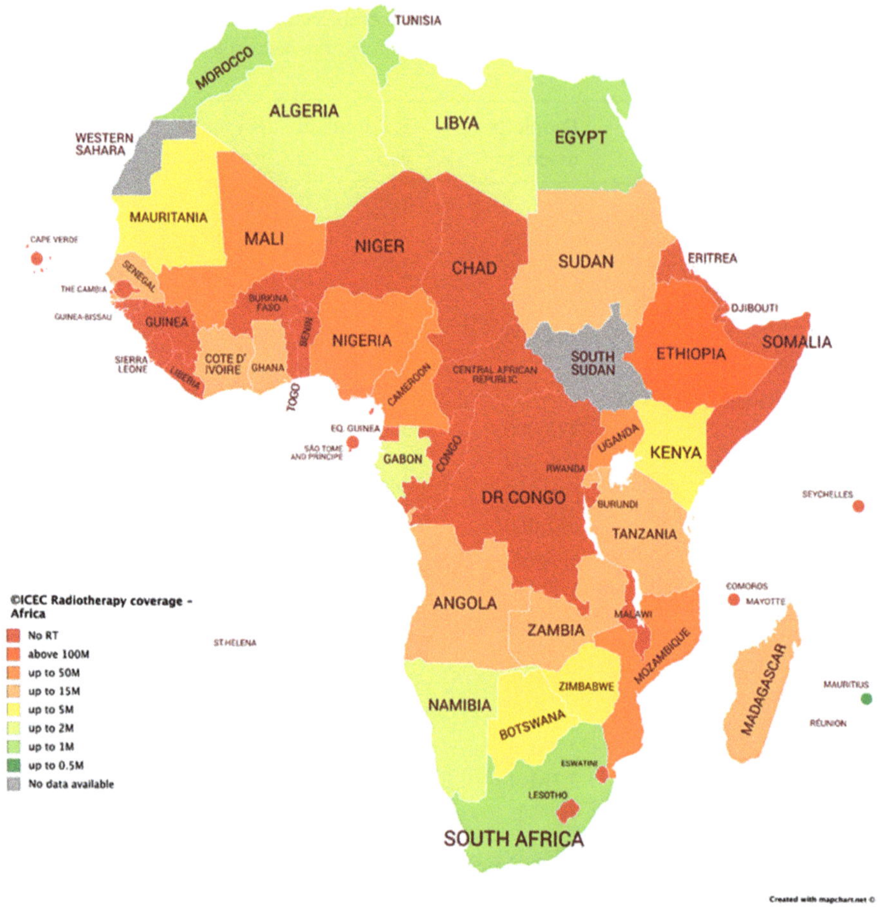

Figure 21.1. is a graphic representation of the data in table 21.1. It shows the variation in RT capacity across Africa, which is especially pronounced in the sub-Saharan region. Figure was prepared with mapchart.net (https://mapchart.net/) by Manjit Dosanjh for ICEC.

participated in the workshop, including accelerator physicists, medical physicists, clinical and radiation oncologists, engineers, policymakers, public health and healthcare systems experts, and representatives from industry. Representatives from LMICs, especially from Africa, participated extensively in a second workshop at CERN in 2017 and additional workshops in the UK and Botswana, partially supported by the UK STFC [15–17]. A review of data from a survey undertaken in 2018 that analyzed the equipment maintenance logs of LINACs in three locations in three countries [18] and discussions at a technical design workshop hosted by ICEC in Washington DC in 2019 showed that there was an absolute need for detailed information from a much larger representation of LMICs describing RT equipment failures, maintenance and service shortcomings, the availability of key personnel and their training, and country-specific healthcare challenges.

The critical team building, the acquisition of baseline data, and the preparation of the questionnaire presented herein are a *sine qua non* for progress. These are now being undertaken through an ITAR grant awarded in 2020 [19, 20].

The informative discussions and consensus building with this critical on-the-ground team at the workshops identified relevant information to be obtained to define design parameters for the LINAC prototype [21]. Among the important questions were:

- Because GNP per capita is generally associated with the extent of healthcare infrastructure and investment [22–24], to what extent is GNP per capita associated with the number of machines available in each country and with LINAC downtime?
- Which environmental factors in LMICs and HICs are most commonly associated with LINAC downtime?
- Which system or subsystem failures are most frequently associated with LINAC downtime (radiation production, power consumption, heat dissipation, automated maintenance, electromechanical collimation, or safety)?
- To what extent is the model and age of the LINAC associated with LINAC downtime?
- To what extent is the method of service and maintenance support associated with LINAC downtime?
- To what extent is training of staff provided?
- To what extent are these associations consistent across LMICs and UICs?

Table 21.2 provides a summary of the information sought from the facilities participating in the survey.

Table 21.2. Survey question categories.

Focus areas	Selected questions
Model	What manufacturer and model? Year of installation?
	What number of treatments is performed per year on each machine?
Environment	What is the temperature and humidity in the area?
	What is the speed and availability of the internet connection?
	How reliable is the electricity supply?
	What is the floor area and ceiling height of the shielded area?
	What photon energy is your shielded area able to safely operate at?
Services	Do you have a service contract? Who provides it? What is the annual cost?
	How often does the machine have maintenance/tuning/calibration?
	What types of failure can you repair locally?
	How many staff are available for in-house repairs? Are staff formally trained?
Sub-systems	How do you identify machine faults? Is it easy?
	Do you have problems with the vacuum system? How often?
	Do you have problems with the vacuum pump? Do you keep spares? Can you repair locally?

	Do you keep spare radio frequency (RF) sources? Can you repair locally?
	Do you have problems with the multileaf collimator? Do you keep spares? Can you repair locally?
	Do you have problems with the electron gun? Do you keep spares? Can you repair locally?
	How much downtime do you experience?
	Do you have any software problems?
Treatment and imaging	Does your hospital have diagnostic computed tomography (CT) near the radiotherapy area?
	Do you use a tilting couch? How important is this feature?
	How important is it for a LINAC to offer electron treatment mode?
	What manufacturer and model? Year of installation?

Because understanding how these environmental and infrastructure conditions in LMICs affect the performance of medical LINAC technology compared to LINAC performance in HICs, the study was expanded to include Jordan as an MIC as well as HIC facilities in Canada, Switzerland, the UK, and the US. In addition to providing input for the technology design, this study will provide information to management and health policy officials on the potential to mitigate some of the factors that affect LINAC downtime. Given the resource limitations in LMICs, the way in which machines are staffed may provide ideas for less expensive staffing models for HICs, a key feature of 'reverse innovation' [25].

21.4 Results

First and foremost, those of us who aim to improve cancer care in LMICs recognize the challenge of obtaining data to address the issues and metrics by which to assess progress and change course. The 'human factor and dedication' are keys to success. The great energy and persistence on the part of co-authors MD and TI enabled responses to be obtained from institutions representing all 28 of the countries in Africa that provide LINAC-based RT services shown in the map of Africa in figure 21.2. The size of this group of countries, the range of their locations, the variation in resource levels, their cancer incidence and mortality, and their healthcare infrastructure provide important inputs that inform a systems solution for a new robust RT system. The inclusion of selected facilities in an MIC and HICs help in determining which of the factors that affect downtime are more universal and the effectiveness of strategies to mitigate them, ensuring greater access for patients.

In figure 21.3, cancer mortality statistics for each county that responded to the survey are compared to their GNP per capita as an example of the effect of variations in resource levels across the countries in the study [26–28]. Using the metric of GNP per capita, the cancer mortality appears to be grouped such that predominantly Northern African countries are separated from Southern and sub-Saharan countries in figure 21.3 and table 21.1.

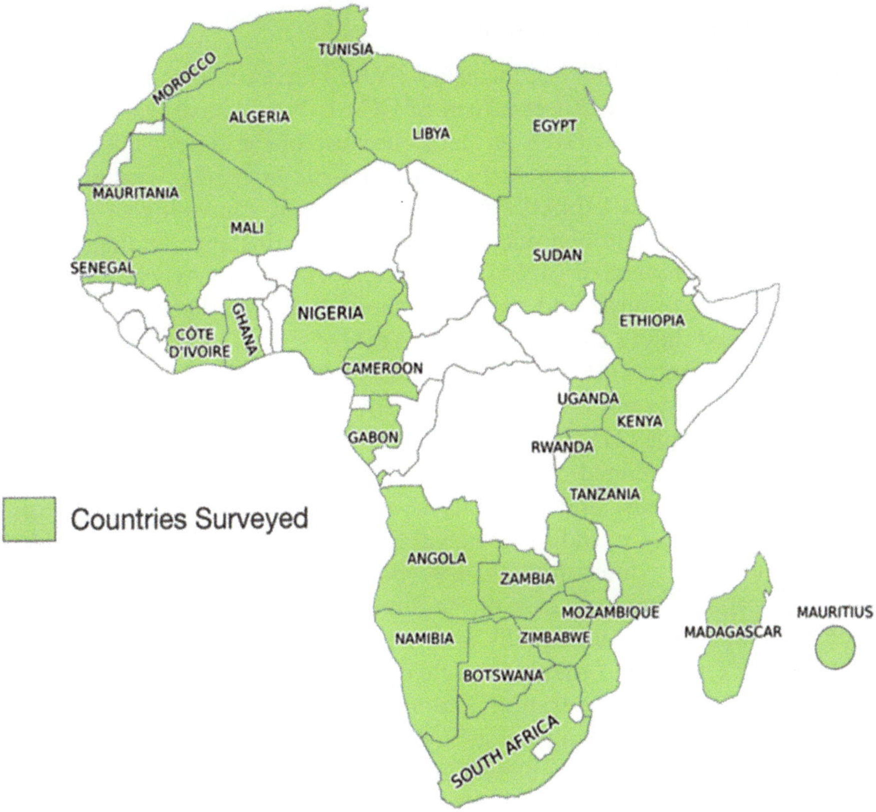

Figure 21.2. Map showing African countries that responded to the survey. Figure was prepared with mapchart.net (https://mapchart.net/) by Manjit Dosanjh for ICEC.

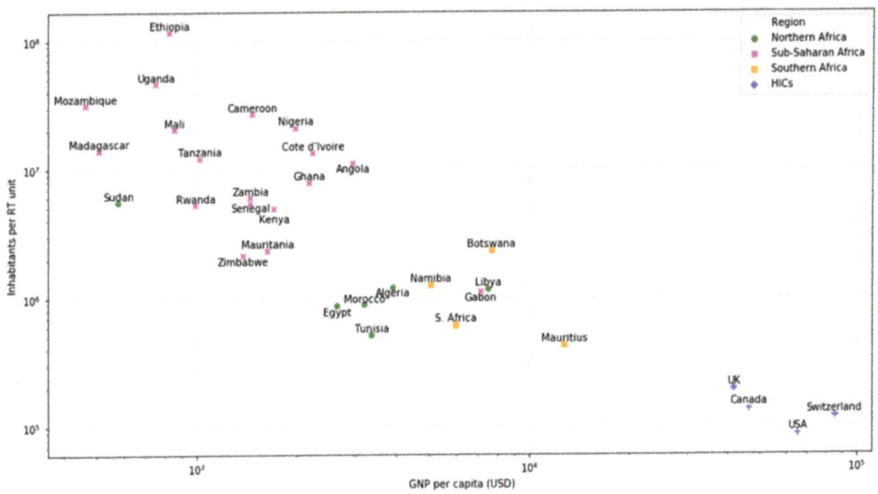

Figure 21.3. Inhabitants per RT unit as a function of GNP per capita.

21.5 Discussion and conclusions

The shortfall in the availability of medical LINACs has been recognized as a major barrier to providing quality cancer care in LMICs. LINACs have greater downtimes in LMICs in Africa than in HICs primarily because of the time it takes to acquire spare parts and the lack of adequately trained on-site or readily available LINAC engineers. It appears that LINAC components in LMICs have higher failure rates than similar components in high-income countries. For instance, in their study that compared the performance of LINACs in the UK with 5 LINACs in Nigeria and 1 LINAC in Botswana, Wroe and associates showed that the vacuum system failed only in LMICs and that in LMICs, the failure rate of six out of twelve other LINAC sub-systems was twice the rate experienced in HICs [18]. In the preliminary review of our survey, vacuum system failures in harsh environments appear to be associated with LINAC downtime [21].

The data being obtained will allow us to move beyond speculating about solutions, such as the ease and reliability of operation, machine self-diagnosis and a prominent display of impending or actual faults, ease of maintenance and repair, insensitivity to power interruptions, low power requirements (and consequent reduced heat production), and ease of modular upgrading. In addition to targeting technological innovations, an equally important aim will be intelligent software for the rest of the RT system to enable the delivery of sophisticated RT treatments with fewer on-site experts for operation and maintenance, especially highly trained personnel such as medical physicists, who are often lacking in LMICs. The comparative data from HICs enables an analysis of whether the absence of resources or environmental factors, or both, most often affect LINAC performance.

In conclusion, the substantial diligence required to build trusted partnerships to obtain the desired critical data cannot be overemphasized. With the data, not only can problems be identified, but solutions may emerge that fall within the concept of 'reverse innovation' [25]. The survey data is literally expected to provide a map with which the shortfall in cancer care can be understood. We have now taken the critical first few steps by which to propose solutions to this dire shortage of cancer care in LMICs.

References

[1] Pistenmaa D A, Dosanjh M and Amaldi U *et al* 2018 Changing the global radiation therapy paradigm *Radiother. Oncol.* **128** 393–9

[2] Hunter D J and Reddy K S 2013 Non-communicable disease *N. Eng. J. Med.* **397** 1336–43

[3] www.cancerresearchuk.org

[4] Global cancer statistics 2018 GLOBOCAN estimates of incidence and mortality worldwide for 36 cancers in 185 countries

[5] Torre L A, Seigel R L and Ward E M *et al* 2016 Global cancer incidence and mortality rates and trends—an update *Cancer Epidemiol. Biomarkers Prev.* **25** 16–27

[6] Sankaranarayanan R 2014 Screening for cancer in low- and middle-income countries *Ann. Glob. Health* **80** 412–7

[7] Plummer M, de Martle C and Vignat J *et al* 2016 Global burden of cancer attributable to infection in 2012: a synthetic analysis *Lancet Glob. Health* **4** e609–16

[8] Abdel-Wahab M, Bourque J-M and Pynda Y *et al* 2013 Status of radiotherapy resources in Africa: An International Energy Agency analysis *Lancet Oncol.* **4** 168–75
[9] Barton M and Jacob S *et al* 2014 Estimating the demand for radiotherapy from the evidence: a review of changes from 2003 to 2012 *Radiother. Oncol.* **112** 140–4
[10] Zubizarreta E, Van Dyk J and Lievens Y 2017 Analysis of global radiotherapy needs and costs by geographic region and income level *Clin. Oncol.* **29** 84e92
[11] Atun R *et al* 2015 Expanding global access to radiotherapy *Lancet Oncol.* **16** 1153–86
[12] Pomper M, Dalnoki-Veress F and Moore G 2016 Treatment, not terror: strategies to enhance external beam therapy in developing countries while permanently reducing the risk of radiological terrorism http://stanleyfoundation.org/publications/report/TreatmentNotTerror212.pdf
[13] United Nations General Assembly. 66th Session. Preservation and control of non-communicable diseases. Report by the Secretary-General A/66/83
[14] https://dirac.iaea.org/Data/CountriesLight
[15] Dosanjh M, Aggarwal A and Pistenmaa D *et al* 2019 Developing innovative, robust and affordable medical linear accelerators for challenging environments *Clin. Oncol.* **31** 352–5
[16] Innovative, robust and affordable medical linear accelerators for challenging environments https://indico.cern.ch/event/661597/overview
[17] Accelerating the future: designing a robust and affordable radiation therapy treatment system for challenging environments https://indico.cern.ch/event/767986/overview
[18] Wroe L, Ige T and Asogwa O *et al* 2020 Comparative analysis of radiotherapy linear accelerator downtime and failure modes in the UK, Nigeria and Botswana *Clin. Oncol.* **32** 111–8
[19] ITAR Project https://iceccancer.org/innovative radiotherapy-technologies
[20] Barksby R 2020 Expanding access to radiotherapy in sub-Saharan Africa *Lancet Oncol.* **21** 1019
[21] Ige T and Jenkins A *et al* Improving access to and technology for cancer care: A collaboration among all 28 African countries that offer LINAC-based RT, Unpublished manuscript
[22] Datta *et al* 2019 Challenges and opportunities to realize 'The 2030 Agenda for Sustainable Development' by the United Nations: implications for radiation therapy infrastructure in low- and middle-income countries *Int. J. Radiat. Oncol. Biol. Phys.* **105** 918–33
[23] Grau *et al* 2014 ESTRO-HERO survey: radiotherapy equipment and departments in the European countries: final results from the ESTRO-HERO survey *Radiother. Oncol.* **112** 155–64
[24] Yap *et al* 2016 Global access to radiotherapy services: have we made progress during the past decade? *J. Glob. Oncol.* **2** 207–15
[25] Crisp N 2015 Co-development, innovation and mutual learning—or how we need to turn the world upside down *Healthc (Amst).* **3** 221–4
[26] World Bank: GNI per capita, PPP (current int. $) August 5, 2020 https://datahelpdesk.worldbank.org/knowledgebase/articles/906519-world-bank-country-and-lending-groups
[27] Bray F, Ferlay J, Soerjomataram I, Siegel R L, Torre L A and Jemal A 2018 Global cancer statistics 2018: GLOBOCAN estimates of incidence and mortality worldwide for 36 cancers in 185 countries *CA Cancer J Clin.* **68** 394–424
[28] International Agency for Research on Cancer data https://gco.iarc.fr/today/data-sources-methods

Chapter 22

Research collaboration to advance cancer prevention and control in Africa

James Alaro

This chapter covers research collaboration, which is crucial for global oncology. It presents examples of opportunities for research collaborations in Africa, implementation science, innovative cancer technologies advancing new frontiers in cancer knowledge, and the advancement of equity in research collaborations in Africa.

Note: A link to James Alaro's talk presented at the Dana-Farber Cancer Institute at Harvard Medical School during the Global Health Catalyst Summit can be found at https://youtu.be/c9jKxTsTKN8 [1].

22.1 Research collaboration to address the cancer burden in Africa

Cancer poses an increasing health and economic burden globally, but the impact is much more profound in low- and middle-income countries (LMICs), where nearly 70% of all deaths occur. Scientific advancements have resulted in substantial progress in the battle against cancer in high-income countries (HICs), where cancer incidence and deaths continue to decline and/or are stable. This progress, however, is yet to translate to LMICs, particularly in Africa, where cancer rates are on the rise. GLOBOCAN predicts that between 2020 and 2040, the greatest relative increases in cancer incidence and deaths will occur in Africa, where the rates are projected to rise by as much as 89% and 93%, respectively. The looming cancer crisis in Africa cannot be resolved by Africa alone, without the support of the rest of the world, and only through concerted and transformative—not progressive nor tentative—actions will meaningful progress be made. These actions must be evidence-based, priority-driven, and resource-appropriate for Africa. Progress will be more rapidly and efficiently realized through coordinated, sustained, and effective cancer research that integrates perspectives and experiences from within and outside Africa.

Cancer research in Africa has resulted in seminal scientific discoveries that have contributed significantly to our understanding of cancers, and to the development of

doi:10.1088/978-0-7503-3075-6ch22

effective interventions. In stark contrast to HICs, Africa has not benefitted equally from these scientific advancements, partly because cancer research in Africa has not always prioritized the needs and priorities of Africa. Often, research conducted in Africa has involved international collaborations in which funding support is primarily provided by HICs. As a consequence, the research has traditionally emphasized areas driven by external interests, and not Africa's priorities. The research has not always accounted for local cultures, politics, economics, and environment, making it hard to link the findings to applicable and tangible outcomes for Africa. For Africa to benefit from cancer research, deliberate efforts must be made to generate Africa-specific data and knowledge and an evidence base to inform cancer prevention and control in Africa. As research collaborations will be pivotal in addressing Africa's cancer problem, such collaborations must be premised on a win-win model in which all parties involved benefit from the research endeavor. There are several opportunities to strengthen mutually beneficial collaborations between African scientists and their HIC counterparts to accelerate the development of cross-cutting and broadly applicable solutions to address the cancer burden in Africa and beyond.

22.2 Opportunities for research collaboration in Africa

The rising burden of cancer in Africa is largely driven by preventable/modifiable risk factors that include environmental exposures, a high burden of cancer-causing infections, increasing rates of tobacco and alcohol use, late-stage presentation of cases, and lack of/poor access to screening, diagnostics, and treatment services. A focus on addressing these well-established determinants has led to a significant reduction in cancer incidence and deaths in HICs. Collaborative research rooted in a deep understanding of the local settings, cultures, and health systems in Africa has the potential to drive similar, if not better success, not only in Africa but also in other low-resource settings around the world. We highlight a few areas in which impactful research collaboration might lead to an immediate impact in Africa and beyond.

22.3 Implementation science

Noticeably, several evidence-based cancer prevention and control interventions and strategies exist, but their application in Africa remains inadequate and rather inconsistent. For instance, despite overwhelming evidence which shows that it is feasible to introduce and attain high vaccine coverage in Africa, only a small percentage of the populations in Africa have been fully vaccinated against cancer-causing infections, such as human papilloma virus (HPV—a causal agent in cervical cancer) and the hepatitis B virus (HBV—associated with liver cancer). Similarly, the many proven and cost-effective cancer screening modalities and tobacco cessation strategies that continue to drive down the cancer burden in HICs have not been completely applied in Africa. Part of the challenge is that most of the existing evidence base has been developed in HICs and/or for HICs, without giving much consideration to implementation and structural barriers in Africa. As it is unlikely that the same implementation strategies that worked in HICs will work in Africa, implementation research has the potential to accelerate progress towards developing strategies best suited for Africa. Collaborative research informed by a deeper understanding of the contextual differences in Africa will most likely lead to the development of interventions and strategies that would not only be applicable locally, but also broadly across diverse settings in Africa and beyond. As the field of implementation science grows in Africa, the research community ought to interrogate current frameworks, methodologies, and measures to ensure suitability/applicability in Africa.

22.4 Cancer health disparities

Cancer-related health disparities present a global problem that, to a greater or lesser extent, affects all populations around the world, yet cancer disparities in Africa remain poorly understood. Striking health disparities in terms of exposure to preventable/modifiable cancer risk factors are observed between HICs and Africa. Cancer-related health disparities are also observed across Africa with considerable heterogeneity, not only between countries but also within countries. Broadly, the causes implicated in cancer-related health disparities are multifactorial and multilevel, including a set of complex and interrelated biological factors (such as genetic predisposition and risk factor profiles) and non-biological factors (such as socioeconomic factors, access to healthcare, culture, politics, lifestyle/health habits, and discrimination). Collaborative research in Africa and on African populations offers an opportunity for large comparative studies that will illuminate how these factors contribute to disparities in cancer risks and outcomes in Africa. Expanding research to include global populations and perspectives would enhance our understanding of how biological, environmental, lifestyle, and cultural factors contribute to the observed disparities. Ultimately, eliminating cancer-related health disparities will not only result from a deeper understanding of the causes and the local context in which they occur, but also from developing and implementing innovative interventions that are better targeted/tailored for the populations and settings for which they are designed. Addressing cancer-related health disparities and advancing health equity in Africa is surely going to be an arduous task, particularly given the incredible heterogeneity of African populations. Cancer-related health disparities must be taken into consideration in the design, execution, and evaluation of all cancer programs. To guide meaningful research on cancer-related health disparities, the research community needs to come together and develop an operational definition that fully incorporates the causes of cancer-related health disparities in Africa, as well as a conceptual framework, and standardized measures.

22.5 Innovative cancer technology

A number of the technologies developed and used to control cancer in HICs have great potential for application in Africa. However, the widespread application of these technologies in Africa has been hampered by the associated high costs and/or a dependency on an elaborate healthcare infrastructure, among other factors.

Research collaborations in Africa will help to bridge this gap by accelerating either the adaptation of some of these technologies or the development of new innovative technologies better suited for application in Africa and other low-resource settings around the world (examples of adaptations and new technologies). The proliferation of cellular phones and hand-held devices in Africa provides further opportunities to develop a new generation of technology-driven cancer prevention and control measures in the continent. Importantly however, Africa must not be left behind in the ongoing research to develop new technologies for cancer control. At present, an explosion of research into innovative and cutting-edge technologies is mostly being undertaken by institutions in HICs, including research into immunotherapy, liquid biopsy techniques, artificial intelligence technologies, lab-on-a-chip, and portable ablative devices. This research much be extended to include Africa and other low-resource settings to ensure the development of user-friendly, affordable technologies for preventing, detecting, diagnosing, and/or treating cancers in diverse low-resource settings worldwide.

22.6 Advancing new frontiers in cancer knowledge

Significant opportunities exist in Africa for basic and applied research collaborations to advance our understanding of, and address cancers that are prevalent in the continent, such as prostate, cervical, and colorectal cancers, Burkitt's lymphoma, liver cancer, and esophageal cancer. There is increasing evidence which shows that many of these cancers exhibit unique manifestations and natural histories. Collaborative research in Africa affords a platform to better understand the different etiologies and unique patterns of cancers in ways that would otherwise not be possible. Studies in Africa also offer great opportunities to understand the unique environmental exposures associated with cancers, such as indoor air pollution. The diverse populations, health systems, and geographic settings in Africa offer a great platform to explore modern innovations in delivering care (including chemotherapy and radiotherapy) and to evaluate new interventions for cancer prevention and control globally.

22.7 Advancing equity in research collaborations in Africa

Research collaborations in Africa offer opportunities to combine expertise and resources from across the world to answer fundamental scientific questions relevant to cancer problems in Africa. However, research collaborations in Africa remain largely imbalanced, due to the skewed economic and academic resources that favor scientists from HICs. Because of the imbalance, the research agenda in Africa is often driven by researchers from HICs, who end up defining the research questions, study designs, data analyses, and how and where the final research products are applied. The African scientists' role is often reduced to data collection. There have been attempts to address the imbalance, but it persists. As key stakeholders, scientists and research funders can no longer remain quiet, and must discuss these inequities openly. All stakeholders must think seriously about their role in perpetuating these inequities and be intentional in addressing them. Impactful and equitable collaboration will require extensive investments of resources, time, and effort. As COVID-19 continues to teach us, creativity thrives in the face of limited resources; therefore, resource limitation can no longer be an excuse for inaction.

A key consideration of advancing equity in research collaboration in Africa is to empower and increase the voice of African scientists. African scientists have a pivotal role to play in driving the cancer research agenda and ensuring that the research addresses the needs and priorities of Africa. The capacity of African scientists to conduct rigorous cancer research continues to be hampered by several challenges, including poor research infrastructure, a dearth of expertise, and inadequate funding for research. These challenges, while formidable, are not insurmountable and can be addressed by deliberate actions. Funding agencies have a big say in the type of research and by whom research is conducted in Africa. For instance, efforts made by some international research funders that require African scientists to be the lead principal investigators in research projects will go a long way towards harnessing intellectual leadership and increasing the African voice in the research conducted in Africa. There is an urgent need to increase the training of African scientists so that they can take the leadership in cancer research in Africa. Transposing training programs from HICs to Africa is most likely not the way forward, and we must reimagine training programs to suit the present needs for research in Africa. Likewise, more training is needed to equip international scientists with skills for impactful and equitable research collaboration.

Ultimately, for Africans to control their own research agenda and ensure that research in Africa addresses the needs and priorities of Africa, African governments must integrate research into their national strategy and invest more in research. As African governments continue to struggle to meet the basic necessities for their citizenry, many governments have paid less attention to investing in research. There is often a general lack of appreciation of the role of research in driving human and societal development. As observed in Asian countries, including China and South Korea, innovations obtained through high-quality research in Africa will help to lift Africa out of poverty. African scientists and other research stakeholders need to rally African governments to invest more in research as a tool for growth, development, and advancement.

22.8 The future of global cancer research starts NOW!

As science continues to generate and/or refine tools to confront health issues, NOW is the time to be more ambitious, more transformative, and more deliberate in our efforts to address health inequities globally. Let our voices be heard and our actions be seen!

Reference

[1] Alaro J 2019 Research collaboration to advance cancer care and prevention in LMICs 24 May, 2019, GHC Summit, Harvard Medical School, Boston, MA, USA

IOP Publishing

Approaching Global Oncology
The win-win model
Ahmed Elzawawy and Wilfred Ngwa

Chapter 23

Repurposing and repositioning drugs and devices in cancer care

Ahmed Elzawawy

There is no need to repeat in detail that there is skyrocketing rise in the costs of cancer drug therapy and there is an increase in the crisis of lack of affordability of cancer care in the world. One of the several scientific approaches that the Win-Win Movement advocates is to conduct scientific studies of the uses of older drugs, either single, in novel combinations, or for newer indications. This includes terms such as repurposing, repositioning, or reprofiling drugs or indication switching. A considerable reduction in the costs of treatment could be achieved, along with an increase in the discoveries of newer indications of the value of older drugs and devices.

23.1 Introduction

New drug development is not enough, and there is a great need for drug repositioning, particularly in oncology [1]. Using scientific approaches, old approved drugs could have new indications, and therefore offer less expensive treatments [2]. This approach has been termed drug repositioning, drug repurposing, drug reprofiling, therapeutic switching, or indication switching, among which, drug repositioning is the term most frequently used [1, 3]. However, contrary to the notion of using the previous terms as alternative expressions, in this chapter and the next chapter, we see that it is confusing to use 'repurposing' and 'repositioning' with the same or nearly the same meaning. Here, we adhere to the definition of 'repurposed' as stated clearly by Dr Clare Thibodaux (in the next chapter):

– **Repurposing**: finding a new disease indication for a drug, device, or nutraceutical already approved for human use. (Nutraceutical is a pharmacological term meaning 'functional food')
– **Repositioning/rescue**: finding an indication for a compound that is safe for a human but still in the pipeline

doi:10.1088/978-0-7503-3075-6ch23

In recent decades, a great deal of work has been conducted in a very costly search for new oncological therapies; however, cancer remains one of the leading causes of death globally [2]. In addition to the skyrocketing rise of cancer drug therapy costs and the increasing crisis of the lack of affordability of cancer care [2], the creation of new drugs requires large quantities of financial capital. According to analysis by Adams *et al* [4], the costs range between 161 and 1800 million dollars per pharmaceutical product.

Alongside the money spent, extensive experimentation and testing are required to support the innovator's recognition of identifiable targets and justification, the establishment of the principal compound, and subsequent studies of efficacy, pharmacokinetics, and toxicity. After this laborious process, a minimal number of possible oncology drugs reach clinical trials, the fraction is considered to be ~5% [5].

Then, if the three phases of clinical trials are successful, the new compound can be authorized for use in therapeutic settings. It has been estimated that the time required to develop a new drug from beginning to end is 11.4–13.5 years [6].

23.2 Repurposing categories

We propose four repurposing categories, based on a broad notion of repurposing:

I. Drugs—single and in combination—for humans, for different indications including cancer (we focus on this topic in this chapter).
II. Diagnostic devices and procedures.
III. Treatment devices.
IV. Nutraceuticals.

23.3 Examples of scientific approaches used to repurpose drugs related to cancer

According to what we published in 2012 and 2015 [2, 7], we identified several scientific tactics for drug repositioning:

A. **Single old drugs**

(1) Old cancer drugs with new uses in cancer and potential new profits.
(2) Old non-cancer drugs with new uses in cancer and potential new profits.
(3) Old cancer drugs with new uses in non-cancer indications and potential new profits.

B. **Newer combinations of older cancer drugs with new indications and benefits in cancer.**

23.3.1 Old cancer drugs with new uses in cancer and new profits

This implies the exploration of new indications or different methods and administration schedules of older (and relatively cheaper) previously approved cancer drugs that could be beneficial in cancer. The following sections give examples.

23.3.1.1 Cisplatin

The relatively old and inexpensive cancer drug Cisplatin has been shown to be useful in the treatment of triple-negative (estrogen receptor, progesterone receptor, HER2/neu 0, 1) breast cancer [8].

Recent studies are investigating whether platinum salts used in the treatment of BRCA-associated breast cancer could be considered as true targeted chemotherapy or not. A randomized triple-negative breast cancer trial showed a significant benefit for carboplatin vs. docetaxel in terms of response rate and progression-free survival (PFS), specifically in patients with advanced gene- (gBRCA1/2) associated tumors [9].

23.3.1.2 Metronomic oral therapy

The metronomic use of prolonged, low oral doses of the old and cheap drugs cyclophosphamide and methotrexate is used as a palliative treatment for metastatic breast cancer [10].

23.3.1.3 Estradiol

(a) **Estradiol in aromatase inhibitor–resistant, hormone receptor–positive advanced breast cancer:** in a phase II trial, low-dose (6 mg per day) oral estradiol achieved the same response as the usual high dose (30 mg per day) of estradiol in approximately 30% of patients with fewer adverse events than with the usual dose in postmenopausal women with aromatase inhibitor–resistant, hormone receptor–positive advanced breast cancer [11].

(b) **Estradiol in triple-negative breast cancer**

Estradiol is a potential treatment for a subset of triple-negative breast cancers. A second form of the estrogen receptor, known as estrogen receptor β, is expressed in approximately 25% of triple-negative breast cancer tumors. When estradiol binds with estrogen receptor β in triple-negative breast cancer, it stimulates the expression of a group of proteins called cystatins, which exhibit tumor-suppressing effects on neighboring and distant cancer cells [12].

23.3.2 Old non-cancer drugs with new uses in cancer and potential new profits

This implies that we have an old, safe molecule of an old non-cancer drug that may have an unexpected use in cancer prevention or cancer treatment.

23.3.2.1 Thirty examples of non-cancer drugs repositioned for the treatment of cancer

Pantziarka *et al* 2018 [13] stated that in oncology, there is an increased level of activity associated with examining the use of non-cancer drugs as possible cancer treatments.

In a recent study published in 2020 in Nature Cancer [14], researchers found dozens of non-oncology drugs approved for diabetes, inflammation, alcoholism, arthritis, and even for lowering cholesterol and other non-cancer indications that also kill cancer cells.

They analyzed thousands of already developed drugs and discovered nearly 50 new (previously unrecognized) anticancer actions. The team at the Massachusetts Institute of Technology (MIT), Harvard University, and other institutions tested all the compounds in the Drug Repurposing Hub on 578 human cancer cell lines from Broad's Cancer Cell Line Encyclopedia (CCLE). What is also exciting is that most of these non-cancer drugs hit new unrecognized molecular targets. These findings could lead to the identification of biomarkers and patients who are more likely to respond. This study could stimulate many future studies.

We present here examples of published studies of non-cancer drugs that could be beneficial in treating cancer:

23.3.2.2 Metformin

Metformin is a biguanide widely used by type 2 diabetics who overproduce insulin. It is an inexpensive oral drug taken as a tablet. It shows significant growth inhibitory effects in several cancer cells in mouse tumor models. In cell culture, metformin inhibits the proliferation of a range of cancer cells including those of the breast, prostate, colon, lung, endometrium, and ovary as well as gliomas [15, 16]. Despite encouraging *in vitro* and epidemiological data for different tumor types, the results of randomized clinical trials of metformin are mostly unsatisfactory [17]. With the use of metformin, it is postulated that there is enhanced antineoplastic activity of the kinase inhibitor [18].

There is still enthusiasm to understand the role of metformin in cancer via ongoing clinical research [19].

It is worth noting that each tablet costs around 20–25 cents. Tablets are taken twice daily. Despite the low price, the cost of running a clinical trial, which involves collecting blood samples, could cost millions of USD [14]. At the moment, more than 80 actively recruiting clinical trials are open; details can be found in a publication by Saraei *et al* 2019 [20].

One of the new exciting studies [21] is that metformin has been shown to directly inhibit the sonic hedgehog pathway, a key pathway in basal cell carcinoma (BCC) pathogenesis; in addition, it has general anticarcinogenic effects. Hence, it may reduce BCC risk. The GHC Win-Win initiative's point of view is: this effect of metformin on BCC could be tested and subjected to more trials, as it could be of valuable benefits for white-skinned people, particularly in countries such as Australia and South Africa.

23.3.2.3 Anti-depressant drug paroxetine

A recent study by researchers at the Karolinska Institute in Sweden and the MD Anderson Cancer Centre in Texas [22] has found that a known anti-depressant drug paroxetine, which impairs a serotonin reuptake receptor, may stop the growth of childhood Ewing sarcoma, at least in mice and laboratory cell experiments. This offers hope that it can be translated to clinical use in humans.

The study explored commonalities between two large groups of cell surface receptors, the so-called G protein-coupled receptors (GPCRs) and the receptor tyrosine kinases (RTKs). GPCRs are targeted by more than half of all the developed drugs used to treat conditions such as allergies, asthma, depression, anxiety, and hypertension, but have so far not been widely used to treat cancers. Paroxetine is part of the GPCR-family. RTKs, on the other hand, are targeted by drugs against cancers, such as breast and colon cancers, due to their implication in a variety of cellular abnormalities.

The study reveals a rational design or repurposing of drugs to selectively cross-target IGF-1R or other RTKs. Therefore, it demonstrates what could be described as 'system bias' or 'biased signalling' [23] as an effective anticancer approach for drug repositioning. The researchers plan to conduct further studies of multiple TRKs and clinical research into Ewing sarcoma. This may be extended to explore possible actions on other tumors such as breast and colon cancers. This represents a new era for a class of cancer-relevant RTKs. It could be the beginning of a rational design of specific drugs for other cancer types using known old drugs that are in clinical use, at a lower cost.

23.3.2.4 A combination of doxycycline, azithromycin, and vitamin C (DAV) as a potent therapy for targeting mitochondria and eradicating cancer stem cells

Previous studies have shown that cancer stem-like cells are the root cause of chemotherapy resistance. Research conducted by a team from the University of Salford, UK, led by Michael Lisanti [24], showed that the two Food and Drug Administration (FDA)-approved antibiotics doxycycline and azithromycin could be used to target the production of 13 key proteins, hence, they stop energy supply in the stem cells. Vitamin C could act as a mild pro-oxidant and consequently amplify the effects. They found that the new inexpensive non-cancer drug combo could reduce stem cell growth by more than 90% in laboratory tests.

23.3.3 New uses for chemotherapy drugs in nonmalignant indications

23.3.3.1 Gemcitabine

Perhaps many may not remember that, previously, Gemcitabine was shown to be effective as an antiviral drug [25]. Gemcitabine is used for cancer chemotherapy alone or in combination with other drugs for various types of cancers, including pancreatic, bladder, lung, and uterine cervical cancers.

Gemcitabine has been the subject of various repurposing studies. It has been found that Gemcitabine is active against 19 different strains of methicillin-resistant *Staphylococcus aureus*. It was found to be effective against glycopeptide-intermediate *Staphylococcus aureus*, a strain resistant to all glycopeptide antibiotics, including vancomycin. Resistance to gemcitabine could develop in treated *Staphylococcus aureus*. However, gemcitabine was found to have a synergistic action with gentamicin, and, if used in combination, the emergence of resistance to these drugs may be slowed [26, 27].

23.3.3.1.1 Imatinib in tuberculosis (TB)

According to the World Health Organization (WHO), it is estimated that nearly two billion people are infected with *Mycobacterium tuberculosis*. Almost one and half million die from the disease each year. Some strains of the bacteria have become resistant to many or all of the available antibiotics. In 2019, close to half a million people worldwide developed rifampicin-resistant TB (RR-TB), among which, 78% had multidrug-resistant TB (MDR-TB) [28].

The drug imatinib is widely used in the treatment of chronic myelogenous leukemia (CML) and gastrointestinal stromal tumors (GISTs). It inhibits the constitutive tyrosine kinase activity of the BCR-ABL protein. Imatinib is a potential host-directed therapeutic (HDT) for drug-resistant TB infections and HIV/TB co-infections (at less than one tenth of the dose used in CML). By targeting the host—not the mycobacteria itself—researchers were able to reduce the host's mycobacterial load and even target antibiotic-resistant strains while enhancing the effectiveness of front-line antibiotics. Moreover, a phase II trial is currently assessing the capacity of low-dose imatinib to induce myelopoiesis and enhance host antimicrobial immunity against tuberculosis [29, 30].

23.3.3.1.2 Imatinib may slow the course of type-1 diabetes

Imatinib may help to preserve beta-cell function in people with recently diagnosed type-1 diabetes. Findings from a phase 2 study [31] have shown that imatinib prevents diabetes and induces remission of recent-onset diabetes in preclinical studies.

Once again, we emphasise the GHC Win-Win initiative point of view: the idea of finding wider uses of an expensive cancer drug such as imatinib in different repurposing, evidenced based indications, could be a smart and scientific way to achieve the wider use and sales of a drug and potentially to increase access to cancer treatment. This is in addition to increasing the value of a drug and beneficial indications that serve patients with different diseases.

23.3.4 Old cancer drugs, new uses in non-cancer cases, potential new profits

23.3.4.1 The action of fluorouracil in repairing skin wrinkles and sun damage

Sachs *et al* [32] showed that the cancer drug fluorouracil could be used as a skin cream to help repair sun damage and skin wrinkles on the face. When used topically, it causes epidermal injury that enhances wound healing and dermal remodeling, resulting in better appearance. The mechanism of topical fluorouracil in photoaged skin is comparable to that used in the laser treatment of photoaging.

23.3.5 Newer combinations of older cancer drugs with new indications and benefits in cancer

One of the most exciting scientific explorations is that of repurposed new combinations of older drugs [2, 7]. Researchers performed 300,000 experiments to test 5000 different combinations of 100 approved cancer drugs on each of 60 cell lines developed by the National Cancer Institute (NCI). The new repository of data will be made available to the public in the NCI's Development Therapeutics Program, in the hope that it will provide investigators insight into potential drug combinations to target or avoid. The NCI hopes to accelerate the advancement of new therapeutic combinations that demonstrate minimum side effects and maximum benefits. If confirmed, this will form a basis for future clinical trials of such combinations [33].

23.4 Opportunities and future directions

The re-establishment of intellectual property for repositioned drugs may solve major problems with their practical use. The repositioning of drugs could pave the way for new and more effective treatments for patients with cancer; hence, more research is needed. Masuda *et al* compared these repurposing searches to finding a baseball player's talent in an active soccer player [34].

The European Medicines Agency (EMA) in Europe, the National Institute of Health (NIH) and the FDA in the USA have already launched programs to identify new uses for existing drugs developed by the pharmaceutical industry [35, 36].

The ReDO project is an international collaboration initiated by several researchers, clinicians, and patient advocates. It has focused exclusively on the potential use of approved non-cancer medications as sources of new anticancer treatment. Information about the project is available online via http://www.redo-project.org/db. This website will be periodically updated to make information available to oncologists as new drugs are added to the database or as new data become available for drugs listed in the database [37, 38].

In Japan, three Japanese pharmaceutical companies have started joint implementation of a drug discovery program, Joint Open Innovation of Drug Repositioning (JOINUS), using a drug repositioning compound library constructed by these companies in 2017 [39].

Philanthropic foundations such as Cures Within Reach (CWR) in the USA (www.cureswithinreach.org) have funded over 90 projects at more than 50 different institutions worldwide that cover drugs in general (including cancer drugs), devices and nutraceutical repurposing research [40]. In the next chapter of this book, Clare Thibodeaux (Vice President of Scientific Affairs of CWR) reveals opportunities for research projects in LMICs. It is hoped that researchers from LMICs will contribute more to the scientific movement. It is a win-win situation [41].

Although this chapter focuses on presenting examples of drug repurposing related to cancer, repurposing includes drugs in general, nutraceuticals, diagnostic procedures, and treatment devices.

As an example, we cite here one of the exciting publications about the repurposing of devices and procedures. Cosmetic lasers may boost the effectiveness of certain anticancer therapies, for example, in melanoma. Immune checkpoint inhibitors (ICIs) have revolutionized treatment for patients with melanoma, although not all patients respond. A cosmetic laser is also known as a fractional laser. When Massachusetts General Hospital (MGH) applied it to a tumor, it was able to induce a form of local inflammation that imitated the presence of mutations, strongly enhancing immune attacks against nonmutated tumor proteins, thereby curing many mice of tumors that otherwise did not respond to immunotherapy. Moreover, the researchers found that exposing the melanoma cells to ultraviolet radiation caused them to mutate more [42].

The repositioning of drugs, according to the definition cited in the beginning of this chapter, deserves scientific studies, but should not be confused in terms of either definition or regulations with the repurposing of drugs and devices.

23.5 Required actions

Based on all the abovementioned examples of publications and resources, we present a brief proposal for a call to action. As indicated in the win-win notions, this proposal is presented to all readers and stakeholders who can modify or adopt it. Once again, we stress that the GHC Win-Win Movement with all its channels, including this book, belongs to all stakeholders.

23.5.1 An international campaign for the repurposing and repositioning of drugs, nutraceuticals, procedures, and devices

The following are needed: an international campaign for information, increased awareness of the importance of these approaches, and collaboration. This is aligned with the proposed global win-win efforts and campaign to increase access to healthcare. We support the notion that the topics of repurposing and repositioning should be a part of the interests of all cancer organizations and big cancer societies, and their conferences, publications, and journals

23.5.2 Global repository for projects, new ideas, and proposals for repurposing and repositioning drugs and devices

In the last chapter of this book (chapter 45), we propose the formation of a 'think tank' for approaches that could lead to increased affordability of better-value cancer care in the world. One of the scientific approaches that needs a web-based repository is the repurposing and repositioning of drugs and devices for diagnosis and treatment.

As mentioned above, the ReDO project is a very important and leading project in this field. Another example is that of Cure Within Reach (CWR)—introduced in the next chapter—which has its Cure Accelerator platform where repurposing stakeholders can read hundreds of public abstracts for research projects submitted to CWR. According to the concepts of the GHC Win-Win Movement, we are completing and not challenging or replacing any. These previous projects could be important resources for a global virtual repository where researchers, industries, and stakeholders could submit their ideas; be inspired freely by published findings, new scientific ideas, and preliminary proposals for research or approaches for funding; or search online, exchange views, and potentially collaborate or form partnerships. Alternatively, our proposal could simply be adopted or taken by one of the existing repurposing data projects and extended to include a virtual global forum for repurposing and repositioning medicines, procedures, and devices. Our clear objective is that we are not seeking any credit for ourselves but wish to see remarkable progress in effective efforts to increase the affordability of cancer care for patients in the world, regardless of who the doers are.

The notion of the win-win movement implies that this initiative does not aim to prevent the manufacturers of new drugs and devices from gaining and flourishing; to the contrary, all would win [2].

It is doubtful that the big pharmaceutical firms will be able to follow their goals in the future using the old model of developing exclusive new drugs that can be sold at high prices. In addition to the economic impact of COVID-19 and the potential for post-pandemic challenges, numerous drugs will be coming off patent in the next few years, opening the way for generics and eliminating an important source of the industry's profits. Hence, there is a need to search for innovative strategic actions that can position a company as a continuous winner [43, 44].

It will be mandatory that all levels of management, particularly the top strategic planning level, will carry out the extraordinary task of creating innovative strategic actions and of preparing and informing all of their company's human resources in using innovative tactics and strategies [44]. One of the many approaches that we see is that it could be beneficial for some industries to invest in research for the repurposing of their products, hence, increasing the chance of gaining more from an increase in sales due to different indications and uses in the forthcoming years. On the other hand, from the point of view of the win-win global model, this could be one of several smart methods for increasing access to some expensive treatments within a global win-win campaign and not as a dispersed or solitary endeavor that could be undertaken for opportunistic and very short-term benefits [2].

At the end of the chapter, we say to all readers, stakeholders, and key players in the world:

> We stress again that this chapter, this book, and the win-win movement will only grow remarkably because of you and for you all. Please feel free to modify, to suggest, to adopt, and to implement what you see convenient. It is yours!

References

[1] Langedijk J, Mantel-Teeuwisse A K and Slijkerman D S *et al* 2015 Drug repositioning and repurposing: terminology and definitions in literature *Drug Discov. Today* **20** 1027–34

[2] Elzawawy A 2012 Science and affordability of cancer drugs and radiotherapy in the world: win-win scenarios *Advances in Cancer Management* ed R Moran (Rijeka: InTech) http://intechopen.com/articles/show/title/science-and-affordability-of-cancer-drugs-and-radio-therapy-in-the-world

[3] Armando R G and Mengual Gómez D L *et al* 2020 New drugs are not enough-drug repositioning in oncology: an update *Int. J. Oncol.* **56** 651–84

[4] Adams C P and Brantner V V 2006 Estimating the cost of new drug development: Is it really 802 million dollars? *Health Aff. (Millwood)* **25** 420–8

[5] Gupta S C, Sung B, Prasad S, Webb L J and Aggarwal B B 2013 Cancer drug discovery by repurposing: teaching new tricks to old dogs *Trends Pharmacol. Sci.* **34** 508–17

[6] Paul S M *et al* 2010 How to improve R&D productivity: the pharmaceutical industry's grand challenge *Nat. Rev. Drug Discov.* **9** 203–14

[7] Elzawawy A 2015 The shortage of essential cancer drugs and generics in the United States of America: global brain storming directions for the world *Int. J. Cancer Clin. Res.* **2** 016
[8] Gronwald J, Byrski T and Huzarski T 2009 Neoadjuvant therapy with cisplatin in *BRCA1*-positive breast cancer patients *J. Clin. Oncol.* **27** 502
[9] Torrisia R, Zuradellia M and Agostinettoa E *et al* 2019 Platinum salts in the treatment of *BRCA*-associated breast cancer: a true targeted chemotherapy? *Critic. Rev. Oncol./Hematol.* **135** 66–75
[10] Colleoni M, Rocca A and Sandri M T *et al* 2002 Low-dose oral methotrexate and cyclophosphamide in metastatic breast cancer: antitumor activity and correlation with vascular endothelial growth factor levels *Ann. Oncol.* **13** 73–80
[11] Ellis M J, Gao F and Dehdashti F *et al* 2009 Lower-dose vs high-dose oral estradiol therapy of hormone receptor–positive, aromatase inhibitor–resistant advanced breast cancer: a phase 2 randomized study *JAMA* **302** 774–80
[12] Reese J, Bruinsma E and Nelson A *et al* 2018 ERβ-mediated induction of cystatins results in suppression of TGFβ signaling and inhibition of triple-negative breast cancer metastasis *PNAS* **115** E9580–9
[13] Pantziarka P, Verbaanderd C and Sukhatme V *et al* 2018 ReDO_DB: the repurposing drugs in oncology database *ecancer Med. Sci.* **12** 886
[14] Corsello S M and Nagari R T *et al* 2020 Discovering the anticancer potential of non-oncology drugs by systematic viability profiling *Nat. Cancer* **1** 235–48
[15] Dowling R J, Goodwin P J and Stambolic V 2011 Understanding the benefit of metformin use in cancer treatment *BMC Med.* **9** 33
[16] Dowling R J, Niraula S and Chang M C *et al* 2015 Changes in insulin receptor signaling underlie neoadjuvant metformin administration in breast cancer: a prospective window of opportunity neoadjuvant study *Breast Cancer Res.* **17** 32
[17] Del Barco S, Vazquez–Martin A and Cufi S *et al* 2011 Metformin: multi–faceted protection against cancer *Oncotarget* **2** 896–917
[18] Haq R and Fisher D E 2013 Improving apoptotic responses to targeted therapy *Oncotarget* **4** 1331
[19] Heckman–Stoddard B M *et al* 2017 Repurposing metformin for the prevention of cancer and cancer recurrence *Diabetologia* **60** 1639–47
[20] Saraei P *et al* 2019 The beneficial effects of metformin on cancer prevention and therapy: a comprehensive review of recent advances *Cancer Manag. Res.* **11** 3295–313
[21] Adalsteinsson J A, Muzumdar S and Waldman R *et al* 2021 Metformin is associated with decreased risk of basal cell carcinoma: a whole-population case-control study from Iceland *J. Am. Acad. Dermatol.* **85** 56–61
[22] Crudden C, Shibano T and Song D *et al* 2021 Inhibition of G protein-coupled receptor kinase 2 promotes unbiased downregulation of IGF1 receptor and restrains malignant cell growth *Cancer Res.* **81** 501–14
[23] Smith J S, Lefkowitz R J and Rajagopal S 2018 Biased signalling: from simple switches to allosteric microprocessors *Nat. Rev. Drug Discovery* **17** 243–60
[24] Fiorillo M, Tóth F, Sotgia F and Lisanti M P 2019 Doxycycline, Azithromycin and Vitamin C (DAV): a potent combination therapy for targeting mitochondria and eradicating cancer stem cells (CSCs) *Aging (Albany NY).* **11** 2202–16
[25] Lee K, Kim D E and Jang K S *et al* 2017 Gemcitabine, a broad-spectrum antiviral drug, suppresses enterovirus infections through innate immunity induced by the inhibition of pyrimidine biosynthesis and nucleotide depletion *Oncotarget.* **8** 115315

[26] Jordheim L P, Ben Larbi S and Fendrich O *et al* 2012 Gemcitabine is active against clinical multiresistant *Staphylococcus aureus* strains and is synergistic with gentamicin *Int. J. Antimicrob. Agents* **39** 444–7
[27] Thomson J M and Lamont I L 2019 Nucleoside analogues as antibacterial agents *Front. Microbiol.* **10** 952
[28] World Health Organization 2020 WHO global tuberculosis report 2020 https://who.int/publications/i/item/9789240013131
[29] Napier R, Rafi W and Cheruvu M *et al* 2011 Imatinib-sensitive tyrosine kinases regulate mycobacterial pathogenesis and represent therapeutic targets against tuberculosis *Cell Host Microbe.* **10** 475–85
[30] Giver C, Shaw P and Fletcher H *et al* 2019 IMPACT-TB: a phase II trial assessing the capacity of low dose imatinib to induce myelopoiesis and enhance host anti-microbial immunity against tuberculosis *Blood* **134** 1050
[31] Gitelman S E, Bundy B N and Ferrannini E *et al* 2021 Imatinib therapy for patients with recent-onset type 1 diabetes: a multicentre, randomised, double-blind, placebo-controlled, phase 2 trial *Lancet Diabetes Endocrinol.* **9** 502–14
[32] Sachs L, Kang S and Hammerberg C *et al* 2009 Topical fluorouracil for actinic keratoses and photoaging. a clinical and molecular analysis *Arch. Dermatol.* **145** 659–66
[33] Holbeck S Cell-based screens of drug combinations at NCI http://deainfo.nci.nih.gov/advisory/ctac/1114/5%20-%20Holbeck.pdf
[34] Masuda T, Tsuruda Y and Matsumoto Y *et al* 2020 Drug repositioning in cancer: the current situation in Japan *Cancer Sci.* **111** 1039–46
[35] Nowak-Sliwinska P, Scapozza L and Altaba A R I 2019 Drug repurposing in oncology: compounds, pathways, phenotypes and computational approaches for colorectal cancer *Biochim. Biophys. Acta, Rev. Cancer* **1871** 434–54
[36] Allison M 2012 NCATS launches drug repurposing program *Nat. Biotechnol.* **30** 571–2
[37] Pantziarka P, Bouche G and Meheus L *et al* 2014 The repurposing drugs in oncology (ReDO) project *Ecancermedicalscience* **8** 442
[38] Pantziarka P, Capistrano I R and De Potter A *et al* 2021 An open access database of licensed cancer drugs *Front. Pharmacol.* **12** 627574
[39] Nishimura Y, Tagawa M, Ito H and Tsuruma K *et al* 2017 Overcoming obstacles to drug repositioning in Japan *Front. Pharmacol.* **8** 729
[40] Thibodeaux C 2019 Repurposing researches: drugs, devices and diagnostic tests already approved for human uses. A Lecture Presented in Global Health Catalyst Summit, Win-Win session. 24 May, 2019 at Harvard Medical School, Boston, MA https://youtu.be/n5F2NfG9THo
[41] Elzawawy A M 2015 Could African and low- and middle-income countries contribute scientifically to global cancer care? *J. Glob. Oncol.* **1** 49–53
[42] Lo J A, Kawakubo M, Juneja V R and Su M Y *et al* Epitope spreading toward wild-type melanocyte-lineage antigens rescues suboptimal immune checkpoint blockade responses *Sci. Transl. Med.* **13** eabd8636
[43] Humer F B 2005 *Innovation in the pharmaceutical industry—future prospects* F. Hoffmann-La Roche Ltd 1–8
[44] Karamehic J, Ridic O and Ridic G *et al* 2013 Financial aspects and the future of the pharmaceutical industry in the United States of America *Mater. Sociomed.* **25** 286–90

Chapter 24

The opportunity to repurpose research in low- and lower–middle-income countries

Clare Thibodeaux PhD

Until recently, the process of repurposing drugs to treat patients with unsolved medical needs was well-known to healthcare stakeholders, but not to the general public. Now, the recent COVID-19 pandemic has brought repurposing into the public eye more than ever. This chapter presents the opportunities presented by repurposing research in low- and middle-income countries (LMICs).

24.1 Introduction

The news frequently contains stories about repurposed therapies that are being investigated for use in the treatment of COVID-19, from the steroid dexamethasone to the century-old BCG vaccine for tuberculosis. In fact, more than 1,000 clinical trials have tested repurposed drugs for the treatment of COVID-19 [1]. Clinicians and researchers who are turning to repurposing to treat COVID-19 are learning what other doctors and patients have known for years: drug repurposing can drive treatments to patients more quickly and less expensively than new drug development [2].

In the United States, doctors can prescribe any FDA-approved drug for their patients, regardless of whether that drug has been approved to treat the patient's condition. Such practice is called off-label use. Approximately 20% of all prescriptions written in the United States are written for an indication other than the approved indication [3], and off-label use is more common in the areas of mental health, pediatrics, and cancer [4]. Repurposing research from randomized controlled trials provides data for physicians and patients to consider when making decisions about off-label drug use. It can also help to generate the data necessary for regulatory agencies to approve a drug for a new indication, when appropriate.

Cures Within Reach (CWR) (www.cureswithinreach.org) is a philanthropic leader in leveraging the speed, safety, and cost-effectiveness of medical repurposing

doi:10.1088/978-0-7503-3075-6ch24

research, driving more treatments to more patients more quickly. Since 2009, CWR has been specifically focused on supporting drug, device, and nutraceutical repurposing research, funding over 100 projects at more than 60 different institutions worldwide. CWR is indifferent to geography, disease, and commercial value when it comes to funding repurposing research, and CWR works with its donors to focus on their specific interests.

CWR defines drug repurposing as testing therapies that have been approved by a regulatory agency for human use in a new indication. Regulatory agencies can include the U.S. Food and Drug Administration, the European Medicines Agency, or another such governmental body. On the other hand, CWR defines drug repositioning or rescue as finding a new use for a human-safe compound that has not yet gained regulatory approval.

While CWR funds repurposing research in any disease area, more than one-third of all its funded research has been in oncology, including brain, lung, prostate, blood, pancreatic, and thyroid cancers, in both adult and pediatric patients. In 2020 alone, CWR approved funding for five oncology repurposing projects, three in rare blood cancers, one in osteosarcoma and one in ovarian cancer. CWR's support of cancer repurposing goes beyond funding research. CWR has honored repurposing leaders in oncology through our annual Global Health Repurposing Awards and held events focused on patient education and bringing cancer research to the public.

Prior to 2019, CWR's funding supported research in North America and Europe. At the suggestion of one of its pharmaceutical company partners, CWR began to expand its repurposing model to diseases impacting LMICs, specifically to build capacity for clinical trial research in LMICs via repurposing. CWR began this initiative by holding a CureAccelerator Live! for the Developing World philanthropic pitch event in May 2019, in which researchers presented their repurposing clinical trials involving patients in LMICs. Five finalists were selected to participate in the event, and CWR funded both the winning project and the runner-up, which relate to malnutrition and dengue fever, respectively. CWR held CureAccelerator Live! for the Developing World the evening before Harvard's 2019 Global Health Catalyst Summit, and on the first day of the Summit, CWR shared its plans for the *Re*purposing *G*rants for the *R*est of the *W*orld (ReGRoW) funding program [5].

The need for ReGRoW stems from 'the 10/90 gap': fewer than 10% of global resources are dedicated to health problems that impact 90% of people worldwide [6]. In addition, only a small portion of global medical research funding is directed to LMICs [6]. CWR and its partners developed ReGRoW to provide repurposing research grants to clinicians and researchers in LMICs to build the capacity for clinical research *from within* the developing world and to find treatments *for* the developing world.

Finding repurposed drugs to treat unmet medical needs is especially important in LMICs, where access to medicines can be limited. For LMIC cancer patients in particular, this limited access leads to poorer quality of life and increased mortality [7]. Finding treatments that are inexpensive and available in-country is critical, not only for cancer patients but for patients of all diseases, and providing funding directly to LMICs allows researchers to solve local health problems locally.

CWR launched its pilot ReGRoW funding opportunity for repurposing clinical trials in December 2019. Researchers from any LMIC (as defined by the World Bank [8]) and at any career stage were eligible to apply. CWR sought investigator-initiated clinical trials utilizing off-patent drugs, nutraceuticals, or indigenous medicines with a budget of up to US$50,000. Submissions could investigate an unmet medical need in any disease area, and researchers were able to submit multiple applications.

As ReGRoW was the first time CWR actively engaged with researchers and institutions in the developing world, CWR worked with a number of organizations already engaged with LMICs to help with outreach. As a result, even with the ongoing COVID-19 pandemic, CWR received more than three times the number of expected proposal submissions, from 14 different countries spread over four continents. One-quarter of the submissions were in the field of cancer, the second most common disease area after infectious diseases. Following a review cycle of the initial proposals, the top-rated submissions, which included oncology projects, were invited to submit applications for full grants.

In August 2020, CWR selected the first three ReGRoW projects for funding. As of March 2021, CWR has begun funding these projects: 'Treating Tuberculosis with the Lipid-Lowering Drug Atorvastatin in Nigeria,' 'Testing the Safety of a Metal Poisoning Drug to Treat Snakebite in Kenya', and 'Improving Outcomes for the Rare Liver Disease Biliary Atresia with a Cancer Drug in Vietnam'. Although no oncology projects were selected for funding in the pilot ReGRoW phase, CWR has seen the opportunity repurposing research can bring to cancer patients in LMICs. In fact, one third of the proposal submissions CWR received in 2021 for Year 2 of ReGRoW were in oncology, more than any other disease area. CWR selected three ReGRoW projects for funding in Year 2, and CWR expects to select additional projects in late 2022 during Year 3 of ReGRoW. CWR looks forward to seeing more oncology submissions for ReGRoW, as well as any other eligible CWR calls for proposals.

Notes from the Editors:

- A video of a lecture 'Repurposing Researches: Drugs, Devices and Diagnostic tests already approved for human uses' presented by Clare Thibodeaux in the Global Health Catalyst Summit, Win-Win session. 24 May, 2019 at Harvard Medical School, Boston, MA, USA is available at: https://youtu.be/n5F2NfG9THo.
- To learn more about CWR funding opportunities or other CWR programs in the field of cancer, please visit the CWR website at https://cureswithinreach.org.

References

[1] Pantziarka P, Vandeborne L, Meheus L and Bouche G 2020 Covid19db – An online database of trials of medicinal products to prevent or treat COVID-19, with a specific focus on drug repurposing MedRxiv DOI: https://doi.org/10.1101/2020.05.27.20114371

[2] Pizzorno A, Padey B, Terrier O and Rosa-Calatrava M 2019 Drug repurposing approaches for the treatment of influenza viral infection: reviving old drugs to fight against a long-lived enemy *Front. Immunol.* **10** 531

[3] Wittich C, Burkle C and Lanier W 2012 ten common questions (and their answers) about off-label drug use *Mayo Clin. Proc.* **87** 982–90

[4] Saiyed M M, Ong P S and Chew L 2017 Off-label drug use in oncology: a systematic review of literature *J. Clin. Pharm. Ther.* **42** 251–8

[5] 2020 Repurposing Researches: Drugs, Devices and Diagnostic tests already approved for human uses https://youtu.be/n5F2NfG9THo

[6] Vidyasagar D 2006 Global notes: the 10/90 gap disparities in global health research *J. Perinatol.* **26** 55–6

[7] Ruff P, Al-Sukhun S, Blanchard C and Shulman L 2016 Access to cancer therapeutics in low- and middle-income countries *Am. Soc. Clin. Oncol. Educ. Book.* **35** 58–65

[8] 2020 The World Bank - The World by Income and Region http://datatopics.worldbank.org/world-development-indicators/the-world-by-income-and-region.html

IOP Publishing

Approaching Global Oncology
The win-win model
Ahmed Elzawawy and Wilfred Ngwa

Chapter 25

PredictCARE: personalized complication risk prediction tool

Elizabeth Charlotte Moser and Gayatri Nayaran

This chapter covers the use of promising technology toolkits in breast cancer care coordination and symptom management.

No breast cancer patient today receives only one treatment. Depending on her biological subtype, stage, age, co-morbidities, and family history, each patient has her own personalised journey in front of her, designed using pathology, surgery, radiation, drug treatment. Comprehensive breast cancer care is complex, making communication essential among all the different care providers. Digital tools can help to guide patients and their care teams, reducing waiting times and errors. Different tools are available for patients, administration, and medical staff; they can even involve family and friends. All tools can also create information overload; therefore, selection, repositioning, and guidance is needed for the right interpretation.

For patients, tools need to provide communication in two ways: their input results in the provision of advice or better planning. For care providers, tools need to give structured and weighted advice, reducing information overload. For caregivers, tools can help to organize appointments and information; however, patient decisions should be always respected.

Given the complexity of care, automatic AI-driven planning can facilitate scheduling; however, human intervention is still needed for psychosocial support and to tackle unexpected urgency.

In the complexity of information streams, AI can structure datasets, provide evidence-based decision tools, and guide personalized medicine and diagnostics; however, these are based on Western countries' care, as well as a relatively fit patient population. The translation of this technology to local populations requires the integration of local data insights into access to care.

doi:10.1088/978-0-7503-3075-6ch25

More research is needed to bring AI modeling into clinical practice and drive well-coordinated, patient-centered cancer care in the complex web of modern healthcare today.

This work was presented at the Global Health Catalyst Summit at Harvard Medical School, Boston, Ma, USA. The reader can view a video of the event at: https://youtu.be/hfKESocLapo.

Some notes

(1) Most cancer clinical trials and studies are conducted in Western countries.
(2) Most of these studies and trials in the US are performed on patients with stage-I and -II cancers and on patients who are fitter than many patients encountered in real daily practice. This is mostly contrary to the stages and fitness of real-life patients in LMICs.
(3) To prescribe a treatment protocol, not only should the responses be considered, but also cost-effectiveness, availability, risks, side-effects, and toxicities.
(4) The published data for treatment outcomes and guidelines focus on survival and disease progression; unfortunately, there is a lack of detailed data on toxicity.
(5) We advocate the need for studies in different communities; therefore, we should know about the side-effects and toxicities of cancer treatments among their patients, including real fitness conditions, disease stages, pathologies, ethnicities, co-morbidities, available healthcare for the management of toxicity, and socio-economic impact.

25.1 Background

Cancer care is complex, involving different diagnostics and treatments for one patient. Appointments need to be scheduled across different departments and clinics and are only found at large distance for many [1]. Patients are emotionally and physically affected by waiting times and communication errors between care providers [3–5]. Many (up to 80%) request a second opinion, involuntarily making their care path even more complex. Also, from the perspective of care providers, information streams are becoming overloaded, and digital tools need to structure information rather than adding to it. Information for patients, care providers, and caregivers can differ in its translation, accessibility, and storage. The development of digital tools requires data access, sharing, and translation for the the user and their context, especially for users outside the US [1, 2].

25.2 Care coordination optimization

To improve individual care coordination and symptom management, we need to unravel breast care management. To capture this in a working model, we simplify it into three facets, as follows: *clinical medicine* (what is needed, evidence-based, for each patient), *the approach to care* (the spectrum of patients' needs) and *system solutions* (human and machine support for the delivery goals) [3, 5].

Clinical medicine: Cancer care involves different types of specialty care and access to expensive diagnostics, drugs, and radiotherapy and surgery facilities. Often, genetic, palliative, and social counselling is required; ideally, all these are centrally discussed. National guidelines are the strong backbone of current tools and clinical practice today. As with all references, they are not always directly translatable to all patients. The integration of AI using local data related to access to certain treatments can tailor these tools further according to patient (local and genetic) profiles. Similar learning loops with local data could tackle the risk of toxicity and the availability of care. The largest datasets today are obtained from clinical trials performed in the US or Europe, as well as in relatively fit patient populations [3].

Approach to care: Translation to an individual patient always needs interpretation of the context and the specifics of that individual, such as social and financial status, which directly interfere with treatment compliance and access to care.

The allocations of treatment and consultations are not only medically driven (timing, sequencing) but also depend on the patient's capacity to understand, consent, travel, and pay [2–5].

System solutions: Automation tools will have to work in a two-way traffic mode that enables the system to consider medical and patient needs, which sometimes affect each other [5]. Information technology (IT) can facilitate this, but needs well-structured datasets to base positioning upon. In principle, IT models using information from historic cohorts can use AI to create planning systems that anticipate medical needs, estimate, and adjust to risks as well as a patient's decision/response facts. Ideally, future tools used for care coordination will take all the above factors into account, while allocating and guiding patients through their most suitable care path. Ideally, the model focuses on maximizing the combinatorial power of IT processing and the socio-psychological judgment of the human director steering the coordination [2].

Human intervention in this process is essential; emotional support as well as interpretation still has significant influence on planning, reporting, and guidance [3].

AI tools can help in estimating the urgency and requirements of exams and consultations to automatically plan care plans and perform allocation. However, scheduled appointments can only be automated to a certain extent; often, access to agendas and overbookings remains a human task [5]. Patient education is essential to retain flexibility and the ability to adapt to unexpected disease and toxicity dynamics.

25.3 Solvable barriers in allocation and timing

Since care coordination is of great interest to the patient him/herself, most existing tools work with a patient portal connected to the different data points. Within one network of care providers, communication and care planning can be streamlined; however, this does not permit the patient to consider opinions, examinations, or treatments that may be faster in neighboring or out-of-center consultations [2, 5].

Overall, good care coordination during active care can be facilitated by telemedicine, centralized data capture, and the alignment of care plans across centers and regional collaboration networks. Data analyses can be performed by creating anonymous cohorts that drive AI decisions and predictive risk tools [6–10]. The analysis of data by AI can uncover patterns of non-compliance, identifying potentially correctable issues with cost or distance (https://youtu.be/hfKESocLapo).

25.4 Symptom management

Poor care coordination during treatment is associated with medical errors, duplicated tests, a lack of supportive care and poor symptom control; high costs are the result [5].

25.4.1 Solvable barriers in symptom monitoring

The risk of toxicity is related to the specifics/dose and the accumulation of different treatments over time, but moreover, it depends on the condition, age, and co-morbidities of each patient. The time is ripe to use these data in AI-driven predictive tools. To keep symptom monitoring manageable, filters are critical. Scaling reported outcomes to cohorts of the same type can highlight severe signs that need urgent intervention [11].

25.5 Cautions

Computers can consider thrombocytopenia as a common factor, as well as distance to the hospital; the medical trade-off involved in weighing the factors that contribute to risk is an art learned over many years of training. AI systems may be overwhelmed with data if self-prediction algorithms run astray due to a software glitch. This issue implies that continuous monitoring of the model should be implemented in clinical practice, since not doing so can have grievous implications for patient care. In general, artificial neural networks are opaque, offering very little information about how they arrive at conclusions through hundreds of layers of information using deep learning. This creates a digital subconscious. Reaching the root cause of an AI problem will involve dismantling the neural network and targeting each nodal decision-making unit, consequently marginalizing patient care during that period. A certain fixed period is required for data collection, a process which is limited to specific patient cohorts in order to generate valuable outcomes using predictive models. Quality care will always need a combination of human intervention to decide upon the direction and a fast computing model to map the complex forest of risk factors that must be navigated [9–11].

25.6 Conclusions

The use of AI in breast cancer care management opens up an exciting research field. Facing a fast-increasing volume of patients, each with their specific traits and risks, we see the first potential of streamlining agendas and securing continuous follow-up. The associated data collection in a secure environment and AI-driven computing risk tools for tailoring treatment are tasks that can be developed further in the coming decade [6–11].

N.B. A video of the event is available at: https://youtu.be/hfKESocLapo [11].

References

[1] Gorin S S, Haggstrom D, Han P K J, Fairfield K M, Krebs P and Clauser S B 2017 Cancer care coordination: a systematic review and meta-analysis of over 30 years of empirical studies *Ann. Behav. Med.* **51** 532–46

[2] Ergu D, Kou G, Shi Y and Shi Y 2014 Analytic network process in risk assessment and decision analysis *Comput. Oper. Res.* **42** 58–74

[3] Clauser S B, Wagner E H, Ajello-Bowles E J, Tuzzio L and Greene S M 2011 Improving modern cancer care through information technology *Amer. J. of Prevent. Med.* **40** S198–S207

[4] Shao J, Rodrigues M, Corter A L and Baxter N N 2019 Multidisciplinary care of breast cancer patients: a scoping review of multidisciplinary styles, processes, and outcomes *Curr. Oncol.* **26** e385–97

[5] Mühlbauer V, Berger-Höger B, Albrecht M, Mühlhauser I and Steckelberg A 2019 Communicating prognosis to women with early breast cancer—overview of prediction tools and the development and pilot testing of a decision aid *BMC Health Serv. Res.* **19** 171

[6] Kukafka R, Fang J, Vanegas A and Silverman T 2018 Crew Pilot study of decision support tools on breast cancer chemoprevention for high-risk women and healthcare providers in the primary care setting *BMC Med. Inform. Decis. Mak.* **18** 134

[7] Collins I M *et al* 2016 iPrevent®: a tailored, web-based, decision support tool for breast cancer risk assessment and management *Breast Cancer Res. Treat.* **156** 171–82

[8] Bejnordi B E *et al* 2017 Diagnostic assessment of deep learning algorithms for detection of lymph node metastases in women with breast cancer *JAMA* **318** 2199–210

[9] Kann B H, Thompson R, Thomas C R, Dicker A and Aneja S 2019 Artificial intelligence in oncology: current applications and future directions *Oncology* **33** 46–53

[10] Kantarjian H and Yu P P 2015 Artificial intelligence, big data, and cancer *JAMA Oncol.* **1** 573–4

[11] Moser E C 2019 PredictCare: personalized complication predictor tool in oncology practice, Global Health Catalyst Summit at Harvard Medical School Boston, MA https://youtu.be/hfKESocLapo

Part IV

Mobilization of different resources, Win-Win collaborations and partnerships

Chapter 26

Engaging the diaspora to advance global health

Lydia Asana, Daivi Rodima-Taylor, Melvin Foote, Sulma Mohammed and Wilfred Ngwa

In recent years, the scientific literature has acknowledged the value that the diaspora brings to global development efforts. Diaspora populations are credited with both tangible and intangible remittances and are recognized as having a vested interest in the initiation, sustainability, and accountability of development projects in their countries of origin. Global health provides boundless opportunities for the diaspora to have a significant impact in saving and enhancing the lives of low- and middle-income country (LMIC) populations and to support the efforts of their adoptive nations, and it fulfils personal, often innate desires to give back to their original nations: a win-win-win. This chapter provides specific reasons for encouraging the diaspora to engage in global health as well as targeted ways in which this can be achieved, based on experiences at the Global Health Catalyst Summits.

For decades, the United States has been a world leader in global health; the government, academic institutions, industry, foundations, and non-profits make major investments in Africa and partner with African countries with considerable success, as shown by the President's Emergency Plan for AIDS Relief (PEPFAR) program [1, 2]. Now as more people survive HIV/AIDs and other diseases in Africa and live longer, non-communicable diseases (NCDs) such as cancer are on the rise and have become the leading cause of death [3]. The dramatic rise in the burden caused by NCDs has been described as a growing health iceberg, one hidden under epidemics of infectious disease that urgently needs to be addressed [4]. Because of this urgency and increasingly limited resources, there is growing need for new approaches to meet these rising challenges in global health. One approach that merits serious consideration is more purposeful engagement and partnership with the diaspora in global health. In this chapter we highlight *why* greater strategic engagement of the diaspora is important, and present key recommendations for *how* greater effective engagement of the African diaspora could turn brain drain and a negative history of slavery into global health gain. These recommendations were

doi:10.1088/978-0-7503-3075-6ch26

developed with the participation of hundreds of American- and European-based diaspora leaders, African ministers of health, ambassadors, and other global health leaders during global health meetings at Harvard Medical School from 2015–2019.

The rationale for engaging the diaspora in global health is multifold. First, diasporans are inherently transnational [5, 6]. Collaborative transnational action [7] is at the crux of global health's priority of improving health and achieving health equity for all people worldwide [8]. Arguably, no one is better suited for such transnational action than diasporans who simultaneously straddle two or more communities in localities across the globe and who leverage the necessary competencies, knowledge, and networks [6, 9] in ways that can significantly benefit both host and originating nations. For policymakers, this transnational attribute is a significant asset that can be harnessed to support more effective global health policies.

Moreover, for many diasporans, global health is intimately personal and local, as it is tied to identity, ancestry, and communal survival. Diasporans are affected in every global health crisis, and this is particularly true for Africans for whom *ubuntu* is part of their culture [10, 11]. Popularized worldwide by African Nobel Prize winners Desmond Tutu and Nelson Mandela, *ubuntu* signifies the idea that 'I am because we are', or human connectedness. The quintessence of this *ubuntu* in global health was evident at the height of the West African Ebola crisis in 2014 [12, 13]. When foreign nationals heeded prudent calls by their governments to leave Africa, many diaspora Africans living in the USA and Europe instead headed to Africa to support their original communities.

Furthermore, culture has been identified as a key challenge in global health [14]. Diasporans can be highly valuable here, proffering a greater appreciation of both host and sending country cultures. The intentional involvement of diaspora health professionals in global health offers opportunities to attend to such factors as cultural context, knowledge of local customs, and access to community gatekeepers. This can greatly influence local community buy-in, significantly enhancing global health projects. As an example, culture was critical in addressing the global health crisis of the African Ebola epidemic. In order to introduce safer mourning and burial practices, communication required sensitivity to the local culture, language, and religions of multiple localities to facilitate buy-in by affected communities [15].

Another challenge identified by global health leaders is that of financial resources. The diaspora can also be a major asset here, with tremendous financial potential that can be harnessed for global health. According to the World Bank Migration and Remittances Factsheet, over $595 billion was globally remitted before the last quarter of 2017, exceeding the $574 billion of 2016; almost 80% of all remittances flowed to LMICs [16]. For Africa, the value of the remittances from Africans in Diaspora (AiD) is greater than that of all foreign aid combined. Greater strategic engagement with the diaspora can direct more financial resources towards sustainable healthcare.

Beyond its financial potential, the diaspora is highly skilled; the African is diaspora recognized as one of the most educated populations in the USA. While these skills are evident in their communities of settlement, research also documents the application of these skills to social (intangible) remittances, as seen in leading philanthropic efforts serving their originating communities. For example, in a qualitative study of nonprofit organizations in Florida working in Africa, nearly one third of the leaders interviewed (CEOs, COOs, Directors) were diaspora Africans. The challenges identified by the participating nonprofit leaders included a lack of awareness of the local diaspora, a lack of diaspora representation within their networks, and minimal diaspora engagement in their work. However, among the most highly sought-after skills and traits were travel experience, cultural experience, high skill levels, genuine interest in, and commitment to the work of the organizations in Africa [17]. These are all qualities that abound amongst diaspora populations.

Given the above rationale for diaspora engagement in global health, participants at the Harvard Medical School meeting actively considered *how* such an engagement might be conceived, developed, and implemented. Table 26.1 highlights key recommendations from these meetings, along with the rationale and examples that show why the strategic implementation of such recommendations could have a significant impact in advancing global health.

26.1 Inviting diasporans to have a say in global health policy and programs affecting their original countries

According to Kerry *et al* [18], global health is largely an unappreciated partner of diplomacy or foreign policy. One recommendation put forward was that the diaspora be more actively engaged in shaping global health policies that affect their original communities. Such engagement should include government entities such as the United States House Foreign Affairs Subcommittee for the different regions. Currently, the Subcommittee for Africa covers Global Health, Global Human Rights, and International Organizations. A former member of the U.S. Congress participating in the Harvard meeting highlighted PEPFAR, as an idea that developed with significant input from the diaspora during his tenure in Congress. We recommend that more of this type of engagement should take place in the USA and other countries. Since such policies can be country specific, the USA and other high-income country (HIC) global health initiatives at the government level are also encouraged to more actively partner with the diaspora of the specific LMIC countries. This level of strategic diaspora engagement in global health could lead to other high-impact initiatives similar to 'PEPFAR' for cancer and other NCDs, which are currently tearing through Africa [19].

26.2 Using an entrepreneurial model for diaspora engagement in global health

Another recommendation put forward was that ministries of health in disaspora-originating countries should incentivize diaspora participation in strengthening healthcare systems and engage the diaspora in public–private partnerships (PPP). At the Harvard meeting, potential areas for PPP discussed included a universal

Table 26.1. Recommendations for greater effective diaspora engagement in global health.

Recommendations for greater effective diaspora engagement in global health	Rationale	Examples of replication, improvement, or scale-up
Inviting diaspora input in global health policy and programs affecting their original countries	• The diaspora is inherently transnational, with a better appreciation of both host and original country interests and culture	United States House Foreign Affairs Subcommittee on Africa, Global Health, Global Human Rights, and International Organizations engaging the diaspora
Using an entrepreneurial model for diaspora engagement in global health	• Win-win-win, profitable for sending countries, host countries, and the diaspora • Sustainable global health and development	DHI in Nigeria allows AiD to purchase a designated health insurance plan for family
Purposeful involvement of the diaspora in global health activities: events, funding, multicentre clinical trials, disease prevention	• Increased global health partners, funding, impact • Increased trust, diversity, and participation in clinical trials or disease prevention activity with LMICs	USA institutions involving diaspora professors in their institutions in culturally sensitive cancer prevention awareness education
Publish *au courant* searchable diaspora databases with diaspora organization profiles and global health opportunities	• Getting to know diaspora global health stakeholders • Making it easy to find and connect with diaspora organizations with similar global health interests	IdEA's interactive searchable database by USAID, which elevates and supports the work of diaspora communities around the world.
Increase collaboration between the ministries of health (and their embassies) and the diaspora and HIC global health programs	• Continuous dialogue with the diaspora to build trust and set common global health collaboration goals	Rwanda Ministry of Health working with USA embassy has lead to increased opportunities and global health support for Rwanda
Use ICT to engage the diaspora and facilitate their participation in telemedicine, online education, and co-mentored e-research	• Bridge space–time barriers to global health • Increased participation in global health • Turn brain drain to global health gain	American institutions/hospitals in continuous medical education online courses and task-shifted telemedicine with LMIC institutions involving diaspora

AiD=Africans in Diaspora; IdEA=International diaspora Engagement Alliance; USAID=U.S. Agency for International Development; DHI=Diaspora Health Initiative; ICT=information and communications technology; HIC=high-income country.

Health Insurance Scheme that involves AiD in partnership with their ministries of health. This would allow diasporans to pay the premiums for beneficiaries (e.g., family members or friends) in Africa, and make such a scheme more viable for quality healthcare for all. Initiatives such as Diaspora Health Services (DHI) in Nigeria and UAP-connect have emerged to provide the opportunity for diaspora Africans in the USA, Canada, UK, and other HICs to purchase a designated health insurance plan for family members in their home countries. It is recommended that such schemes be encouraged and enhanced by working with the ministries of health. This would increase impact and sustainability and could include life insurance as well as covering telemedicine, as further discussed below.

Another PPP area discussed was that of diaspora bonds, which have been proposed by the Lancet Oncology Commission as a potential avenue to support the establishment of start-up cost-intensive radiotherapy services needed for the treatment of more than 50% of cancer patients in LMICs [20]. New PPP areas of global health that could significantly benefit both LMICs and HICs include phytomedicines. PPPs to develop this sector would enable the development of new low-cost medicines with consequential increased access to medicines. As an example, a collaboration with USA-based institutions is developing plant-derived cannabinoids delivered using smart biomaterials to avoid the psychotic side-effects that have hampered clinical translation [21]. Many agree that such collaborations could allow the development of the increased effective use and adoption of low-cost phytomedicines in closing disparities such as the global pain divide [22].

26.3 Purposeful involvement of the diaspora in global health activities

A challenge identified by global health leaders is that of finding appropriate partners to work with in LMICs. A recommendation was that global health programs in the USA and other HICs should purposefully engage diaspora organizations in their local regions, invite diaspora leaders/celebrities to global health events and funding proposals benefiting their original countries. Global health event participation provides opportunities for diaspora leaders to share, network, and collaborate with others from academic institutions, industry, and other global health organizations with which their interests or mission statements align. Win-win collaborations could include joint funding proposals. Diaspora-crowdfunded global health research projects and training fellowships have already been reported as outcomes of engagement between the diaspora and some American institutions [14]. Purposefully including diaspora health professionals in multicenter clinical trials and disease prevention programs that involve their original LMICs is also encouraged.

26.4 Establish *au courant* searchable databases with diaspora organization profiles and global health opportunities

Another recommendation is to develop searchable databases on global health program websites with profiles of diaspora organizations from specific LMICs with interests in global health areas. This could be synergized with that of the International diaspora Engagement Alliance (IdEA), a USAID-supported organization that promotes diaspora-centered initiatives in countries and regions of diaspora origin [23]. The availability of such a resource that would provide an interactive map of who does what and where would be very valuable in advancing global health collaborations.

26.5 Developing regular communication between ministries of health and embassies, academic institutions, and diaspora groups

A further recommendation is for LMIC ministries of health and their corresponding embassies abroad to engage high-income country institutions and their diaspora in ongoing dialogue to identify areas in which they could continually work together, and also recruit their participation in strengthening the healthcare system. The annual Global Health Catalyst summit has provided a platform for such global health dialogue. An excellent recent example is that of Rwanda, where diaspora leaders worked together with the Rwandan Embassy in Washington and the Rwandan Ministry of Health on global health that benefits Rwanda, including commitments from American and German Institutions to train oncology health professionals in Rwanda over the next five years, participation in ICT-powered multicenter clinical trials, support for the new Rwanda Military Hospital's clinical oncology, and other global health activities. Regular communication will build trust and should employ multiple media, such as social media, radio, churches, and other worship centers in medical missions for global health [24, 25]. In a laudable initiative, the African Union Mission in Washington has recently launched a radio station for communications with diasporans and American institution leaders [26]. This provides an opportunity for communications and the active engagement of diasporans in global health.

26.6 Employing advanced information and communications technology

A sixth recommendation is to invest significantly in the use of advanced information and communications technology (ICT) to engage the diaspora and leverage their contribution to global health. Like many healthcare professionals at American institutions, many diasporans desire to participate in global health but may not be able to travel to LMICs for reasons of distance and time. However, they may have one hour a week to teach a course online, consult a patient, provide a second opinion, or participate in research. The use of ICTs can overcome these distance–time barriers and allow for the major pooling of a substantial diaspora contribution in global health through task-shifted telemedicine, online education, and ICT-powered research and advocacy. The approach of using ICT to bridge space–time barriers in global health provides an enormous opportunity to allow the highly educated/skilled diaspora to more easily contribute to their originating countries, turning brain drain to global health gain. Already there is effort to involve diaspora

African health professionals in the USA and Europe in a major tele-oncology initiative that could significantly increase access to quality cancer care, research, and education in Africa.

In perspective, as cancer and other NCDs tear through Africa, it is time to seriously ponder a more purposeful and strategic engagement of the diaspora as a major global health stakeholder and a part of global health policy. In so doing, the potential loss of opportunities, resources, and most importantly lives can be mitigated. As seen in the successful engagement and sustained involvement of the diaspora in the Global Health Catalyst endeavors, the intentional engagement of the diaspora can support, enhance, and sustain independent diaspora efforts, contribute to effective implementation of collaborative initiatives, provide a sustained improvement in the quality of life, and ultimately save lives for LMIC populations served. In short, the purposeful engagement of the diaspora results in win-win-win outcomes with gains for the diaspora; for policy, institutional, industrial, and organizational partners; and for the at risk populations at the heart of global health efforts. The recommendations highlighted in this chapter provide a reference for developing such engagement in the USA and other HICs to advance global health, reducing global health disparities and saving lives.

Conflicts of interest

We declare that we have no conflicts of interest.

Note from the Editors:

For further relevant reading on how diaspora is one of the present resources for Africa; chapter 5 in the book: *Mobilization of Resources for Cancer Care Services in Low- and Middle-Income Countries and Africa: Myths, Realities, and Hopes* by Ahmed Elzawawy.

References

[1] Katz I T, Bassett I V and Wright A A 2013 PEPFAR in transition—implications for HIV care in South Africa *N. Engl. J. Med.* **369** 1385–7

[2] Dzau V, Fuster V, Frazer J and Snair M 2017 Investing in global health for our future *N. Engl. J. Med.* **377** 1292–6

[3] Nyirenda M J 2016 Non-communicable diseases in sub-Saharan Africa: understanding the drivers of the epidemic to inform intervention strategies *Int. Heal.* **8** 157–8

[4] Naghavi M and Forouzanfar M H 2013 Burden of non-communicable diseases in sub-Saharan Africa in 1990 and 2010: Global Burden of Diseases, Injuries, and Risk Factors Study 2010 *Lancet* **381** S95

[5] Brinkerhoff J M 2009 *Digital Diasporas: Identity and Transnational Engagement* (Cambridge: Cambridge University Press)

[6] Mahroum S and De Guchteneire P 2006 Transnational knowledge through diaspora networks editorial *Int. J. Multicult. Soc.* **8** 1–3 www.unesco.org/shs/ijms/vol8/issue1/ed

[7] Beaglehole R and Bonita R 2010 What is global health? *Glob. Health Action* **3** 1–2

[8] Koplan J P, Bond T C and Merson M H *et al* 2009 Towards a common definition of global health *Lancet* **373** 1993–5

[9] Wojczewski S, Poppe A and Hoffmann K *et al* 2015 Diaspora engagement of African migrant health workers – examples from five destination countries *Glob. Health Action* **8** 29210

[10] Falola T and Essien K (ed) 2013 *Pan-Africanism, and the Politics of African Citizenship and Identity* (Abingdon: Routledge)

[11] Ngwa W, Ngoma T and Zietman A *et al* 2016 Closing the cancer divide through ubuntu: information and communication technology-powered models for global radiation oncology *Int. J. Radiat. Oncol. Biol. Phys.* **94** 440–9

[12] WHO Ebola Response Team 2014 Ebola virus disease in West Africa—the first 9 months of the epidemic and forward projections *N. Engl. J. Med.* **371** 1481–95

[13] Dzau V J and Rodin J 2015 Creating a global health risk framework *N. Engl. J. Med.* **373** 991–3

[14] Ngwa W and Ngoma T 2016 *Emerging Models for Global Health in Radiation Oncology.* (Bristol, UK and Philadelphia, PA: IOP Publishing)

[15] Frieden T R and Damon I K 2015 Ebola in West Africa—CDC's role in epidemic detection, control, and prevention *Emerg. Infect. Dis.* **21** 1897–905

[16] The World Bank 2017 Migration and remittances data https://www.worldbank.org/en/topic/migrationremittancesdiasporaissues/brief/migration-remittances-data

[17] Asana L 2018 Inclusion of the African diaspora in florida nonprofit organizations *PhD Dissertation* Walden University https://scholarworks.waldenu.edu/dissertations/4905/

[18] Bradford Kerry V, Auld S and Farmer P 2010 An international service corps for health—an unconventional prescription for diplomacy *N. Engl. J. Med.* **363** 1199–201

[19] McNeil D 2017 As cancer tears through Africa, drug makers draw up a battle plan *New York Times* https://nytimes.com/2017/10/07/health/africa-cancer-drugs.html

[20] Atun R, Jarrray D A, Barton M B and Bray F *et al* 2015 Expanding global access to radiotherapy *Lancet Oncol.* **16** 1153–86

[21] Ngwa W, Kumar R, Moreau M, Dabney R and Herman A 2017 Nanoparticle drones to target lung cancer with radiosensitizers and cannabinoids *Front. Oncol.* **7** 208

[22] Knaul F M, Farmer P E, Bhadelia A, Berman P and Horton R 2015 Closing the divide: the Harvard Global Equity Initiative-Lancet Commission on global access to pain control and palliative care *Lancet* **386** 722–4

[23] Wittingen K 2016 Engaging diasporas in development and diplomacy https://businessfightspoverty.org/engaging-diaspora-in-development-and-diplomacy/

[24] Dodson J E 2011 African diaspora studies and religion *OFO: J. Transatl. Stud.* **1** 3–26 https://www.bgsu.edu/content/dam/BGSU/college-of-arts-and-sciences/africana-studies/documents/ofo-volume-1-number-1.pdf

[25] Adogame A 2010 *Religion Crossing Boundaries: Transnational Religious and Social Dynamics in Africa and the New African Diaspora* ed J V Spickard (Leiden: Brill)

[26] African U 2018 African Union Washington https://au.int/en/washingtonmission

IOP Publishing

Approaching Global Oncology
The win-win model
Ahmed Elzawawy and Wilfred Ngwa

Chapter 27

Win-win in Latin America. Collaboration with the Latin American and Caribbean Society of Medical Oncology. Partnerships and projects

Eduardo Cazap

Multifaceted cancer control systems are often lacking or poorly developed in resource-poor settings, despite the fact that such systems can play a vital role in the prevention and management of the ever-growing cancer burden for their populations. With the advent of COVID-19, initiatives aiming to establish collaborative cancer control programs have been hampered. This chapter chronicles the collaborative efforts in Latin America to establish cancer control parameters and highlights the added burden that COVID-19 has imposed on cancer control efforts.

27.1 Introduction

The Latin American and Caribbean Society of Medical Oncology (SLACOM) is an academic entity that consists of different cancer control specialists who have a comprehensive vision for combatting cancer, which includes acknowledging the multifaceted nature of the problem and understanding that the current international approach requires the problem to be faced from diverse perspectives, including education, research, primary prevention, secondary prevention, correct and timely diagnosis and appropriate treatment, as well as palliative care, access to morphine, end-of-life care, and survivorship.

These aspects must be strongly integrated with health systems and the appropriate public policies in the Latin American region. SLACOM acts as an integrated network of centres, experts, public and private institutions, and leaders in the region, together with civil society as a whole, to reduce the incidence and increase the curability of human cancers [1].

The win-win initiative is a leading-edge collaborative initiative pioneered by Professor Ahmed Elzawawy as a model for successful collaborations in which all stakeholders win, especially patients [2]

doi:10.1088/978-0-7503-3075-6ch27

After initial development in African countries and with a strong partnership with the Global Health Catalyst (GHC) summit, the Win-Win Initiative launched an expansion into the Latin American region.

SLACOM developed a series of projects, aligned with the win-win objectives, which we describe in the following examples. These cases demonstrate that coordinated action, working in conjunction with national, regional, or international organizations, can be implemented in underserved regions for the improvement of cancer control. Moreover, such examples can be extrapolated to other countries or regions of the world with similar capabilities and challenges.

27.1.1 The Integrated Cancer Control Initiative in Latin America

Launched in 2019, the Integrated Cancer Control Initiative in Latin America (ICCI-LA) is a first-of-its kind comprehensive policy study of health systems' responses to cancer control in four countries in Latin America—Argentina, Brazil, Chile, and Colombia.

This project is a joint effort of the Harvard T. H. Chan School of Public Health, Boston, USA; the Princess Margaret Cancer Centre, Canada; the Institute of the Americas, University of Miami; the Union for International Cancer Control (UICC), Geneva, Switzerland; and SLACOM (the Sociedad Latinoamericana y del Caribe de Oncología Médica).

In the first case study, the aim of the Integrated Cancer Control Initiative in Latin America (ICCI-LA) is to help improve Argentina's response to the rising burden of cancer, as part of its constitutional commitment to health as a human right and as part of the international push for universal health coverage. A final report discusses the overall context of the Argentinian health system as it relates to cancer, presents the major health system challenges identified by stakeholders, and identifies policy options proposed by the leading experts involved in the ICCI-LA study [3].

The highest-priority recommendations of the study include:

1. Develop and enact a comprehensive National Cancer Law (policies).
2. Strengthen the entities responsible for developing cancer policies, conducting evaluations, and implementing the national cancer plan.
3. Conduct transparent cost-effectiveness analysis to better delineate cancer policy goals and allocated resources for cancer services.

27.1.2 The Network of Latin American Cancer Institutes and Institutions–SLACOM partnership

Cancer is a challenge for most societies and governments in the Latin American region. This situation is becoming increasingly complex and relevant due to the disease's increasing incidence and mortality, mainly in low- and middle-income populations.

In addition to this, the current pandemic crisis related to COVID-19 severely affects healthcare systems and economies, making many cancer control actions even more challenging to implement or causing costly, and in some cases life-threatening, delays.

Under this changing scenario, it is imperative to develop rapid and efficient responses, coordinate actions, implement the proper strategies to adapt cancer programs, and create new ones that can feasibly be to put into practice in real-world scenarios at the country level, with coherent and scientifically valid regional considerations.

The integration of an outstanding group of experts with the collaboration of leading cancer institutions of the region in a coordinated strategy will increase capabilities, develop and implement regional programs and projects, and promote better cancer control at the country and regional levels.

In this partnership, the Network of Latin American Cancer Institutes and Institutions (RINC) provides its network of leading institutions and cancer experts and SLACOM provides a centralized operating office, a strategic plan, and partnerships with the leading international cancer organizations.

27.1.3 The Latin American and Caribbean code against cancer—developing evidence-based recommendations to reduce the risk of cancer in the region

In order to develop evidence-based recommendations to reduce the risk of cancer in Latin America and the Caribbean (LAC), recommendations from the 4th edition of the European Code against Cancer (http://cancer-code-europe.iarc.fr/index.php/en/) will serve as the foundation for adapting, updating, and creating new recommendations tailored to the LAC region, taking into account specific risk factors and the cancer burden, regional settings, and health systems [4]. The recommendations will have two levels:

LEVEL 1—A set of region-specific recommendations targeted to the individual and the community but linked to known cost-effective policies that need to be in place to comply with the recommendations, making the policymakers an indirect target group of the LAC Code (with reference to worldwide authoritative sources of cancer prevention policies such as the WHO Best Buys, the World Cancer report, the Disease Control Priorities report—DCP3—, the International Agency for Research on Cancer (IARC)/WHO Global Report on Cancer, and Pan-American Health Organization (PAHO) Country situation analysis reports).

LEVEL 2—Online training for health professionals in the topics covered by the recommendations.

For the LAC adaptation of the cancer prevention recommendations, a coalition of Latin American institutions, including the RINC, the SLACOM, and the Asociación Latina e Ibérica Contra el Cáncer (ALICC), together with international organizations (the PAHO/WHO and IARC/WHO), united to work for cancer prevention and promote collaborations in the region, will collaborate on a joint project to collect, analyse, and promote the scientific evidence and significance of the cancer prevention recommendations as a package that is appropriate for the LAC context. The IARC methodology will be used to develop the recommendations [5].

27.1.4 Latin American Report about the COVID-19 pandemic and the impact on cancer control

The COVID-19 pandemic has challenged health services worldwide. The difficulties of both affected and unaffected populations in facing the COVID-19 pandemic have negative consequences for some aspects of the population's health. Moreover, the negative effects, direct and indirect, sectoral (health) and intersectoral, affect the overall health of the population.

The necessary measures implemented by health providers to reduce the risks associated with attending health centers have involved postponing health controls, including screening studies for early detection, face-to-face consultations and treatments due to the risks of infection complications or potential critical care requirements. In addition, physical isolation measures can have destructive effects on healthy habits and behaviors, resulting in the 'unlearning' or 'decoupling' of healthy lifestyles. This can also lead to serious economic effects due to the generation of poverty, a key determinant of disease. This may indicate that the morbidity and mortality of cancer—and other non-communicable diseases—will skyrocket in the coming months and will far outnumber the evils of the pandemic itself. Likewise, as a consequence of diagnoses in more advanced stages of the disease, the costs of care are very likely to increase significantly. From the intersectoral point of view, it is worth noting the possible absence of a resurgence of public transport when considering the accessibility of the most vulnerable people to health services.

The impact and variability of these determinants in Latin American countries is unknown, as is the damage they may generate. The objective of the report is to discover whether the COVID-19 pandemic has changed the morbidity, mortality, monitoring and control of cancer in selected countries in Latin America. To this end, an observational study is designed to quantify the temporal variations in indicators of the level of cancer control in eight Latin American countries.

Argentina, Brazil, Chile, Colombia, Honduras México, Perú and Uruguay participated and each country provided a team of epidemiologists, policymakers, health economists, and clinicians.The report was due to be finalized in September 2020 [6].

References

[1] Slacom home page https://www.slacom.org

[2] The GHC win-win initiative www.icedoc.org/winwin.htm and www.icedoc.net/winwin.htm

[3] UICC, Novartis 2020 Addressing the rising burden of cancer in Argentina: Challenges & opportunities https://www.uicc.org/resources/addressing-rising-burden-cancer-argentina-challenges-opportunities

[4] Espina C *et al* 2018 Toward the world code against cancer *J. Glob. Oncol.* **4** 1–8

[5] Cazap E *et al* 2019 Latin America and the Caribbean code against cancer *J. Glob. Oncol.* **5** 1–3

[6] Cazap E Personal communication—unpublished

IOP Publishing

Approaching Global Oncology
The win-win model
Ahmed Elzawawy and Wilfred Ngwa

Chapter 28

Collaboration with the European Society of Surgical Oncology

Riccardo A Audisio and Tibor Kovacs

The role of surgery in oncology is not an independent alternative to other modes of treatment. Rather, it is best employed alongside an understanding of the other clinical oncology avenues with the best outcomes stemming from collaborative interactions with diverse teams of stakeholders, including the patient and caregivers. Similarly, surgical oncology as a discipline is not meant to be a standalone discipline of study, but one that is interwoven with research that includes contextual considerations. This chapter further develops these ideas, based on the experiences and recommendations of the *European Society of Surgical Oncology* (ESSO).

ESSO has been supporting the science and practice of surgical oncology since 1981, for the benefit of cancer patients.

This has been delivered through a number of activities: ESSO organises a range of activities and educational events, including the largest convention on surgical oncology in Europe, which connects a network of 20,000 individuals and corporate members. ESSO provides constant and up-to-date e-learning as well as courses and is the co-owner of the *European Journal of Surgical Oncology* (EJSO). The Journal is very receptive to projects focusing on low- and middle-income countries (LMICs), and scientific advancements from these geographical areas are prioritized [1].

The European Society of Surgical Oncology has been making several fellowship programs available to facilitate cultural exchanges and to forge connections and scientific interactions across countries and continents, offering specific opportunities to young cancer surgeons and surgical colleagues from developing countries to attend the ESSO Congress. When sponsors are available (local/regional, African Royal Colleges, the Merck Foundation, and others), ESSO has committed itself to allocating fellows to training programs with observational facilities at several European centres of excellence. The available network is very broad and covers all disciplines of cancer surgery (upper gastro-intestinal (UGI), breast, colorectal,

doi:10.1088/978-0-7503-3075-6ch28

hepato-ancreatic-biliary (HPB), sarcoma, melanoma, peritoneal disease, thoracic, neuro-oncology, gynae-oncology, and uro-oncology).

It comes as no surprise that ESSO has been extremely supportive of the 'Win-win Collaboration for Global Health', which has the aim of improving the knowledge and practice of cancer surgery internationally and especially in LMICs, where the risk of falling ill with a malignant disease it is nearly the same as the risk of dying from it.

ESSO is keen to contribute in LMICs through the five streams clearly framed in its mission statement [2]. An active research platform is accessible to all its members in order to improve education and advocacy; this is intended to achieve excellence in patient care at an international level (figure 28.1).

Jointly with the Harvard Open University, ESSO has established a series of web-based lectures, followed by question and answer sessions.

Cancer research is the foundation of good clinical practice in oncology. It has undoubtedly been demonstrated that incorporated oncological research is a proxy for better cancer outcomes [3]. Unfortunately, LMICs are insufficiently involved in research; therefore, ESSO is dedicated to bridging the gap and joining forces with countries interested in developing their surgical and research programs. ESSO fosters quality cancer research in LMICs and is committed to providing know-how on this topic. All available funds and research proposals (e.g. AORTIC and others) are encouraged to join with ESSO in order to achieve the most relevant scientific outcomes and highest visibility.

Surgical oncology is not intended to be a particular technical skill; rather, it is up-to-date, evidence-based knowledge which is founded on the true multidisciplinary

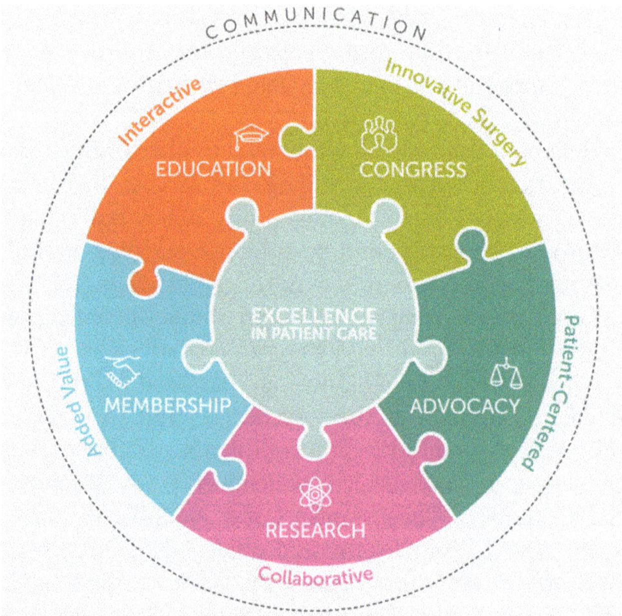

Figure 28.1. ESSO's mission and vision. Adapted from [2]. Copyright 2016 ESSO (European Society of Surgical Oncology).

management of cancer patients. As our curriculum clearly demonstrates [4, 5], the surgical management of cancer patients requires insights into chemo-, immuno-, hormonal- and radiation therapy; plus a deep knowledge of genetics, pathology, palliative care, nursing, and imaging. The incorporation of modern adjuvant curative plans and the administration of pre-operative treatments make a significant difference in terms of long-term prognosis and quality of life.

In addition to the concept of surgical oncology as a general specialty, ESSO has developed specialist training in the fields of peritoneal disease [6] and soft-tissue sarcomas [7]. Recently, ESSO contributed to the establishment of Breast Surgical Oncology (BRESO) project team to bring together all the necessary skills for the education of breast cancer specialists [8]. BRESO is a team within ESSO that works to promote accredited specialist breast surgical care for breast cancer patients and women at high risk of breast cancer.

The vision of BRESO is for all women affected by breast cancer to be treated by specialists trained and accredited in breast surgical oncology, instead of a general surgeon who occasionally practices breast cancer surgery. BRESO promotes the highest quality and most innovative, evidence-based breast cancer care. It intends to develop the highest standards of breast surgical oncology in a multidisciplinary setting, so that women can benefit from the best available care, no matter which country they live in. A partnership with colleagues and societies from LMICs could be extremely helpful.

The ultimate goal of ESSO is to satisfy cancer patients' needs and requests; therefore, patients' representatives and advocates are welcomed to join in and assist in targeting those issues which are most relevant to cancer patients. It has been noted that targets and aims might vary according to geographical and cultural background; it is thus necessary to prioritize research efforts and projects according to the specific needs of each individual background.

References

[1] Wiafe B A, Karekezi C, Jaklitsch M T and Audisio R A 2020 Perspectives on surgical oncology in Africa. *Eur. J. Surg. Oncol.* **46** 3–5

[2] ESSO mission statement essoweb.org

[3] Are C, Yanala U, Malhotra G, Hall B, Smith L, Cummings C, Lecoq C, Wyld L, Audisio R A and Berman R S 2018 Global curriculum in research literacy for the surgical oncologist *Eur. J. Surg. Oncol.* **44** 31–42

[4] Are C, Caniglia A, Malik M, Cummings C, Lecoq C, Berman R, Audisio R and Wyld L 2016 Jun Variations in training of surgical oncologists: proposal for a global curriculum *Ann Surg Oncol.* **23** 1769–81

[5] Van der Hage J, Sandrucci S and Audisio R 2021 The ESSO core curriculum committee update on surgical oncology **47** e1–30

[6] https://www.essoweb.org/school-of-peritoneal-surface-oncology-es/

[7] https://www.essoweb.org/european-school-of-sts/

[8] https://www.essoweb.org/about/breso/

IOP Publishing

Approaching Global Oncology
The win-win model
Ahmed Elzawawy and Wilfred Ngwa

Chapter 29

Partnership with *e*cancer

Eduardo Cazap, Danny Burke, Lara Finan and Katie Foxall

In order to achieve sustainable gains in combatting the growing cancer burden, particularly for low- and middle-income countries (LMICs), it is imperative that diverse sectors not only acknowledge, but also take ownership of impactful ways of contributing to addressing the global cancer challenges within their sectors. In this chapter, *e*cancer illustrates the value and possibilities of this truth by sharing its concerted, collaborative efforts to promote access to global cancer education and credible literary resources in the publication sector and beyond.

29.1 Global oncology is an evolving field with significant implications for world health

New approaches that define how existing health infrastructure can be adapted to resource-appropriate use are needed but mostly unreported. The dissemination of innovative and applicable global cancer information is a fundamental component in the *e*cancer endeavour. As physicians and investigators, it is our responsibility to alert our colleagues and the world to the epidemic of cancer in the coming years and to apply pressure to governments and society as a whole for urgent action to support cancer control [1].

Nevertheless, even sophisticated and highly renowned publications are insufficient to manage the enormous amount of information that exists today. To this end, partnerships are a tool that can increase the visibility of data; in this regard, the development and implementation of innovative and accessible educational platforms is vital to pursue these objectives as well as a means to avoid duplications and gaps.

*e*cancer is a charity whose mission is to raise the standards of care for cancer patients across the world through education. Its ethos is to support global healthcare professionals so that every patient will receive the best possible care. This is achieved by providing free and high-quality educational resources through the website ecancer.org, which includes an open-access peer-reviewed journal, thousands of

doi:10.1088/978-0-7503-3075-6ch29

video interviews with key experts, accredited e-learning, and the latest news. *e*cancer also runs educational meetings, predominantly in LMICs and contributes to international research into the improvement of cancer care.

29.2 *e*cancer recognizes the importance of successful collaboration

*e*cancer is proud to work alongside the Win-Win Initiative, as they share a joint recognition of the importance of successful collaborations. All of *e*cancer's educational initiatives are developed and run in partnership with experts and organisations who provide local expertise and ensure the highest-quality education for different audiences and settings across the world. The organisation's success is based on fruitful collaborations with organisations such as the Union for International Cancer Control (UICC), the African Organisation for Research and Training in Cancer (AORTIC), the National Cancer Grid of India, the Latin American and Caribbean Society of Medical Oncology (SLACOM), and many more.

*e*cancer's open-access peer-reviewed journal, *e*cancermedicalscience, supports oncology professionals worldwide in publishing their research and helps them to access the information they need to get the best outcomes for their patients. The journal particularly focuses on publishing research from under-resourced settings and LMICs, as this group of authors and readers is often marginalised by the international publishing industry. *e*cancer strongly believes that cost should not be a barrier to having research published; therefore, the journal operates a 'pay what you can afford' model in which the costs of publishing are supported by the charity, and actively encourages and supports international collaborations to help increase the number of authors from LMICs.

As an organisation, *e*cancer recognises that there is a major inequity in the availability of high-quality local data and research from LMICs compared to that from high-income countries and wants to lead the way in reducing this imbalance. *e*cancer believes that journal publishers have a duty to work towards increasing the number of authors from LMICs and to ensure that this research is freely available to all. This is vital in order to ensure that governments, organisations, and healthcare professionals across the world have access to high-quality local data and research to develop robust cancer-control policies and treatment guidelines and can make evidence-based decisions to ensure that every patient receives the best possible care.

A survey of oncology professionals from LMICs carried out by *e*cancer in early 2019 found that the majority of the 85 respondents (78%) had faced barriers in getting their research published, due to a lack of funding, inadequate research techniques, geographical bias, or linguistic difficulties. Eighty-five percent had faced problems accessing the latest research and guidelines in order to be able to treat their patients. It is vital to recognise and address these inequalities, especially in the light of their likely expansion in the coming years; as such, the World Cancer Declaration calls for the provision of innovative education and for the training of healthcare professionals to improve significantly, particularly in LMICs [2]. For example, Africa has 25% of the global burden of disease but only 3% of the world's healthcare workforce [3], and 80% of global cancer deaths occur in LMICs but only 5% of total global spending on cancer care is expended in these regions. *e*cancer's aim, in partnership with global organisations, is to increase the number of authors and the volume of research from LMICs, which will help to address any lack of awareness among policymakers and other stakeholders concerning the magnitude of the current and future cancer burden, its expected impact and the best way to tackle these challenges.

As a founding member of the Win-Win initiative and the editor-in-chief of *e*cancermedicalscience, Dr Eduardo Cazap saw an opportunity for the two organisations to work in partnership with each other to realise their common aims. Dr Cazap invited Danny Burke, CEO of *e*cancer, to attend the 2019 Harvard Global Health Catalyst Summit, where he participated in a discussion on the topic of how international journals can support the publication of LMIC research, as well as conducting interviews with the key speakers, which can be found at this link: https://ecancer.org/en/conference/1164-global-health-catalyst-summit-harvard.

*e*cancer will continue to pursue global collaborations to develop free and high-quality educational resources for oncology professionals in LMICs and across the world. If you would like to discuss the opportunities, please get in touch at info@ecancer.org so that we can continue to strive towards a world where every cancer patient receives the best possible care.

References

[1] Cazap E and Anderson B 2016 Vision for the global health and cancer section *Oncologist* **21** 521–2

[2] UICC World Cancer Declaration 2013 https://www.uicc.org/sites/main/files/atoms/files/131119_UICC_WorldCancerDeclaration_2013_1.pdf

[3] Anyangwe S C E and Mtonga C 2007 Inequities in the global health workforce: the greatest impediment to health in sub-Saharan Africa *Int. J. Environ. Res. Public Health* **4** 93–100

IOP Publishing

Approaching Global Oncology
The win-win model
Ahmed Elzawawy and Wilfred Ngwa

Chapter 30

Perspectives from the Balkans

Bashkim Ziberi, Gazmend Nafezi, Ilir Ismaeli, Suzana Manxhuka-Këliu, Ana Ugrinska, Shaban Memeti, Vildane Goga çmega, Arben Bislimi and Wilfred Ngwa

The challenges of establishing robust, cancer care systems are worsened by a lack or shortage of trained professionals, research, sufficient data, and even political and administrative limitations that make the uphill battle against cancer even more arduous in some Balkan countries. Despite their proximity to European Union nations, the experiences of Balkan nations in terms of prevailing cancers, available resources, and access to up-to-date methods and processes differ significantly from those of the EU. This chapter delves into the challenges, realities, and needs of Balkan nations with regards to the growing cancer burden. It also identifies opportunities for improvement, including recently established international collaborations.

Cancer is one of the leading diseases in the world, the main cause of death in many countries, and the second one worldwide [1, 2]. It is a disease that affects both high-income countries (HICs) as well as low- and middle-income countries (LMICs). However, the statistical data of many studies show a large gap in mortality cases vs. incidence rate between HICs and LMICs [3–5]. Although the number of cancer cases is increasing more rapidly in HIC countries (mainly due to longer life expectancy) compared to LMIC countries, the mortality rates are lower than in LMICs. A similar scenario can be observed if we compare the data, summarized in table 30.1, between Balkan countries (belonging to middle-income countries [6]) still waiting to join the European Union, Western European countries, and the European average. In most Balkan countries, the incidence rate is below the European average, while the mortality rate is much higher, reaching almost two thirds of the incidence rate [7]. It should be stated that the Globocan data are estimated, as there are no reliable and consistent sources for Balkan countries.

This discrepancy is due to different reasons related to smaller expenditures on healthcare systems, which is much lower in Balkan countries, ranging from 2.5% in Kosovo to 6.5% in Bosnia and Herzegovina [8], compared to the European Union

doi:10.1088/978-0-7503-3075-6ch30

Table 30.1. Summary of cancer incidence and mortality rates for some Balkan countries compared to the Western European and European averages [7]. There are no mortality data for Kosovo.

Country	Population	Incidence	Incidence rate per 100,000	Mortality rate	Mortality in (%)
Albania	2 934 345	8 294	283	4 693	56.5
Bosnia & Herzegovina	3 503 565	14 385	410	9 012	62.6
Kosovo	1 777 104*	1 500**	84	n.n.	n.n.
Montenegro	629 217	2 366	376	1 287	54.3
North Macedonia	2 085 056	7 807	374	4 116	52.7
Serbia	8 762 022	47 960	547	26 919	56.1
Western Europe	194 072 953	1 370 332	706	548 355	40
Europe	743 837 100	4 229 662	568	1 943 478	45.9

*Kosova Agency of Statistics 2019 *Estimation Kosovo Population in* 2018.
**Oncology Clinical Center of Kosovo, Prishtina, Kosovo.

average of 9.9% [9]. The lack of infrastructure and healthcare professionals, reduced access to quality care and treatment options, the shortage of effective drugs, the lack of a national registry, and the lack of effective and implementable action plans are additional obstacles for qualitative cancer care in the Balkan countries. An important factor is the lack of healthcare professionals, which is partly due to increased migration towards European Union countries [10, 11] and the absence of reliable data based on scientific research [12]. The early detection of cancer cases is very important in order to increase the chance of surviving the disease; it mostly comprises early diagnosis and screening, which requires access to affordable healthcare services. We will discuss the situation in two Balkan countries, North Macedonia, which has made significant investments in increasing treatment capacity and Kosovo, which is in the first stages of establishing a reliable healthcare system for cancer treatment.

North Macedonia had 7573 cancer cases in the year 2018 with a mortality rate of 179.8 per 100 000 inhabitants, an increase in mortality of 6% compared to 2008 [14]. The most common cancer for men is lung cancer, which accounts for 12.99% of the overall number of cases, while for Europeans as a whole, the most common cancer is prostate cancer. For women, breast cancer is the most common type, accounting for 11.32% of the overall incidence. North Macedonia has four clinical centers that are situated in Stip, Bitola, Tetovo, and the main one situated in the capital, Skopje. The Clinical Center for Oncology and Radiotherapy situated at the Mother Teresa University clinical center is the only public center that offers radiotherapy treatment as the most common method for the treatment of cancer cases, either alone, or in combination with other treatments [15]. The oncology center has 29 radiotherapy and oncology specialists, 58 nurses, 25 RTG technicians, 11 medical physicists working with two Varian linacs dating from 2003 (6 MeV, 15 MeV), one Varian TrueBeam, intensity-modulated radiation therapy (IMRT), one computed tomography (CT) simulator, and one high-dose-rate (HDR) brachytherapy machine. The country also has a publicly funded National Center for Positron Emission

Tomography. It is worth mentioning that there are three other linacs in the country, but they have not been functional for more than five years. A very important aspect of decreasing the mortality rate is the early detection of cancer cases, for which the country has organized screening programs for breast and cervical cancer operated by public health centers. However, the participation of women in the screening programs is very low; for example for cervical cancer screening, only 18% of women between 24 and 60 years took part [16], far less than the participation rate in European Union countries, which lies between 70% and 80%. In addition human papilloma virus (HPV) vaccination is mandatory for young girls in North Macedonia; however, only 55% have agreed to be vaccinated. A larger focus should be given to implementing elements related to screening programs in order to increase the participation [17]. Overall, as an imPACT team from IAEA concluded during their visit to cancer diagnosis centers in 2018, the country has sufficient treatment capacity. However, to ensure more effective patient care and the efficient use of available resources, the coordination and integration of cancer services should be enhanced [18].

As the youngest country in Europe, Kosovo only started with the treatment of cancer cases in the last six years. Therefore, the data for the distributions of different cancer cases and the total number of cancer patients in Kosovo was not obtained in a systematic and coordinated way.

In Kosovo, about 1500 new cancer cases are identified every year. All cases are treated in one oncological center, covering about 1.8 million people. The center has about 70 staff members, including oncologists, medical physicists, nurses, internal medicine professionals, radiotherapists, psychologists, and others.

Cancer patient data are obtained from the Oncology Clinical Center of Kosovo and the National Institute of Public Health, however the country still lacks a reliable, well-organized, and sustainable database, and due to the lack of death certificates, it is difficult to determine the number of cancer-related mortalities.

The chemotherapy department receives up to 250 medical visits per day. The number of medical visits per year is up to 40 000 patients. Thirty thousand of these patients are offered cytostatic, target therapy, or hormone therapy services. The medical oncology clinic has 55 beds for outpatient treatment and 15 beds for hospital treatment. The monthly budget for cytostatic drugs provided by the Ministry of Health is €600 000. Many drugs have to be paid for by the patient; for many families, this is a huge financial burden that they cannot afford.

The oncological center of Kosovo also offers external radiotherapy treatment using two Primus Medical linear accelerators with photon energies of 6 MeV and 15 MeV and electron-mode energies of 5 MeV to 14 MeV, in the multileaf collimator mode only. On average, about 60 patients per day are treated using one linac. The physicians, medical physicists, and technicians lack proper continuous training skills, which would lead to higher-quality patient treatment. The Oncology Clinical Center in Kosovo is in the process of purchasing one Elekta linac and also working to develop a brachytherapy unit for cervical cancer cases using an HDR brachytherapy machine, an Elekta Flexitron model with 40 channels that has an iridium-192 radioactive source. Due to unresolved political issues, Kosovo cannot be part of the IAEA and UNESCO training programs, which would increase the treatment quality of cancer-related diseases.

The challenges that the Balkan countries are facing in the treatment of cancer-related diseases are different from those of European Union countries. The lack of national registries, the shortage of physicians, medical physicists, and technicians, the lack of effective implementation of early detection programs, the public unawareness of risk factors such as smoking, obesity, alcohol consumption, the absence of regular screening programs, and the lack of a sustainable strategy and financing in the healthcare sector make it difficult to achieve better quality treatment of cancer patients. Training programs for nurses, medical physicists, oncologists and general practitioners, a program for the follow up and control of patients and survivors, and regular control and evaluation of implemented measures are also needed.

An important activity that can lower the incidence and mortality of cancer-related diseases is international collaboration, in which an exchange of expertise takes place, different and unique approaches and experiences in addressing different challenges are discussed, and new ideas, cooperation, and partnerships are born [13]. In this light, the invited attendance of a group of scientists and physicians from North Macedonia and Kosovo at the Harvard Global Health Catalyst (GHC) summit that is held yearly at leading Harvard-affiliated cancer care institutions and hospitals was significant. The Harvard GHC offers great opportunities through information communications technology (ICT)-based care, education, and research programs such as those for the training of nurses, oncologists, medical physicists, and other professionals through the Global Oncology University [19]. Furthermore, the GHC summit paved the way for cooperation between the oncological centres in Kosovo and North Macedonia and the University Medical Centre, Mannheim in the field of telemedicine and in training professionals for brachytherapy treatments.

References

[1] Cancer - key facts

[2] Bray F, Ferlay J, Soerjomataram I, Siegel L R, Torre A L and Jemal A 2018 Global Cancer Statistics 2018: GLOBOCAN estimates of incidence and mortality worldwide for 36 cancers in 185 countries *CA: Cancer J. Clin.* **68** 394–424

[3] Vrdoliak E *et al* 2016 Cancer control in central and eastern europe: current situation and recommendations for improvement *Oncologist* **21** 1183–90

[4] Znaor A *et al* 2013 Cancer incidence and mortality patterns in South Eastern Europe in the last decade: gaps persist compared with the rest of Europe *Eur. J. Cancer* **49** 1683–91

[5] Carioli G *et al* 2020 European cancer mortality predictions for the year 2020 with a focus on prostate cancer *Ann. Oncology* **31** 650–8

[6] World Bank Country and Lending Groups

[7] Cancer fact sheets

[8] Enlargement countries - health statistics

[9] Healthcare expenditure statistics

[10] Lazarevik V, Kongjonaj A, Krstic M, Malowany M, Tulchinsky T and Neumark Y 2016 Physicians migration from Western Balkan *Eur. J. Public Health* **26** S132–3

[11] Bundesärztekammer, Ergebnisse der Ärztestatistik zum 31. Dezember 2019
[12] Begum M *et al* 2018 Mapping cancer research across Central and Eastern Europe, the Russian Federation and Central Asia: Implications for future national cancer control planning *Eur. J. Cancer* **104** 127–36
[13] Ngwa W and Nguyen P 2017 *Global Oncology Harvard Global Health Catalyst Summit Lecture Notes* (Bristol: IOP Publishing)
[14] Cancer in the Republic of North Macedonia, 2008–18, 2019 Institute of public health of the Republic of North Macedonia
[15] Ngwa W *et al* 2015 Potential for information and communication technologies to catalyze global collaborations in radiation oncology *Int. J. Radiat. Oncol. Biol. Phys.* **91** 444–7
[16] Association for Emancipation, Solidarity and Equality of Women 2011
[17] Davies P and Dimitrievska V 2015 Situation analysis of cancer breast, cervical and prostate cancer screening in Macedonia *Technical Report*
[18] Juric A 2018 The Former Yugoslav Republic of Macedonia to Further Strengthen its Cancer Control Following an IAEA Review (Vienna: IAEA)
[19] Welcome to Global Oncology University https://www.ghcuniversity.org/

IOP Publishing

Approaching Global Oncology
The win-win model
Ahmed Elzawawy and Wilfred Ngwa

Chapter 31

Win-win collaborations with governments

Wilfred Ngwa, Omoruyi Credit Irabor and Diane Gashumba

Global health is an emerging cross-disciplinary field, bringing together the best of science, medicine, and humanity. It is a field which recognizes that in today's world 'global health is local health and local health is global health', a field in which everyone can participate and collaborations are crucial. Highlighting the urgency of collaboration, the recent World Health Organization Cancer Report [15] describes the growing global burden of cancer as alarming and a major obstacle to human development and wellbeing. Since the growing scourge of cancer costs millions of lives and trillions of dollars across the world each year, people are increasingly coming together across institutions, cultures, countries, and continents to work together with a greater sense of purpose and urgency to stop this scourge and reduce the disparities. In the growing field of global oncology, win-win collaborations with governments are crucial, especially for low- and middle-income countries (LMICs) whose healthcare systems are largely state sponsored. In this chapter we highlight the importance of win-win collaborations in global oncology in fields such as policy, public–private partnerships, global oncology diplomacy and socio-economic development.

31.1 Introduction

Global health was front and center as leaders from nearly 50 countries gathered in Washington in early August 2014 for the first-ever US–Africa Leaders' Summit, intended to expand trade and investment, encourage sustainable development, and enhance cooperation on peace and security. At that time, the United States Government's National Institutes of Health was supporting research and training across the African continent through about 1500 grants. During the event, participants discussed global health and how collaborations could accelerate treatment advances, increase access to healthcare, and catalyze global health and economic development. Since then, the Global Health Catalyst (GHC) summit, launched at the Harvard Radcliffe Institute in 2015, has organized sessions hosting

doi:10.1088/978-0-7503-3075-6ch31

government leaders in recognition of the crucial role government has to play in global health and oncology. Collaboration between governments is readily seen when governments address communicable diseases and pandemics such the COVID-19 pandemic. However, it is also crucial as the global burden of cancer surges.

For decades, the United States has been a world leader in global health; the has government partnered with LMICs with considerable success, as demonstrated by the President's Emergency Plan for AIDS Relief (PEPFAR) program [1–3]. Today, as more people survive HIV/AIDs and other diseases and live longer, non-communicable diseases (NCDs) such as cancer are on the rise, and have become the leading cause of death [4, 5]. The dramatic rise in the burden caused by NCDs has been described as a growing health iceberg which urgently needs to be addressed, hidden under epidemics of infectious disease [6]. The role of government in collaborative investment with international institutions and scientists is multifold. Government can debate, further develop, customize, and enact global health policies with high impact. Government, be it local, state, provincial, national, or even a union of nations, has clear roles in the control of cancer. This is particularly crucial for LMICs, whose healthcare systems are largely state sponsored.

According to Kerry *et al* [12] global health is largely an unappreciated partner of diplomacy or foreign policy. Engagement for such diplomacy in oncology by the GHC has included engagement with government entities such as the United States House Foreign Affairs Subcommittee for the different regions. We recommend more of this type of engagement in the USA and other countries. Since such policies can be country specific, engagement with ambassadors from different countries is also encouraged. Areas that are suitable for high-impact collaborative engagement with governments include those of policy, public–private partnerships, diaspora engagement to turn brain drain to global oncology gain, and implementation and dissemination.

31.1.1 Policy

Many many years ago, President John F Kennedy stood before a joint session of the United States Congress and said, 'I believe we should go to the Moon'. It was a call to mankind that inspired a generation in pursuit of science and innovation, one in which science and innovation literally pushed the boundaries of what was possible. In 2016, another USA President, Obama, also stood before Congress to announce the 'moonshot to cure cancer' initiative. The USA government followed this announcement with a two-point execution plan: first, for increased resources, both private and public—to support cancer work, and second, to break down silos and catalyze collaboration and information sharing to 'end cancer as we know it'. Funding for the moonshot initiative was secured on December 7 2016, when the U. S. Senate approved the 21st Century Cures Act. President Obama signed the Act into law and then Vice President Joe Biden led its implementation from a policy perspective and served as a catalyst to facilitate collaboration. This example, along with PEPFAR, highlight the value of engaging governments to enact laws and policy in the fight against cancer. Following the election of Joe Biden as President of the United States, the *Lancet Oncology* has published articles on Cancer moonShot 2.0; many see a momentous opportunity to addressing cancer health disparities, in which we envision Biden as the 'Abraham Lincoln of cancer' in 'abolishing' inequalities. This will require further policy with accountable measures and sustained funding and resources dedicated to innovation and collaboration focused on eliminating cancer inequalities. Biden has already prioritized racial equality, and together with Vice President Harris, has a personal history with cancer. Biden has also demonstrated steadfast support for science and collaboration in the form of robust sustained funding over the years, including that of the cancer moonshot. The GHC is now planning a Global Cancer moonshot summit in 2022 with a major engagement of the American government and LMIC governments and their countries' first ladies. It is time for governments to collaborate in making cancer history. It is time for greater global oncology diplomacy with global win-win collaborations to eliminate global cancer disparities. The World Health Organization recognizes the importance of this and is increasingly making global oncology a priority. The ability of governments to develop effective health and fiscal policy aimed at improving health is directly correlated with the effectiveness of their negotiating capacity and their ability to build a national consensus; global oncology is a similar case.

31.1.2 Public–private partnerships

As well as policy, public–private partnerships for greater investment in sustainable cancer control programming should also be promoted. Public–private partnership for global oncology has been a good model and has been championed by the Pink Ribbon Red Ribbon (PRRR) initiative at the George W Bush Institute. PRRR's leading public–private partnership model aims to reduce deaths from cervical and breast cancer in sub-Saharan Africa and Latin America. This model could be adapted to strengthen global oncology along the continuum of cancer care, and embed it in existing national health systems and funding mechanisms. A number of informed grassroots movements in favor of this emerged from the GHC summit, including public–private partnerships with the diaspora. This included Tanzanians United Against Cancer, Nigerians United Against Cancer, and Cameroonians United Against Cancer. Ministries of health can incentivize diaspora participation in strengthening healthcare systems and engage the diaspora in public–private partnerships (PPPs). At a recent GHC summit meeting at Harvard, potential areas for PPP discussed included a universal Health Insurance Scheme that involves the diaspora in partnership with their ministries of health. This would allow diasporans to pay premiums for beneficiaries (e.g., family members or friends) in their original LMICs, and help such a scheme to support quality healthcare for all. Initiatives such as Diaspora Health Services (DHI) in Nigeria and the UAP-connect have emerged to provide the opportunity for diaspora Africans in the USA, Canada, UK, and other high-income countries (HICs) to purchase a designated health insurance plan for family members in their home countries. It is recommended that such schemes be encouraged and enhanced via win-win collaborations with ministries of health. This would increase impact and sustainability and could include life insurance and telemedicine.

Another PPP discussed at the summit included diaspora bonds, which have been proposed by the *Lancet Oncology* commission as a potential avenue to support the establishment of startup cost-intensive radiotherapy services needed for the treatment of over 50% of the cancer patients in LMICs. New PPP areas of global health that could significantly benefit both LMICs and HICs include phytomedicines in oncology. PPPs to develop this sector would enable the development of new low-cost medicines, thereby increasing access to medicines. A further recommendation is for governments to engage their diasporas in continuous dialogue to identify areas in which they could continually work together, and also recruit their participation in strengthening the healthcare system. The annual Global Health Catalyst summit at Harvard has provided a platform for such global health dialogue. An excellent recent example is that of Rwanda, where diaspora leaders worked together with the Rwandan Embassy in Washington and the Rwandan Ministry of Health in global health that benefits Rwanda, including commitments from American and German institutions to train oncology health professionals in Rwanda over the next five years, participation in ICT-powered multicentre clinical trials, support for the new Rwanda Military Hospital's clinical oncology, and other global health activities. Other examples are the Memorandum of Understanding (MOU) between The Ministry of Health, Rwanda and The GHC, in Kigali, Rwanda, on November 7, 2017 (figure 31.1).

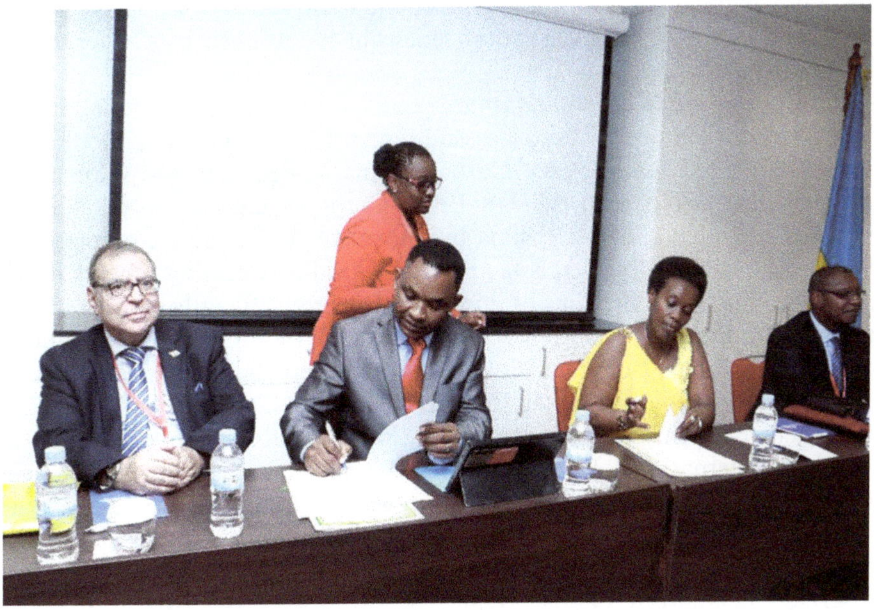

Figure 31.1. November 7, 2017. Kigali, Rwanda. The signing of an MoU between Global Health Catalyst (GHC), Harvard Medical School, USA and the Ministry of Health, Rwanda. From right to left: the Minister of Public Health, Rwanda, Dr Diane Gashumba, the Minister of Health, Rwanda, Professor Wilfred Ngwa, Director GHC, Harvard Medical School, USA, Professor Ahmed Elzawawy, Egypt, Chair of the GHC win-win initiative.

31.1.3 Global health diplomacy

HICs use global health as part of their soft power. Global health diplomacy is a key part of the strategy of the American government and there are tremendous opportunities for win-win collaborations in this area. Global Health Catalysts are quintessential global health diplomats. They work at the intersection of public health and foreign affairs—governments foster critical relationships with multi-lateral organizations, foreign governments, and ministries of health, and represent their countries in key global discussions and negotiations to protect and promote health worldwide. Through global health diplomacy, there are opportunities to apply and receive expertise globally, advance research through collaboration, and contribute to effective global policy. Global health diplomacy also leverages a widely agreed-upon goal—a healthier, safer world—to develop the foundation for diplomatic relations in other sectors. Global health security has never been more critical to the wellbeing of countries such as the United States and its citizens than it is right now. Infectious diseases spread more quickly than they ever have before, as evidenced by COVID-19. COVID-19 was the third leading cause of death in the USA in 2020. However, cancer was the second leading cause of death, and equal importance must be attached to global oncology security. The GHC is one of the leading global health initiatives in building global oncology diplomacy, including Win-Win Initiative ambassadors such as Her Royal Highness Princess Dina Mired, and ministers of health and first ladies in LMICs. They have also helped to catalyze and establish win-win collaborations with country and state governments, which has resulted in initiatives to establish cancer centers in countries such as Nigeria, Kenya, and Cameroon.

Professor Vanessa Kerry at Harvard and founder of Seed Global Health is helping to champion one of the successful global health diplomacy models, which involves the United States Peace Corps. In this model, the Seed Global Health organization partnered with the US Peace Corps to launch the Global Health Service Partnership (GHSP). GHSP is an innovative public–private partnership and global health program that sends faculty to medical and nursing schools in under-resourced settings, with the aims of improving capacity, strengthening global health systems, and ultimately saving lives. The creation of the GHSP was a landmark, since efforts for such a global health initiative had been underway since former U.S. President John F Kennedy created the Peace Corps by Executive Order in 1961 [8]. In 1979, Senator Javits proposed the International Health Act of 1979, which aimed to build an International Health Service program, but it was never passed [9]. PEPFAR, which helped to fund the GHSP, was itself launched by the US Government in 2003, and in 2005, the Institute of Medicine published a report titled 'Healers Abroad: Americans Responding to the Human Resource Crisis in HIV/AIDS', detailing a Global Health Service Corps that would send health professionals to offer clinical, technical, and managerial support to healthcare workers in developing countries [10].

Few global health advocates, political diplomats, and institutions continued advocacy for a GHSP model for international health until the Peace Corps and Seed

Global Health (then called the Global Health Service Corps) launched GHSP in March of 2012. Notable among these advocates are Dr Fitzhugh Mullan, who proposed a model that blended the strengths of the U.S Peace Corps and the National Health Service Corps [11] and chaired the Institute of Medicine (which released reports focusing on the importance of health to international development and diplomacy), Dr Paul Farmer, and Senator Frist.

The GHSP model works through the recruitment and deployment of doctors and nurses to medical and nursing training institutions in low-resource settings, supporting a range of US health professionals to serve as clinical faculty—formally and informally teaching students and house staff through daily patient rounds and separate regularly scheduled didactic sessions and courses [7, 12]. The model aims to enhance existing clinical training systems and structures through the development and implementation of innovative teaching tools, clinical guidelines, treatment protocols, and continuing education programs in partnership with host country faculty [7, 12]. GHSP volunteers work closely with in-country faculty to help to ensure that they integrate into and foster an efficient and culturally sensitive educational environment (see figure 31.2).

The selection process for GHSP placements takes place through a consultative process in partnership with the ministries of health and of higher education, their commitment to strengthening their health care systems, a strong in-country PEPFAR presence, and committed local implementation partners [7, 13, 14].

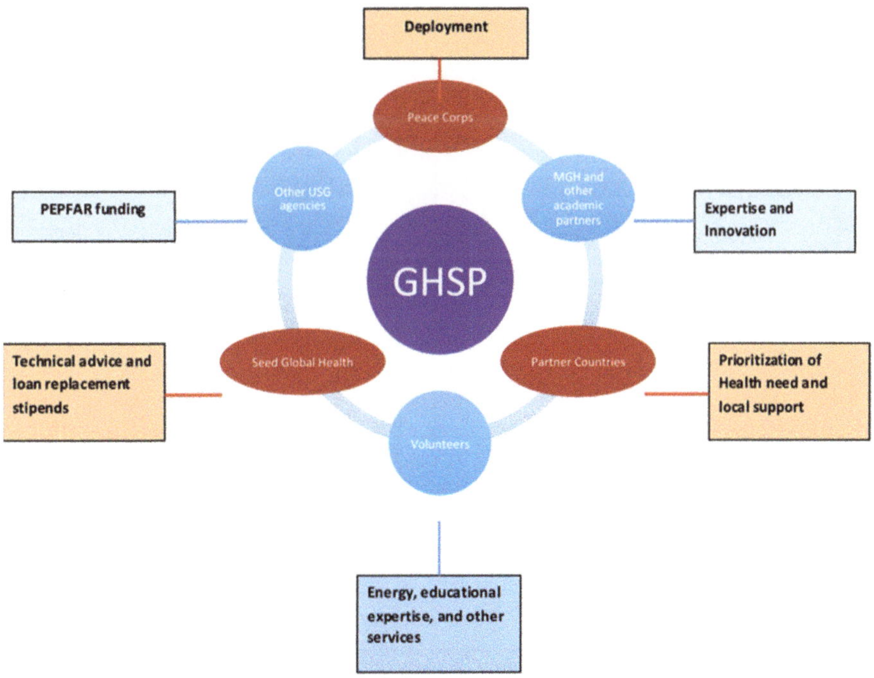

Figure 31.2. The GHSP model. Adapted from [16].

A mapping exercise is undertaken with the US and international partners to reach rapid consensus on priority countries for the roll out of the pilot [13, 14]. The GHSP's aim is to create a continuum of health professionals who can teach in order to address the country's disease burden and can serve as educators in the health and education systems of their countries (see figure 31.3).

Each cohort of health professionals must include board-eligible or board-certified doctors and nurses experienced as educators in core specialties. GHSP volunteers are awarded medical or nursing licenses in the countries where they work to ensure that they are fully qualified and approved. To facilitate the service of health professionals, the GHSP helps to ensure that educational or other debt does not preclude being able to serve. Through private philanthropy raised by Seed, the program provides up to $30,000 of debt repayment for each year served. GHSP also aims to create specific partnerships with academic institutions to create a structured sabbatical program and to help recruit mid-career health professionals [14]. Vanessa Kerry gave one of the keynote addresses at the GHC summit and for the American Society of Radiation Oncology (ASTRO), which included opportunities to extend this model with a main focus on win-win collaborations in global oncology. In conclusion, win-win collaborations involving both HIC and LMIC governments are crucial to advance global oncology.

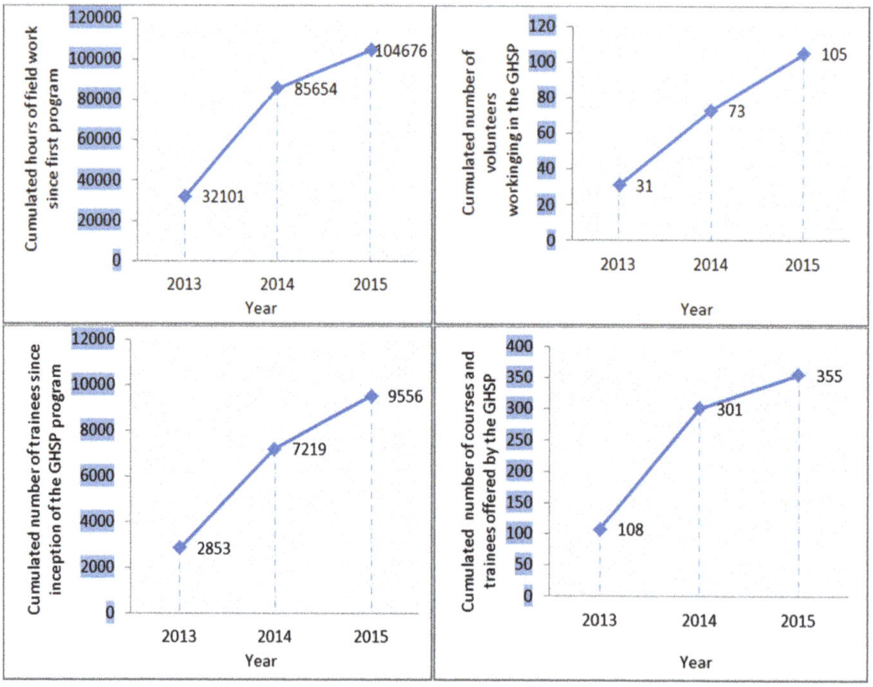

Figure 31.3. Cumulative growth in the number of volunteers, service hours, trainees, and courses offered by the GHSP. Created using information from [16].

References

[1] Katz I T, Bassett I V and Wright A A 2013 PEPFAR in transition—implications for HIV care in South Africa *New Engl. J. Med.* **369** 1385–7

[2] Dzau V, Fuster V, Frazer J and Snair M 2017 Investing in global health for our future *New Engl. J. Med.* **377** 1292–6

[3] Fauci A S and Eisinger R W 2018 PEPFAR—15 years and counting the lives saved *New Engl. J. Med.* **378** 314–6

[4] Nyirenda M J 2016 Non-communicable diseases in sub-Saharan Africa: understanding the drivers of the epidemic to inform intervention strategies *Int. Health* **8** 157–8

[5] Ali M K *et al* 2013 Systems and capacity to address noncommunicable diseases in low- and middle-income countries *Sci. Transl. Med.* **5** 181cm4

[6] Naghavi M and Forouzanfar M H 2013 Burden of non-communicable diseases in sub-Saharan Africa in 1990 and 2010: Global Burden of Diseases, Injuries, and Risk Factors Study 2010 *Lancet* **381** S95

[7] Kerry V B and Mullan F 2014 Global health service partnership: building health professional leadership *Lancet* **383** 1688–91

[8] The White House 1961 Executive Order 10924: establishment of the peace corps

[9] Javits J *et al* 1979 S.1424 - International Health Act of 1979, 96th Congress (1979–1980)

[10] Institute of Medicine 2005 *Healer's Abroad: Americans Responding to the Human Resource Crisis in HIV/AIDS* (Washington, D.C.: National Academies Press)

[11] Mullan F 2007 Responding to the global HIV/AIDS crisis *JAMA* **297** 744

[12] Kerry V B Global health service partnership: a model for global health

[13] Jacobsen L and Kaplan L 2015 Building healthcare capacity: the global health service partnership *Nurs. Pract.* **40** 16–6

[14] Concept paper for the Peace Corps Global Health Service Partnership, Peace Corps Worldwide

[15] World Health Organization 2020 WHO report on cancer: setting priorities, investing wisely, and providing care for all (Geneva: World Health Organization) https://apps.who.int/iris/handle/10665/330745 (Accessed August 23, 2021)

[16] Irabor O C, Kerry V B, Matton J and Ngwa W 2017 Leveraging the Global Health Service Partnership model for workforce development in global radiation oncology *J. Glob. Oncol.* **4** 1–8

Chapter 32

The South Asia Centre for Medical Physics and Cancer Research: its activities and collaboration with the Global Health Catalyst

Mohammad Ullah Shemanto, Hasin Anupama Azhari and Golam Abu Zakaria

This chapter focuses on efforts in South Asia, highlighting the power of collaborative efforts, in particular, in the education and training of cancer care professionals. It details efforts and gains made by the South Asia Centre for Medical Physics and Cancer Research (SCMPCR) through south—south and south–north collaborations, highlighting specific memorandum of understanding (MoU) goals and citing collaborators whose combined efforts are already bearing fruit.

The South Asia Centre for Medical Physics and Cancer Research (SCMPCR), Dhaka, Bangladesh

Globally, the cancer burden is increasing, putting enormous physical, emotional, and financial strain on individuals, families, communities, and health systems. Because health systems in low- and middle-income countries (LMICs) are the least prepared to deal with this load, a huge percentage of cancer patients around the world are unable to receive timely, high-quality diagnosis and treatment.

With 1.9 billion people, the South Asian (SA) region (Afghanistan, Bangladesh, Bhutan, India, Maldives, Nepal, Pakistan, and Sri Lanka) accounts for roughly one-quarter of the world's population. South Asia has some of the world's most severe socioeconomic disparities.

This is especially important in light of the fact that most South Asian (SA) countries have limited healthcare expenditure, an insufficient skilled workforce, and insufficient hospitals.

This region is currently seeing a transition away from infectious diseases and toward non-communicable diseases such as heart disease and cancer. Despite their enormous diversity, the majority of South Asian countries face significant challenges.

doi:10.1088/978-0-7503-3075-6ch32

As a result, a comprehensive collective effort is essential to guarantee that this region has access to high-quality cancer care, as cancer may become an epidemic in SA countries in the next decades.

On the other hand, in today's world, a diversity of updated new technologies are appearing in the healthcare sector. All equipment, from diagnostic to therapeutic approaches, requires regular maintenance and quality standards.

Medical physicists, together with medical doctors and technicians, are required to support these departments according to international standards and regulations. Without specifically qualified medical physicists (QMP), radiotherapy and nuclear medicine departments, as well as diagnostic radiology—in particular, computed tomography (CT) and interventional radiology—cannot be performed precisely and reliably, resulting in mortality or secondary cancer.

To comply with the 2030 Sustainable Development Goals (SDGs) three (Good Health and Wellbeing) and four (Patient Benefit), the slogan is 'Quality Education and Health Science for Patient Benefit' (Quality Education).

To meet the rapidly increasing need for cancer treatment, the SCMPCR works to increase the trained workforce by enlisting international experts and utilizing national and international collaborative approaches.

Germany is a key pioneer in this project, thanks to the support of the Mannheim Medical Centre (UMM) and Heidelberg University, as well as DAAD (German Academic Exchange Service) funding. As a result, other SA countries, such as India, Sri Lanka, and Nepal have engaged with the SCMPCR because they share our objectives and vision (www.scmpcr.org).

In conjunction with national and international organizations and institutions, the SCMPCR hosts three to four authorized hands-on training workshops (HW) for cancer team specialists (doctors, medical physicists, nurses, and other providers) each year. The trainers, vendors, and industries are from both developing and developed countries, while the participants are from various SA countries.

The International Organization of Medical Physics (IOMP) and the European Board for Accreditation in Medical Physics (EBAMP) have accredited these programs, allowing participants to earn certificates with continuing professional development points that will help them further their careers in the future. The SCMPCR also runs an Awareness and Screening Program, which includes the development of self-help groups for cancer patients.

In addition, health education programs are held at various levels in schools, colleges, and universities in both urban and rural locations to teach people how to live a healthy lifestyle and avoid disease. In the near future, the SCMPCR wants to launch residency programs for medical physicists, as well as welfare houses, quality control labs, and research networks.

The SCMPCR also provides in-service training. Training in a foreign nation is frequently less successful than training at home because only a few people can benefit from and afford it. More people can be engaged in hospitals using in-service training, and the everyday routine of hospital-based cases can be experienced utilizing local equipment. Experts provide guidance for better treatment outcomes at the same time.

In order to organize educational events, the SCMPCR also collaborates with Gono University (GU) in Savar, Dhaka, Bangladesh. At present, Gono University is the only university in Bangladesh offering a full master's course in medical physics (https://gonouniversity.edu.bd/mpbme/).

In order to meet the challenge of the next industrial revolution and the digitalization of healthcare technologies, the SCMPCR introduced an e-learning program for medical physicists during the corona pandemic in June 2020. The overwhelmingly positive feedback obtained from over 150 participants from more than 50 countries for this e-learning program confirmed it was a big success. From 2021, the SCMPCR is going to organize accredited e-learning courses three times a year accompanied by a series of lectures by well-known international speakers.

In August 2018, during a combined conference of the GHC and the UMM, a collaboration agreement was signed between the Mannheim Medical Centre and Rwanda in the presence of the honorable health minister of Rwanda, Dr Diane Gashumba, Professor Wilfred Ngwa of the Harvard School of Medicine, Professor Dr Stephen Avery of the University of Pennsylvania, Professor Dr Frederik Wenz, director and Mr Volker Steil, chief medical physicist of the Mannheim Medical Centre (UMM), Heidelberg University, Germany.

Soon after the signing of this MoU, in response to an invitation from the Health Ministry of Rwanda, personnel from the Global Health Catalyst (GHC) and the SCMPCR attended a program in Kigali, Rwanda in November 2018. The chairman of the SCMPCR, Professor G A Zakaria, attended the meeting and comprehensively discussed the prospects of cancer treatment and how to introduce medical physics education in Rwanda (figure 32.1).

Consequently, in May 2019, the Harvard GHC (HGHC) hosted the Global Health Catalyst Summit in Boston, which is a regular yearly event designed to

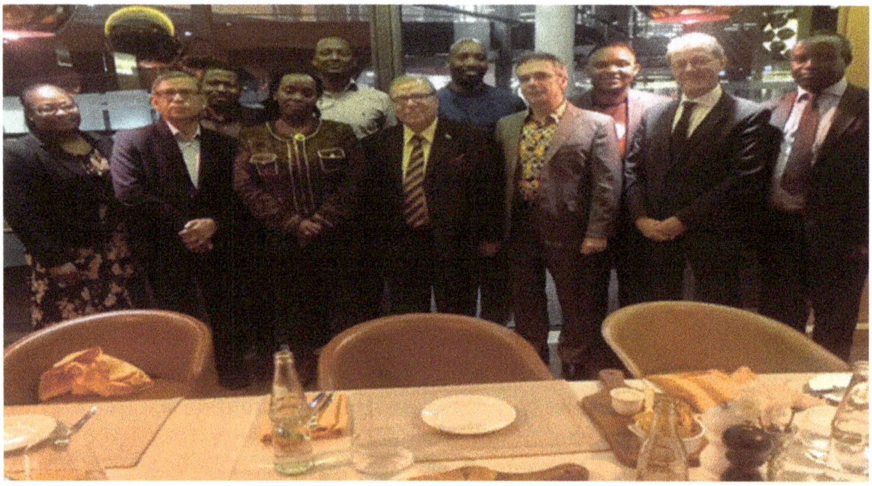

Figure 32.1. Professor Dr Wilfred Ngwa, Professor Dr Luca Incrocci, Dr Johannes Schweizer, Professor Dr Ahmed Elzawawy, Professor Dr Golam Abu Zakaria with the Health Minister of Rwanda Dr Diane Gashumba and her team in November 2018 in Kigali.

catalyze high-impact international collaboration to eliminate global health disparities. This summit mainly focused on cancer, considering the dream that people of all socioeconomic, racial, religious, and cultural backgrounds will have access to quality healthcare one day. On behalf of the SCMPCR, two members, Jobairul Islam and Mr Rashed Al Amin, our Chairman Professor G A Zakaria and Medical Physicist Volker Steil (UMM) attended the seminar and delivered their speeches. We are thankful to the HGHC for providing scholarships (travel and local costs) for our two members (figure 32.2).

During the GHC conference in Mannheim on the 6th September 2019, Professor Dr G A Zakaria was awarded the 'Global Radiation Oncology Distinguished Leader Award 2019' by the Global Health Catalyst of Harvard Medical School for his contribution to radiation medicine education worldwide (figure 32.3).

The Global Health Catalyst (GHC) based in Boston has a very good platform of e-learning programs around the globe, especially for the African continent. The SCMPCR plans to cooperate with the HGHC in providing this e-training to participants from the SA and South-East Asia.

In the meantime, partners from Germany/Bangladesh (Professor Dr G A Zakaria, Dipl.-Ing. Volker Steil, Dr Frank Hensley, Professor Dr Hasin Anupama Azhari); Africa/USA (Professor Dr Wilfred Ngwa, Professor Dr Stephen Avery, Professor Dr Ahmed Elzawawy and Professor Dr Twalib Ngoma) formulated an MoU that provides a framework for collaboration between all parties to achieve the following objectives:

- Education/Training: help to educate a sufficient number of medical physicists (MPs) and train health professionals in oncology, diagnostic radiology, and nuclear medicine as mutually agreed upon with LMIC partners via face-to-face and online learning.
- Research: participate in research collaborations that involve both high-income countries (HICs) and LMIC partner faculties with co-authored research publications.
- Care: collaborate on task-shifted tele-oncology (telemedicine) activities in which complete responsibility is taken by the LMIC partners in areas such as second opinions, remote treatment planning, and quality assurance, powered by

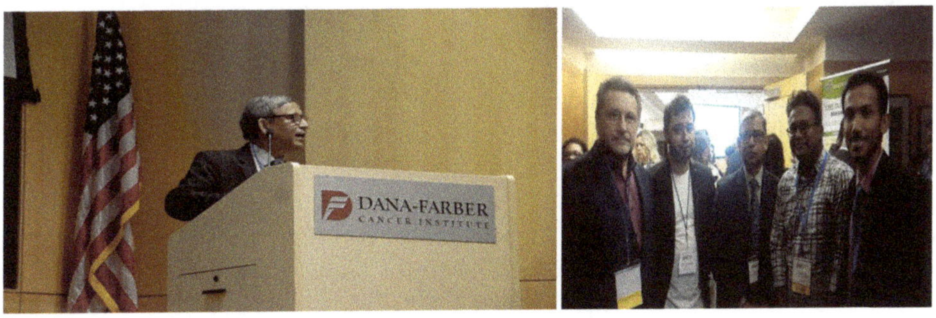

Figure 32.2. (Left) Speech delivered by G A Zakaria at the Global Health Catalyst summit, Harvard GHC in Boston, May 2019; (Right) Participants from Germany (Dipl.-Ing. V Steil, F P Zakaria, Professor Dr G A Zakaria) and Bangladesh (R Amin and J Islam).

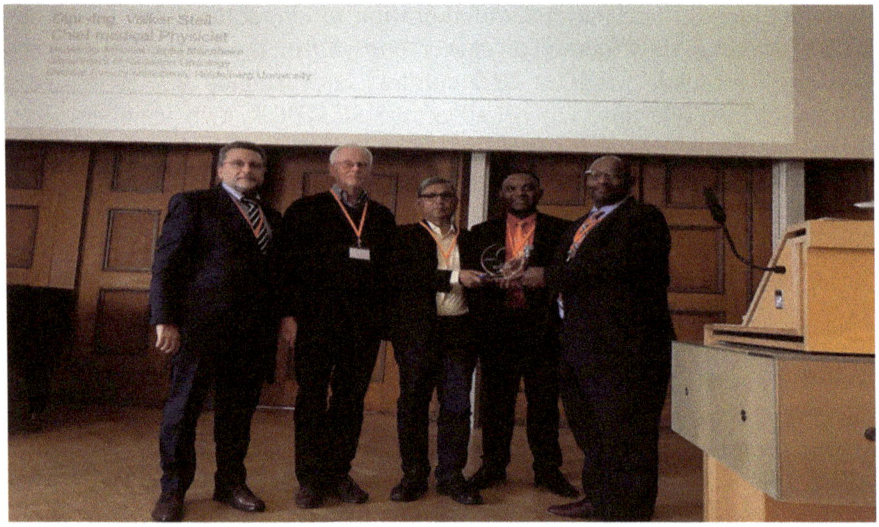

Figure 32.3. The Global Radiation Oncology Distinguished Leader Award 2019 is awarded to Professor Dr G A Zakaria, Mannheim (Germany).

advanced information and communications technology (ICT) or artificial intelligence (AI).

- Resource Mobilization: collaborate in joint funding proposals (e.g. DAAD in Germany and the National Institutes of Health (NIH) in the USA) and also including industry and diaspora organizations.
- Residency Program/Internship: to provide professional certification for QMPs, the residency program will be arranged by mutual agreement.

This project could be a fruitful example of collaboration that promotes global health with LMIC, diaspora, and industrial partners, introducing north–south cooperation. The collaborative partners are:

- The Department of Radiation Oncology, UMM, Heidelberg University
- Gono Bishwabidyalay (University)
- The South Asia Centre for Medical Physics and Cancer Research (SCMPCR)
- The Harvard Global Health Catalyst (HGHC)
- The University of Pennsylvania Radiation Oncology (UPRO)
- Muhimbili University of Health and Allied Sciences (MUHAS)

The first implementation of the program has been initiated by scholarships granted (by Gono University and SCMPCR) for two students from Rwanda in the Department of Medical Physics and Biomedical Engineering (MPBME) at Gono Bishwabidyalay (University), Bangladesh for the master's program (MSc) in medical physics (figure 32.4). These two students, Mr Rangira Laurent and Mr Kamanzi J D'amour, were chosen by the Health Ministry, Rwanda. Our plan is to exchange students and teachers between African universities and Bangladeshi

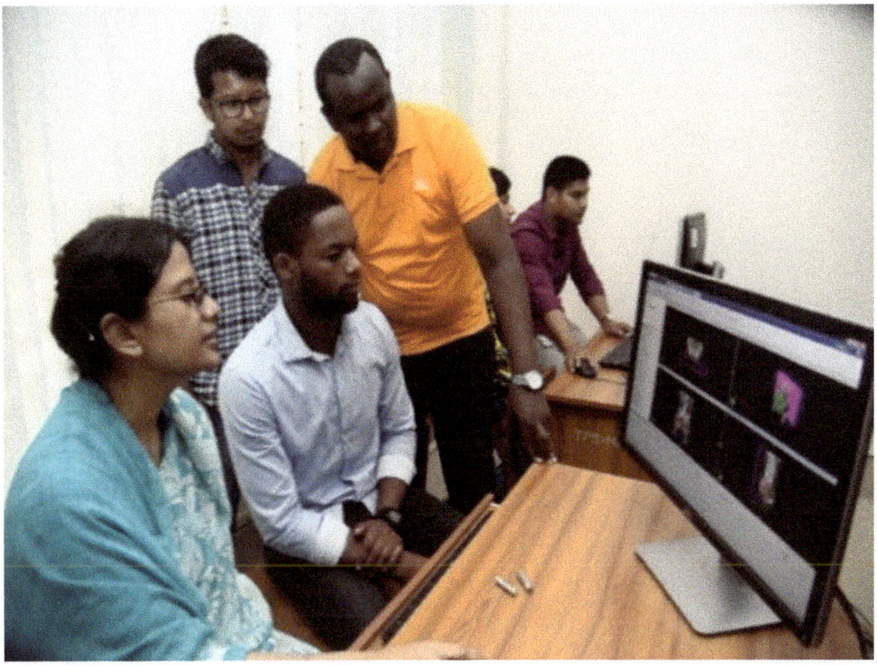

Figure 32.4. Students from Rwanda in the Department of Medical Physics and Biomedical Engineering (MPBME) with the chairman, Professor Dr Hasin Anupama Azhari of MPBME (left) and with classmates (right).

universities in cooperation with SCMPCR and in this way to establish medical physics education in East Africa, in particular, in Rwanda and Tanzania.

To realize this dream, we have adopted a transformative approach rooted in the values of creative and collaborative work. This approach focuses on building partnerships, leveraging ICT using lower-cost technologies, and unprecedented outreach partnerships. The SCMPCR and the GHC will hopefully play an important role in producing manpower to meet the challenges of 21st century medicine.

N.B. An additional source for the readers of chapter 31 is the AAPM Newsletter May/June 2020 vol. 45 no. 3 by aapmdocs (https://issuu.com/aapmdocs/docs/4503).

Part V

Perspectives of leading industries of equipment of radiation therapy and informatics systems and the win-win movement

Chapter 33

Perspectives of Varian, a Siemens Healthineers Company as a leading manufacturer of radiation therapy equipment

Dow Wilson, Andy Whitman, Kevin Massoudi, Julia Sheely-Chan and Valerie Sinden

In the win-win movement, we stress the inclusion of all stakeholders and consider their contributions. Stakeholders in the industrial space offer valuable incentives in order to create remarkable increases in the affordability of better-value cancer treatment in the real world. As such, the perspectives of leading industries are essential. Our intent is not to promote certain companies, but the representation of this sector supports the expansion of clinical oncology services in the world, particularly in the underserved regions in Africa and indeed in low- and middle-income country (LMICs) all over the world. The first major section of this chapter is inspired by the keynote speech made by Mr Dow Wilson, president and CEO of Varian Medical Systems, at the Global Health Summit on the 24th May, 2019 at Harvard Medical School, Boston, MA, USA. The second part briefly addresses the potential for industry contributions and identifies key areas of focus for gains against cancer in the coming years.

33.1 Increasing value-based radiotherapy in LMICs—a sustainable partnership for Africa

To the organizers of the Global Health Catalyst, to our host the Dana-Farber Cancer Institute, Brigham and Women's Hospital, Harvard Medical School, and to all of you our honorable guests, as we say in Africa (all protocols observed): thank you for the invitation to talk to you about increasing value-based radiotherapy in lower- and middle-income countries. As Dr Ahmed Elzawawy [2] outlined, this is a multi-year journey which will take the efforts of all of us to provide better access to care. There is some inspiring evidence that we are making

doi:10.1088/978-0-7503-3075-6ch33

a big contribution to this improvement and slowly starting to see better care models in sub-Saharan Africa as well as in many other emerging markets throughout the world. We will have a chance to talk a little bit about some of those today. I'm going to try not to make this too much of a marketing message for Varian Medical Systems, but I will acknowledge it is the experience I have and so that's what I will talk about for context.

I will discuss Varian and Varian's solutions, give an overview of cancer in Africa, and discuss some key procurement considerations that people should be thinking about as they think about radiation therapy. It is very important for governments to consider some technological solutions for Africa and celebrate successful partnerships in Africa. There is not one business model that is going to work for all; rather, it is a combination and variety of models. I will show some business models that have been successful so far, and conclude with a discussion about sustainability, especially from an education and training point of view.

33.2. An introduction to Varian and Varian solutions

Our company's vision is one that we like waking up to every morning: you know there's one of the unique things we have in the world of healthcare and that is being purpose-led. You know that we join you as caregivers, as governments, as NGOS, and as companies in the space.

We love being inspired by a vision that is fun to get up to everyday—a vision of 'a world without fear of cancer.' In our family, that means a lot to us. My wife is a stage III B breast cancer survivor, and she wouldn't be here without the tools and training of people in our field.

Our mission is to combine the ingenuity of people: our own people, our customers, partners, and scientists, with the power of data and technology to achieve new victories against cancer.

Varian has an installed base of over 8000 machines. For several years, this was kind of a replacement cycle in which we stayed at a consistent level. We'd ship new machines every year, but they were mostly just replacements. Now, we are seeing dramatic growth in the installed base. In 2019 alone, the net installed base of our own machines will grow by about 400 machines.

To grow the installed base by about 5% a year globally is a pretty big deal. Most of that growth is in emerging markets. Over half of our business is outside of the USA and we see that trend continuing. We believe that over the next 10 years that 70% of our business will be outside of the USA.

For the past 70 years, we envisioned the accelerator as the center of our strategy. Our strategy was characterized by 'how can we accessorize and put something new on that accelerator'. Today, we are pivoting toward the future and putting the patient and healthcare providers in the center of our strategy and thinking about what the products and services are, especially from an information technology point of view. One of the things we can bring, along with artificial intelligence, is to deliver on a vision where any patient in the world can get the best possible care. Using these innovative technologies, we can provide access to care, whether you are in a village in India or Africa, and provide the same level care a patient might get in downtown Boston.

In this vision, we will dramatically increase the patients we touch each year. This year, we will treat about 3.5 million patients with our technology and services. By 2027, we would like to be treating 20 million patients.

One of the most inspiring things we have seen across the world today is the number of survivals in the last decade. These patients are looking for ways to interact with caregivers and companies as they manage their post treatment survivorship.

33.3 Overview: cancer in Africa

Cancer is the second leading cause of death globally, and was responsible for an estimated 9.6 million deaths in 2018. Globally, about 1 in 6 deaths is due to cancer. Approximately 70% of deaths from cancer occur in low- and middle-income countries. [3] In the most affluent countries in the world, it is now number one. [4] Cancer is also fast becoming a leading cause of deaths in Africa, with almost 700 000 deaths in 2018 [5]. The interesting thing is that LMICs have a mix of infectious and non-communicable diseases. In 2016, the infectious disease burden was still more than half of the mortality burden. In 2045, cancer is projected to account for between two-thirds and three-quarters of the mortality burden.

As ministers of health wrestle with this shift, they must change their approach to how they invest. This approach has been embraced across Africa and in many other emerging markets. There is a gap that is well known and studied which was published in the *Lancet Oncology* [6]. It shows the installed base of radiation oncology centers and linear accelerators in 2015 and the projection of what is needed. If we project the current usage rates to 2035, you'll see that we need about 21800 linear accelerators by 2035.

Perhaps more significant than the capital resource is the significant increased need for radiation oncologists, physicists, and technologists. This burden is often overlooked. We talk about the struggle to acquire equipment and build services, but there are several cases where equipment has been installed but is not functioning because people don't have the training that they need to use that equipment. Solving this problem is critical to the future of cancer care, and we are working to bend this curve with data science, machine learning, and artificial intelligence.

There are over a million new cancer cases in Africa. In 2016, breast, cervical, prostate, liver, and colorectal cancers tended to be the big burden and were the most common cancers in Africa. Depending on the country, what we are seeing is a disease burden that is oriented to treatment by radiation therapy. 55%–80% of cancer patients, depending on the country, need radiation therapy as part of their treatment. Today, there are around 300 linear accelerators in Africa. Only less than 10% of patients have access to radiation therapy in low-income countries and in Africa. The population of Africa on Tuesday August 11, 2020, the day of editing this section, was 1 343 899 185 based on United Nations estimates [7]. In Africa alone, we estimate that at least a thousand plus linear accelerators will be required to address the known disease of today. Just to give you a benchmark for that, in China, it is about 20 to 28% of patients that have access to radiotherapy [7] https://www.worldometers.info/world-population/africa-population/.

33.4 Key procurement considerations

Radiation therapy requires vaults to house linear accelerators and protect service providers from excess radiation exposure. These vaults often exist at hospitals and cancer centers, but some have turned these spaces into storage for medical records and inventory due to a lack of funding. When funding can be secured, we are able to partner with governments to facilitate this process. In Kenya, a vault was built as part of a visionary future for the Moi Teaching and Referral Hospital (MTRH). Alternatively, in Sierra Leone, secondhand cobalt was purchased. We see a lot of secondhand equipment going into LMICs and often these machines don't work. These often cause problems, because they are poorly installed, poorly supported, and poorly maintained. It sets all of us back when things such as this happen. But gradually things are improving. While the Lancet Oncology report [6] identified challenges, such as limited resources, infrastructure, funding, human resources, lack of awareness, prevention, lack of diagnosis and high patient incidence numbers, procurement challenges also exist, such as price-based tender requirements that are often outdated and very specification oriented. Guidance from traditional entities and tender communities often lacks technical and clinical expertise. I am sure my competitors would say the same thing. New technology can address many of the common LMIC challenges.

This is the paradox: LMICs would benefit the most from a value-based procurement approach, but are most likely to rely on traditional procurement and evaluation methods. It is a reasonable goal to change the procurement conversation from technical components to an outcome oriented approach. If the goal is included in the tender, we can educate providers about value, as Dr Ahmed Elzawawy stated [1], hence create value-based tenders to drive clinical care. One of the most exciting things about radiotherapy—especially as it relates to advocacy with governments—is that our cost per patient is one of the lowest of any therapy in cancer. It is not a radiation vs. surgery vs. chemotherapy conversation; rather, we all work together. Yet too often, in the Health Minister's office, it's a conversation about what the drugs cost.

A combination of high patient volumes and short fractionation schemes means that the cost per patient can, in fact, be quite low. The cost per patient of delivering radiotherapy is a huge advantage compared to the cost of chemotherapy or surgery. Sometimes people are afraid of the upfront equipment cost and don't realize that the actual investment in drugs is equal to the number of units times price. This means that they could end up spending a lot more money on other approaches, when radiation therapy is actually the appropriate treatment technology. There have been a few recent papers published on this. We will provide these to the organizers. We need to do a better job of advocating for the value of radiation therapy and its cost-effectiveness per patient.

33.5 New solutions for Africa

I am not going to do marketing here, as you know, but suffice to say that we have introduced a new product focused on delivering the best IMRT in a very safe way at high volumes. This helps to bring the cost down and improve the patient experience, it is very easy on patients, and it is very easy to use.. One of our first customers on this project was treating 100 patients per day within 3 weeks using image-guided intensity-modulated radiotherapy (IMRT). It is also a product that will go into nearly any cobalt room, with not much additional shielding and requires about half the electricity of historical machines.

These are some of the things we must do for emerging markets to make it easier for folks to get in. Dr Ahmed Elzawawy asked 'What is the challenge in the last 12 months in Africa?' There is a 10% increase in Africa alone in terms of installed-base growth of radiotherapy linear accelerators. This is not year-over-year growth. It is the contribution to the installed base. This is probably the most significant change in any installed base we have seen in several decades at a country/geographical continent level.

33.6 Celebrating successes: partnerships to add value to RT procurement

We should celebrate these successes. Morocco, South Africa, Nigeria, and Kenya have ordered the 'Halcyon' product I mentioned above. What is just as inspiring is to see is that countries have embraced radiation therapy that haven't had it before. We have had the first radiation therapy in the Ivory Coast and the first non-cobalt machines in Tanzania and Senegal, all building partially on early positive experiences in Senegal and Sierra Leone. We have had the first reliable therapy after years of breakdown in Sudan, Nigeria, and the Republic of Congo.

Another example we are particularly proud of is Nigeria's NSIA-LUTH cancer center [2]. There is a lot of medical tourism outside of Nigeria. There are 115 000 new cancer patients in Nigeria annually. Most of the patients went to India or Europe prior to this cancer center opening. There were only six machines in Nigeria, and many were nonfunctional or only provided palliative care. A new public–private partnership was set up and the NSIA-LUTH cancer center operates with some of their own staff plus external operators. The tender, which was a cobalt-to-linear-accelerator transition included extensive training and education and was launched in February of 2019 by President Buhari. This has got off to a good start treating lots of patients where patients either had to leave the country or not get cured at all.

In Uganda, we had an in-country partnership with the African Development Bank, where they financed the construction and equipment for the Uganda Cancer Center Institute. This was another transition from cobalt to a linear accelerator. One important aspect of this partnership was a grant by the United States Trade and Development Agency (USTDA), which provided a training and education grant for three weeks of in-classroom training at Groot Schuur Hospital in South Africa, one month of onsite training by the University of California, San Diego, and a ten-week

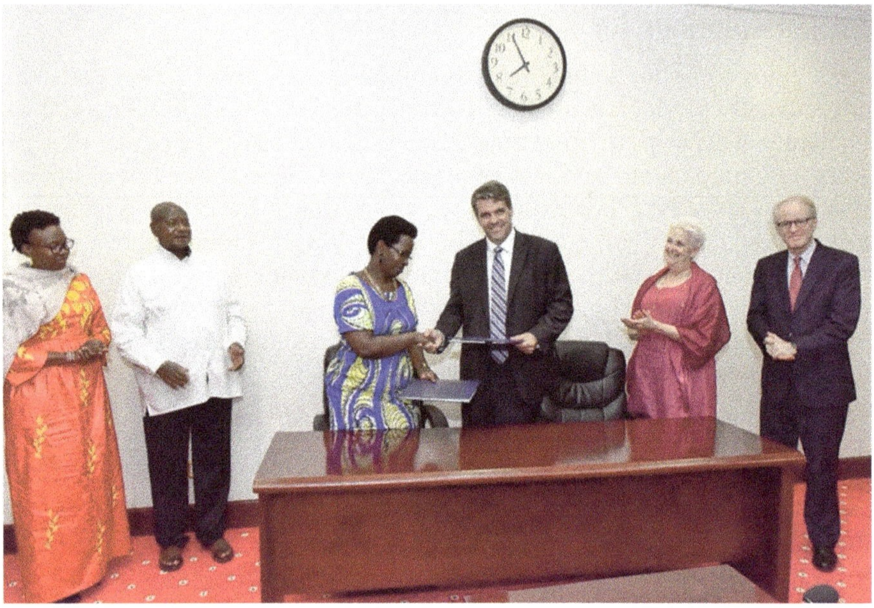

Figure 33.1. The President of Uganda along with the Minister of Health shaking hands with the director of USAID. To the right, Mr Dow Wilson, CEO and president of Varian Medical Systems (Siemens Healthineers).

remote mentoring period and transition from 2D to 3D conformal radiotherapy techniques for local radiation therapists (figure 31.1).

In Kenya, the government encouraged the private sector to address the cancer burden, and in doing so they developed a comprehensive reimbursement system to increase access to care. The Kenyan government provided coverage for radiation therapy to the private sector to increase access to care and development. The first 'Halcyon' at Nairobi West Hospital and the Mediheal Group of Hospitals was procured based on the reimbursement coverage provided by the government. The Mediheal Group has signed a partnership agreement for five linear accelerators; two of the five are very close to being turned on. The Kenyan government provided the ecosystem, so to speak, for the industry to grow.

As I mentioned before, Sierra Leone, based on what they saw in their neighbor Senegal, was encouraged to sign a Memorandum of Understanding (MoU) to establish the first radiation centre in the country. Financing was provided for a center and an enduring gap was filled in Sierra Leone.

33.7 Toward a more sustainable future

The Varian Medical Systems Foundation was established in 2007 to manage the company's philanthropy and charitable giving. The Varian Medical Systems Foundation makes grants, donations, and gifts to non-profit organizations that provide information and services involving the prevention, detection, and treatment of cancer, with a special emphasis on funding programs that address the role of radiation therapy in treating cancer. The Varian Medical Systems Foundation is an advised charitable fund managed by the Silicon Valley Community Foundation [8].

To help achieve our patient-centric vision, we acquired Cancer Treatment Services International (CTSI) in 2018. CTSI is an oncology solutions company dedicated to delivering high-quality cancer treatment around the world. CTSI emerged out of the University of Pittsburgh Medical Center (UPMC). They perform dosimetry and treatment planning services in the United States, and have a footprint of eleven cancer centers in India. They provide standardized evidence-based care based on the UPMC care pathway. We are very interested in developing the insights from these centers, and then pushing technology-enabled services to help emerging marketing customers to get into the field faster, with more expertise, and less need for both capital and operating resources. As noted before, there is a large gap in professional services that needs physicists, physicians, and therapists, and can we provide some of these services in these markets to help people get into the business faster. We are very excited about this and the data that comes with it and using the data not only in radiation therapy but across the cancer enterprise to help inform how we can treat cancer better and more effectively and also help us through this scale gap.

In 2019, the Global Access to Cancer Care Foundation (GACCF) was also launched. The GACCF offers training, technology, access, and hope; specifically, LMICs in South America, Africa, and South and East Asia. The foundation's cancer care professionals help to implement and oversee training courses and workshops in collaboration with local partners, such as universities, hospitals, or governmental institutions that enhance cancer treatment through radiotherapy treatment. Many Varian employees and many companies are participants in this foundation to help bring education, training, and capability to markets where they are especially difficult issues [9].

33.8 Spotlight on the outlook for the 3rd decade of the 21st century, particularly after the COVID-19 pandemic

Towards a historic increase of access to better-value radiotherapy and clinical oncology care in the real world.

33.9 The burden

As we look forward to the next 20 years, we are at a key point in the story of cancer mortality in Africa. If the current trajectory continues, forecasts estimate that cancer mortality will increase significantly to over 1.4 million deaths per year by 2040. To put this into perspective, current WHO estimates for combined HIV-, TB-, and malaria-related deaths by 2040 are estimated to total approximately 300 000. The success in addressing these diseases should be celebrated, but the gravity of the cancer burden should not be ignored [10].

A strong contributor to this success is global health financing; the majority of all financing dollars is spent on these three diseases. Of the approximately $13 billion spent in 2018 across sub-Saharan Africa alone, less than 1% was spent across all non-communicable diseases [11].

As such, governments need to not only increase their awareness of the current and future cancer burden but also start to take action, prioritize their cancer programs, and invest in their cancer systems. We, as the global cancer community, need to support LMICs that are still developing the infrastructure, expertise, and capability to create and execute their cancer plans.

33.10 Taking action

Several of the elements already outlined above need to be adopted across LMICs to drive sustainable cancer systems—most notably, national reimbursement models. Most high-income countries have established reimbursement models which support a sustainable radiotherapy ecosystem and encourage private-led investment, which is thus far absent in the vast majority of African countries. Whilst most global reimbursement is driven by fee-for-service models, Africa also has the opportunity to adopt a value-based approach from the onset.

Reimbursement will stimulate the local ecosystem and improve radiotherapy access, but to accelerate this process, there is a need for new innovative models which leverage regional consolidated purchasing power and innovative and blended financing. Multistakeholder engagement and alignment is critical to drive this, as many African countries are yet to have a comprehensive cancer plan, let alone a radiotherapy strategy.

There is also an opportunity for the radiotherapy community to adopt some best practices and innovative approaches that other industries have implemented across the region. One such initiative is the Cancer Access Partnership, which is improving access to 'chemotherapies and endocrine therapies aligned to evidence-based guidelines harmonized for sub-Saharan Africa' [12].

33.11 Technology

As the radiotherapy industry continues to innovate, it will incorporate more artificial intelligence and automation and this will in turn support task-shifting, minimize the prerequisite limitations to setting up cancer centers and in turn making their running easier and more efficient. It is important that the cancer community encourages these new technologies and innovations to be properly evaluated and considered, as Africa will benefit significantly from these. Governments should place importance on innovation and assess the impact that newer technologies can have on their cancer burden and both the quality and cost-effectiveness of these improvements.

33.12 Capacity building

Finally, whilst technological advancements will support radiotherapy access, it is still necessary to ensure that clinical and technical capacity building are supported in each country. The long-term sustainability of cancer delivery is dependent on local expertise and capacity. It is also important that key leadership roles are identified and filled by experts who are empowered to drive meaningful, transformational change and bend the cancer mortality curve before it materializes [9].

Note from the Editors:

- Varian Medical Systems was acquired by Siemens Healthineers on April 15, 2021. This transformative combination accelerated Siemens Healthineers' impact on global healthcare and establishes a strong partner for customers and patients along the entire cancer care continuum.
- As we mentioned, this book is presented as a 'living book', hence, the reader is invited to access the video of the speech by clicking on [1]: https://www.youtube.com/watch?v=6r6icocR26o&feature=youtu.be.
- Moreover, for all readers, the links for book feedback, suggestions, and ideas can be found at:
  http://icedoc.net/feedback.html
  http://icedoc.org/feedback.html
- Once again, we welcome all. The challenge is huge and it needs all.

References

[1] Wilson D Increasing value-based radiotherapy in LMICs. Sustainable partnership for Africa. Global Health Summit, 24th May, 2019 at Harvard Medical School, Boston, MA, USA https://youtube.com/watch?v=6r6icocR26o&feature=youtu.be

[2] Elzawawy A Harvard global health win-win initiative. Where we are? Where we go. Global Health Summit, 24th May, 2019 at Harvard Medical School, Boston, MA, USA https://youtu.be/gPnfjY8kqyA

[3] World Health Organization. Key facts https://who.int/news-room/fact-sheets/detail/cancer#:~:text=Cancer%20is%20a%20leading%20cause,Lung%20(2.09%20million%20case

[4] World Health Organization Global health observatory data repository http://who.int/gho/database/en/

[5] The global cancer observatory. World Health Organization https://gco.iarc.fr/today/data/factsheets/populations/903-africa-fact-sheets.pdf

[6] Atun R, Jaffray D A and Barton M B 2015 Expanding global access to radiotherapy *Lancet Oncol.* 2015 Sep **16** 1153–86

[7] Worldmeters. World population https://worldometers.info/world-population/africa-population/

[8] Varian Medical Systems Foundation https://varian.com/about-varian/corporate-citizenship/giving/varian-medical-systems-foundation

[9] Global access to cancer care foundation (GACCF) https://globalaccf.org/

[10] Projections of mortality and causes of death, 2016 to 2060 https://who.int/healthinfo/global_burden_disease/projections/en/

[11] Financing global health https://vizhub.healthdata.org/fgh/

[12] New agreements to lower prices and increase access to lifesaving cancer treatment in sub-Saharan Africa https://clintonhealthaccess.org/agreements-to-increase-access-to-cancer-treatment-in-africa/

Chapter 34

Cancer does not discriminate between the rich and the poor: precision radiation medicine for everyone everywhere

Habib Nehme

This chapter shares another industry perspective echoing the need for collaboration, increased access to needed precision radiotherapy treatment, and concerted policy efforts to guard against discriminate access to cancer treatments, especially in resource-poor settings. Solutions currently adopted by ELEKTA are also shared.

Cancer does not discriminate between rich and poor, but good treatment does. However, there is no reason to have such inequalities in cancer treatment between countries. Our collective aim is that healthcare policy shapers, suppliers, and academic and financial institutions will align all the elements of holistic solutions to fight cancer. This starts with prevention, adapting lifestyles, early detection, fast diagnostics, precise treatment planning, precision treatment, and continuous control. The question is how to get all these solutions in countries that sometimes lack the basics of highly functional healthcare systems and even the fundamental means of economic survival.

At ELEKTA, we believe that part of our corporate and social responsibility in treating patients with cancer is to enable and find all the elements of the solution by localizing human capital and building the backbone of sustainable local precision radiation medicine.

Almost 43% of the global population, 3.3 billion inhabitants, live in the 79 African, Middle Eastern, and Indian countries covered by my team. We believe that cancer incidence will be more than 3.8 million new patients annually by 2025. In these regions, 7.2 million people suffer from cancer and 50% or more of them should have access to radiation therapy. This number is overwhelming, as it means that 3.6 million persons should be treated by the existing linear accelerators per year, which are only 1200 in number. A rough calculation shows that the region would need at least four times more linear accelerators and the associated human resources to

doi:10.1088/978-0-7503-3075-6ch34

accommodate this number of patients. (*Human resources*: radiation oncologists, medical physicists, radiation technologists, and administrators)

Many solutions are currently being pursued to accelerate access to precision radiation medicine in developing and emerging markets:

1. ***Localisation: the more we know, the more we dare.***

   We should build local backbones of organizations capable of implementing radiotherapy techniques not only for palliative cases but for all stages. These local solutions will allow the transfer of technical clinical knowledge to qualify needs and sustain the good use of radiation therapy and other methodologies in cancer treatment.

   Moreover, the pandemic is showing us that that we are in reverse globalization, as countries should be self-sufficient enough to treat cancer locally. Patients are less mobile and digital platforms could be used extensively to provide planning remotely and treatment locally.
2. As company, we have a responsibility to ***partner with health ministries*** to develop national cancer plans and enable equal access to radiation therapy treatment in all regions of these countries, urban and rural. The productivity and continuity of the overall circle of treatment is key; therefore, we should advise governments how to alleviate the hurdle of the transportation of patients to cancer care centres. We should bring the treatment to the patient, not the opposite.

   We should help governments to develop and prioritize budgets for cancer treatment and support them in understanding the trade-offs between radiation therapy, chemotherapy, and/or surgery. Engaging the private sector and outsourcing cancer treatment to global clinical operators would accelerate and improve clinical outcomes.
3. ***Comprehensive Education and training programs*** are key to building local human capital through continuous or academic training. From 'get me started' to 'make me an expert', companies and academies should join efforts to design the full range of curricula from pregraduation to postgraduation and to locally nurture knowledge of medical physics and radiation oncology.
4. ***Innovative***, fast, easy to use adapted technology would accelerate the adoption of radiation therapy. Siting, reliability, and high serviceability would make solutions sustainable in countries where operating expenses are scarce.

Finally, we believe that each country, regardless of the level of the economic ladder at which it is situated, could, and deserves to, have radiotherapy solutions, either internal or external beams. Economic reasons could slow down the implementation of these solutions in some poor countries, but they are not enough to stop it. Our objective should be more about overall healthcare systems, about know-how, and the sustainability of the solutions. ELEKTA, as a global precision radiation therapy company, is ready to contribute to the fulfilment of the vision and the mission.

Note from the Editors:

The reader can view a video of the talk presented by Habib NEHME, vice president of Elekta entitled 'We are here till cancer not' at The Global Health Summit, May 24–26, 2019 at Harvard Medical School, Boston, MA, USA [1] at the following link: https://www.youtube.com/watch?v=cA5HfRagz-Q.

Reference

[1] Nehme H 2020 We are here till cancer is not! Mr Habib Nehme, Executive Vice President of Elekta for emerging Markets, Presented in GHC Summit May 25, 2019, Harvard Medical School, Boston, MA

Part VI

Examples of initiatives and actions

Chapter 35

The International Cancer Expert Corps (ICEC): a 'Win^n' model solution with the exponential growth necessary for global cancer care

C Norman Coleman, Manjit Dosanjh, Donna O'Brien and Miles A Pomper

ICEC's '**Win^n**' approach can transform global cancer care. The many terrific non-government organizations such as the Union for International Cancer Care and its members (https://www.uicc.org/) and the efforts of the Health Campus of the International Atomic Energy Agency (https://humanhealth.iaea.org/hhw/) demonstrate that there is an interest and reasonable data with which to address the shortage of global cancer care. It seems somewhat obvious that the pace of developing cancer care can build from these programs but requires the exponential growth of the ICEC '**Win^n**' solution. We can create a paradigm shift built on the African proverb: 'If you want to go fast, go alone. If you want to go far, go together'. Is it too hard, or not worth the effort, or someone else's problem? Hogwash! The need is clear. The scope of the required cancer care and the systems to accomplish it are largely well-known in the HIC world. What makes it possible to overcome this challenge is the new generation interested in social change that addresses longstanding inequality issues. Cancer, a diagnosis that has the urgency of an infectious disease, which requires attention to prevention and etiology and involves both infectious and noncommunicable diseases, is the ideal template upon which to develop the sustainable, on-the-ground expertise that constitutes the ICEC model. Collaborators, participants, supporters, advocates, and those who seek life-transforming challenges: welcome to the **Win^n** team!

Disclaimer: This article reflects the authors' personal opinions regarding global health disparities and does not represent the opinion or policy of the companies, non-governmental organizations, or federal agencies (C N Coleman, CNC) through which they are employed. The International Cancer Expert Corps (ICEC) is an 'official outside activity' of CNC.

35.1 Introduction—the problem to be solved

There is no reason why people with cancer should not have access to at least a basic effective level of cancer care. There are excuses and explanations as to why some do not, often based on the assumption that meeting this need would be 'too expensive', stealing resources needed for other basic healthcare services. We have carefully considered these assumptions, comparing what is available for cancer care in high-income countries (HICs), low- and middle-income countries (LMICs), and geographically remote regions in HICs, often involving the aboriginal and indigenous populations (which the ICEC has dubbed 'local–global'), examined disease burdens in these areas, looked at the potential economic gains of proper cancer care [1], and concluded that these explanations are 'hogwash'! Doctors Elzawawy and Ngwa's basic premise in 'Approaching global oncology: The win-win model' is not only logical but essential. In the era of COVID and visible exponential growth, the global cancer care solution can and should be a '**Win^n**' (i.e., a Win to the *n*th power).

35.2 Why the ICEC was established

The roots of the ICEC date back many decades (to the 1960s) but also jibe with a recognition of the damage caused by inequality damage, which is currently being expressed in the social unrest of Black Lives Matter and similar movements around the globe. The ICEC's approach to healthcare system solutions is built on cancer care, which has required us to not only address societal inequality but also the opinions of a variety of policymakers and experts as to what aspects of healthcare are 'affordable'. In the field of global cancer care, some emphasize that only some aspects of cancer care are reasonable (or another such term), such as prevention or palliative care, because effective treatment is too expensive for populations in LMICs and the 'local–global' whose access issues are similar to those of LMICs. We strongly support prevention but reject this approach in that it is not acceptable in HICs and should not be in LMICs.

35.3 Broad impact for global oncology

Built on the decades-long experience of many of ICEC's founders and members (www.iceccancer.org), the non-government, not-for-profit entity was formally established in 2013, incorporated in the US but global in origin. The program needed to be built from the ground up using knowledge from 'top-down' experience, articulated by Love, Ginsburg, and Coleman as 'Public Health Oncology' [2]. In an ICEC paper in *JAMA Oncology*, 2019 [3], Coleman *et al* described 'a System Approach to Global Oncology'; six program components are interrelated in a complex system with achievements that provide patient-centered global oncology care. (This is illustrated in [3].)

Program components for patient-centered global oncology:

(i) Expertise beyond healthcare; radiation scientists, economists, educators, and sociologists;

(ii) Expertise in healthcare; clinicians, allied healthcare professionals, trainees, mentors;
(iii) Disease treatment; infectious and non-communicable diseases;
(iv) Research and development; academia and industry;
(v) Novel technological approaches;
(vi) Funding and support; visionaries, donors, entrepreneurs.

Achievements:
- Catalytic innovation to address intractable problems;
- Encouragement of global collaboration;
- Public/private partnerships and social engagement;
- Promotion of broader societal benefit;
- Novel partnerships to advance goals;
- Healthcare delivery innovation;
- Capturing the wisdom of senior and retiring experts;
- Academic and private sector global health career paths;
- Comprehensive cancer care including infectious and noncommunicable diseases;
- Implementation of accepted research;
- Disruptive innovation;
- Reverse innovation and knowledge sharing.

The above program represents our vision of patient-centered global oncology [3]. We are endeavoring to establish our '**Win**^{n}' and then address some of the challenges in global health that require the win-win approach.

35.4 Expertise in healthcare

The essence of the ICEC solution for global cancer care is to have the necessary, sustainable onsite expertise built through local champions and local or country-based investment. The broad expertise required includes medical care delivery, scientific expertise, and supporting care. (See the ICEC table at www.iceccancer.org). Not only is proper education and training critical to expert care, but also the ability to remain up-to-date in a world of rapidly advancing science. The ICEC uses a mentorship model that extends from trainees to mid-career staffers to senior leaders to retirees, built on twinning relationships between hubs (cancer centers, professional societies, and community practitioners) and ICEC centres (LMIC-based and 'local–global') coordinated by a central network to ensure broad global interaction and ultimately a corps of experts available to achieve the '**Win**^{n}' outcome.

35.5 Disease treatment

Global health often opts to compartmentalize one disease versus another. This is understandable to some extent and reflects the various charities and causes in HICs. However, it is counterproductive, as systems solutions are needed that build healthcare capacity versus disease-specific programs that reflect available expertise. Cancer is a complex disease that requires the management of care across a continuum: from prevention and screening through diagnosis and treatment, surveillance, and palliative and end-of-life care as well as understanding cancer's relationship to infectious diseases (such as viruses that cause cancer) and the immunosuppression caused by cancer treatment. As Harvey Fineberg, former President of the Institute of Medicine (now the National Academy of Medicine) has said, 'if we can solve the problems of cancer care, we have the key to solving healthcare more broadly' [4]. Cancer is a disease for which healthcare management has recognized that there is a benefit to health system investment [5].

The ICEC is promoting local investment in infrastructure to support cancer care and access to expertise; among its goals are sustainable programs for cancer that also strengthen healthcare overall.

35.6 Technology

The current LINAC technology used to deliver radiation therapy (RT) requires a large number of expert professional staff (including radiation oncologists, medical physicists, dosimetrists, service engineers, and radiation therapy technologists) to treat patients and to maintain the equipment. In most LMICs, there is a shortage of machines, frequent breakdowns, and too few engineers to keep the machines working.

Therefore, we need technological development to produce a modular, robust machine suited for harsher environmental conditions and often poorer infrastructures while requiring fewer qualified experts. The RT system needs to be user- and patient-centered and incorporate artificial intelligence (AI) and machine learning (ML) throughout all processes to help reduce both clinician effort and the need for costly and scarce technical support personnel. The use of modular design in conjunction with remote monitoring and fault analysis will expedite maintenance and repairs, lessening the need for specialized personnel and shortening downtime.

In order to meet these challenging but essential goals, the ICEC and CERN hosted a dialogue between multistakeholder collaborators consisting of clinicians, accelerator physicists, AI experts, and public health and healthcare system experts to kick off this ambitious effort of bringing the high-energy physics community's broad expertise in global networking, technology innovation, and open-source knowledge to the benefit of all. The project to implement radiation therapy in resource-limited settings is now well underway [6].

35.7 Expertise beyond healthcare

Support for the development of such machines has also gained support from stakeholders in the security community, who are concerned that the cobalt-60 machines that still provide external radiation treatment could be a source of material for a terrorist 'dirty bomb' or other radiological weapon [7]. The provision of the new LINACs better suited for these countries, therefore, could be a win-win, providing improved treatment and decreasing the risk of terrorism.

35.8 Aspects of the challenges to creating Win^n solutions for collaboration:

The ICEC model used to develop expertise is largely centred on people who have the time to build expertise and technological systems. Ideally, medical professionals would be able to do this as part of their job, but doing so often requires some additional commitment. To encourage and enable participation, individuals and institutions need: (a) appropriate recognition for their contribution as part of a larger effort, (b) support for global health as a bona fide part of a career, even as performance metrics are often tied to revenue generation, (c) a career path including academic promotion [8] that values contribution and continual growth through and including retirement and a grant/funding system that rewards collaboration and enables a continual expansion of capacity and (d) appreciation of the scope of a solution for cancer care for all. Exponential growth is essential in that commissioning one well-staffed LINAC per week would require a century to fill the *current gap o*f 5000 and probably twice that number to address the WHO Sustainable Development Goals (https://www.who.int/sdg/en/).

Healthcare is the sector that can lead the way, because the common goals are obvious, as clearly demonstrated most recently by COVID-19 and in the past with the introduction of the Medicare program, which required an end to segregation in U.S. hospitals [9]. We involved in addressing inequity in global cancer care have an enormously important opportunity to build the teamwork, network and collaborations to help solve a problem of human suffering the solution for which others inappropriately deem as 'to hard'.

References

[1] Atun R, Jaffray D A, Barton M B *et al* 2015 Expanding global access to radiotherapy *Lancet Oncol.* **16** 1153–86

[2] Love R R, Ginsburg O M and Coleman C N 2012 Public health oncology: a framework for progress in low- and middle-income countries *Ann Oncol.* **23** 3040–5

[3] Coleman C N, Wendling E N and Pistenmaa D A 2019 A broad impact for global oncology *JAMA Oncol.* **5** 1397–8

[4] Fineberg H and Institute of Medicine 2013 *Delivering Affordable Cancer Care in the 21st Century: Workshop Summary* (Washington, DC: National Academies Press (U.S.)) p 3

[5] Holden D J, Reiter K, O'Brien D and Dalton K 2015 The strategic case for establishing public-private partnerships in cancer care *Health Res. Policy Syst.* **13** 44

[6] Dosanjh M, Aggarwal A,Pistenmaa D *et al* 2019 Developing innovative, robust and affordable medical linear accelerators for challenging environments *Clin. Oncol. (R Coll. Radiol.).* **31** 352–5

[7] Pomper M A, Dalnoki-Veress F and Moore G M 2016 Treatment, not terror. Strategies to enhance external beam cancer therapy in developing countries while permanently reducing the risk of radiological terrorism (Monterey, CA: James Martin Center for Nonproliferation Studies)

[8] Rodin D, Yap M L, Grover S *et al* 2017 Global health in radiation oncology: the emergence of a new career pathway *Semin. Radiat. Oncol.* **27** 118–23

[9] Smith D B 2016 The power to heal: civil right, medicare, and the struggle to transform America's health care system (Nashville: Vanderbilt University Press)

IOP Publishing

Approaching Global Oncology
The win-win model
Ahmed Elzawawy and Wilfred Ngwa

Chapter 36

Solar-powered radiotherapy

Ralf Müller-Polyzou and Holger Wirtz

One necessary but sometimes unanticipated challenge in establishing and maintaining radiotherapy and other technology- and equipment-reliant components of cancer care is the lack of, limited, or high-cost sources of energy needed to power these machines. Meanwhile, many LMICs benefit from significant amounts of sunshine for much of the year. This chapter makes the case for investing in solar-powered radiotherapy, utilizing the example of a pilot project in Africa, referencing an established facility in Europe, and providing details of the potential and necessary considerations for such an endeavor.

36.1 Introduction

Only a few years remain to fulfill the 17 global goals defined by world leaders in 2015 in order to create a better world by 2030 [1]. Many of the Sustainable Development Goals (SDGs) and corresponding targets relate to the challenges and minimum requirements for radiotherapy (RT) in low- and middle income countries (LMICs) [2, 3]. However, three goals stand out in particular: (1) SDG3, which relates to good health and wellbeing; (2) SDG7, which relates to affordable and clean energy; and (3) SDG9, which relates to industry, innovation, and infrastructure. The SDG targets that are directly or indirectly linked to RT practice are listed in table 36.1. These three SDGs guide us in formalizing our proposed win-win-win partnership to accelerate solar-powered RT in LMICs.

Pioneering inventions shaped the development of RT over decades. Electrification was the prerequisite for x-ray tubes and modern linear accelerators. Computerization and the increase in processing power enabled computed tomography (CT), magnetic resonance imaging (MRI), and complex radiation planning. State-of-the-art RT, sometimes referred to as Radiotherapy 4.0, is based on integrated systems and information and communications technology (ICT) [4]. Today, electrical energy is a prerequisite for modern RT practice worldwide.

The demand for electricity at healthcare facilities can be satisfied or be reduced using renewable energy sources [5–7]. Franco *et al* presented a comprehensive review

doi:10.1088/978-0-7503-3075-6ch36

Table 36.1. Three sustainable development goals and their radiotherapy-related targets.

SDG3: good health and wellbeing	SDG7: affordable and clean energy	SDG9: industry, innovation, and infrastructure
3.4 Reduce mortality from non-communicable diseases. 3.8 Achieve universal health coverage 3.A Implement the WHO framework convention on tobacco control. 3.C Increase health financing and support the health workforce in developing countries	7.1 Universal access to modern energy. 7.2 Increase global percentage of renewable energy. 7.3 Double the improvement in energy efficiency. 7.A Promote access to research, technology, and investments in clean energy 7.B Expand and upgrade energy services for developing countries	9.3 Increase access to financial services and markets. 9.4. Upgrade all industries and infrastructures for sustainability. 9.A Facilitate sustainable infrastructure development for developing countries. 9.C Universal access to information and communications technologies

of sustainable energy sources and technologies for healthcare facilities in the Global South. They estimated the energy needs, analyzed different technologies and presented implementation projects. Access to stable electricity is identified as the main energy challenge for healthcare facilities in the Global South. Unstable electricity, including power outages and voltage surges, causes damage to medical devices and products. Photovoltaics (PV) is a green energy source that combines many advantages. The technology is mature, robust, scalable, almost maintenance free, and can be installed by a local workforce. The investment costs have declined due to mass production, while the operational cost over the typical lifetime of 20–25 years is low. Furthermore, PV technology is flexible and can be deployed in hybrid systems that include wind turbines, battery storage, and fuel-based support generators [8]. Finally, PV systems can be established as independent off-grid or grid-connected systems [9]. The overall PV capacity installed worldwide is constantly increasing, according to the figures reported by the International Renewable Energy Agency (IRENA) for both off-grid and grid-connected systems [10, 11].

PV energy is the preferred choice for RT. The Global Solar Atlas provided free of charge by the World Bank Group can be used to analyze the Sun's irradiation and anticipated PV electricity production for worldwide locations [12]. Figure 36.1 shows a direct comparison of the expected PV output versus RT availability according to the DIrectory of RAdiotherapy Centres (DIRAC) [13]. Electricity production of more than 4 kWh per installed 1 kWp of PV power is possible in many regions that are currently underserved with RT.

However, installation-specific conditions must be considered for PV. The available space, roof orientation, shadow obstacles, and distance to the grid network influence the electricity output and PV system cost. A structural analysis must also be performed in

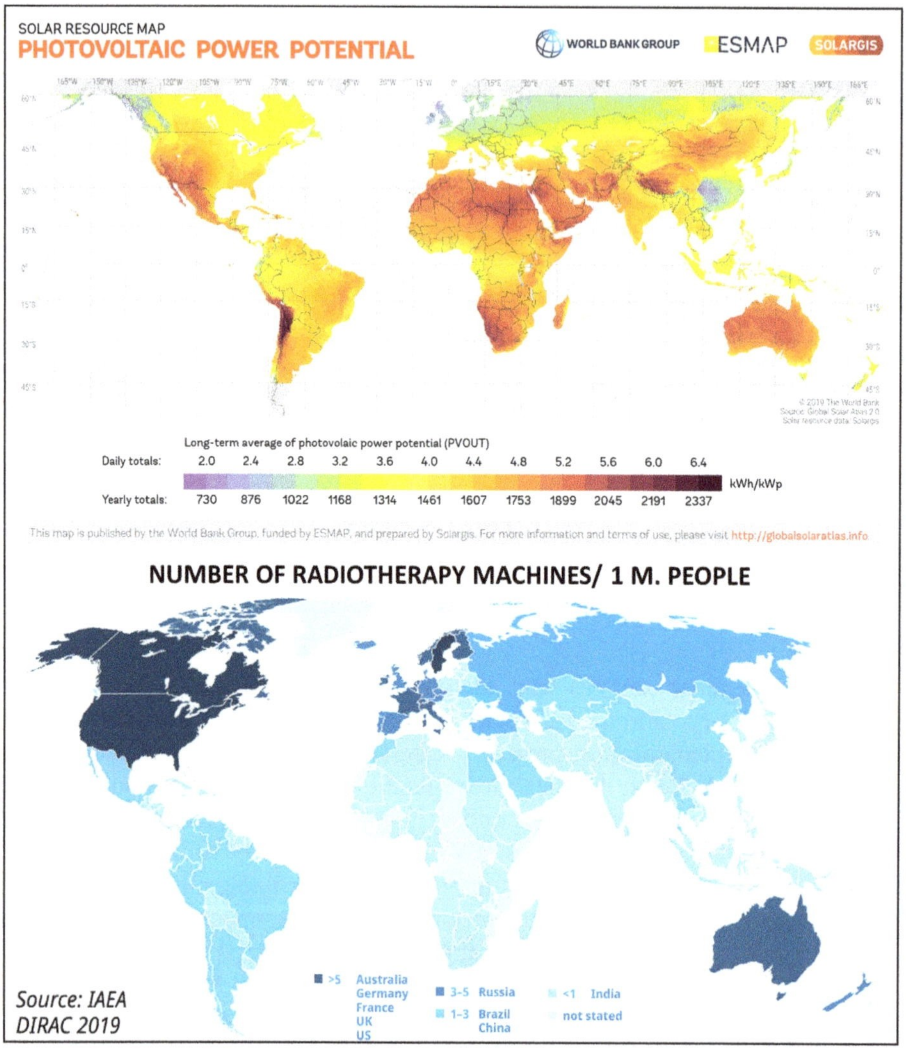

Figure 36.1. Comparison of the expected PV output (reprinted with permisson from [25], copyright The World Bank/CC BY 4.0) and RT availability worldwide (reprinted with permission from [13], copyright 2022 International Atomic Energy Agency).

many cases due to the weight and wind loads of PV installations—particularly on roofs. Thus, PV systems are dimensioned by experts using professional software tools [14].

The Lake Constance Radiation Oncology Center in Germany partly operates two linear accelerators, one CT scanner, and advanced ICT and cooling systems. The PV system is grid-connected and started operating in 2011. It consists of 232 photovoltaic modules in 400 m^2 with a total installed power of 55.68 kWp and three non-central inverters [15]. Energy storage in the form of batteries could be added to the system, as shown in figure 36.2.

A PV study for RT has been conducted by the Deutsche Gesellschaft für Internationale Zusammenarbeit (GiZ) for an RT center in Ghana. The optimum PV

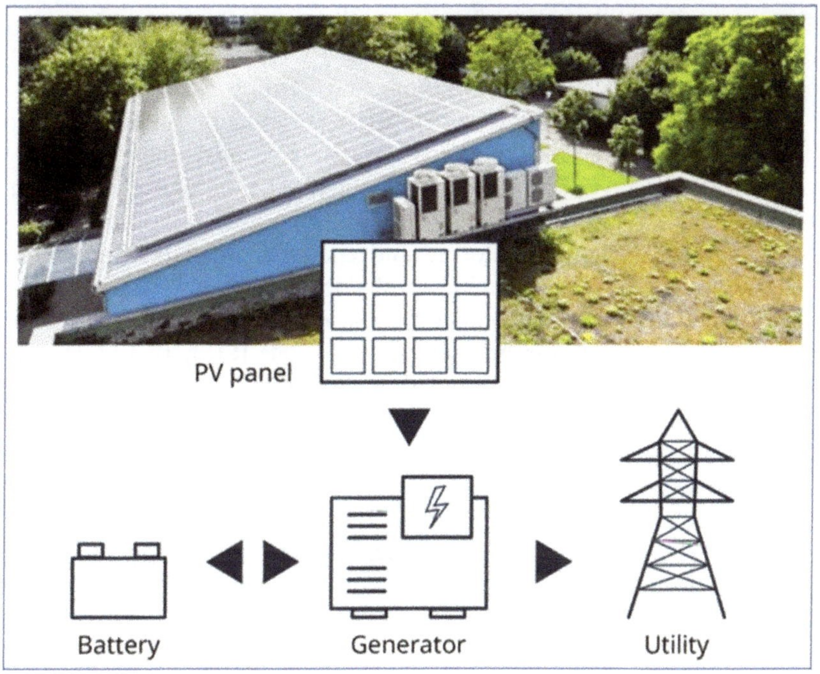

Figure 36.2. PV rooftop installation at the Lake Constance Radiation Oncology Center in Germany.

panel size, the optimum energy storage system (ESS), the load profile, and the local installation conditions have been evaluated. The study shows that a well-designed PV system with short-term energy storage reduces the average cost of energy [16, 17]. The study of the power replacement of an existing RT center started with load measurements during the day and at night. The peak load was measured at noon, when the patient workload is high and cooling systems operate at their maximum. On the contrary, load requirements are low at night, as linear accelerators and CT scanners are normally switched off. MRI scanners, however, remain constantly powered because of their coils. The mid-size RT center in Ghana is equipped with one linear accelerator, one CT scanner and one MRI scanner. In total, 35 configurations have been evaluated for PV power ratings of up to 300 kWp and ESS sizes of 0 to 400 kWh. The ESS systems were able to support the required load of 120 kW for the RT department, considering the balance between the production and consumption of energy during a full day. Based on the study, a standard RT site located near the equator requires a PV system of approximately 150 kWp, an ESS of 120 kW/140 kVA, and 100 kWh. The PV field has a size of approximately 1500 m^2. For an investment of €375 000, a payback time of five years can be achieved. Introducing energy efficiency measures, such as replacing light bulbs with light-emitting diodes (LEDs) would have a further positive impact. A project design, including potential expansions, is mandatory and should be performed by experts.

PV systems are conveniently monitored and controlled using web portals that visualize yield data, energy flows from the grid/batteries, system status, and overall performance. Even weather information such as sun irradiation, temperature, and wind speed are collected locally and stored in the cloud. Soon, energy management systems will control loads according to the PV system's capability and user requirements. Cooling systems, ventilation, and lighting will be intelligently controlled to optimize consumption, lower energy costs, increase self-consumption, and avoid load peaks. The required information could be provided straight from the medical devices or by external energy meters. The energy requirements and availability could even be considered in therapy and appointment planning. Therefore, both PV system monitoring and energy management systems require an internet connection. Additionally, a reliable internet connection of sufficient bandwidth would support tele-oncology opportunities, such as e-consultation, second opinion, remote tumor boards, and even tele-RT networks [18, 19]. The importance and potential of ICT for RT, including its possible catalyzing role for global collaboration, has been outlined in [23].

The SDGs provide a global framework that international companies apply to their corporate sustainability and responsibility activities. These companies include the leading manufacturers of RT, PV, and ICT equipment, such as Elekta, Ericsson, Microsoft, and others [24, 25]. SDG17 challenges us to revitalize global partnerships for sustainable development. We believe that a true win-win-win partnership for solar-powered RT can be created based on common interests between the leading manufacturers in the RT, PV, and ICT fields. The incorporation of nonprofit organizations [24] can further strengthen partnerships to provide better value cancer care worldwide. Table 36.2 presents an overview of common and special contributions as well as essential benefits for companies.

The win-win-win partnership for solar-powered RT in LMICs can succeed, considering the common and special interests of the involved stakeholders. It is not so much a question of technology, but rather a matter of developing the right partnership model. The challenges are great and increasing, but so will the strength of the partnership companies and their resources. With this article, we launch a call to international companies to build such partnerships in the short term, in the interest of all.

Note from the Editors:

In some African and other LMICs, one of the problems is the interruption to, or the inefficiency of, the electricity supply. This hinders the establishment of radiation oncology units. One proposal is to use solar-powered radiotherapy. It could also be an energy supply source for neighboring services or locations. This could be an option in some business models to produce income that serves in making the establishment of a radiotherapy unit more cost-effective, even in such situations. In the Win-Win movement, we do not impose any proposal as a sole solution for the stakeholders and decision makers, but we call for a continuous search for smart approaches. We stress the concept that implies that as far as possible, whatever the challenges, stakeholders should not surrender easily to the saying 'good-quality radiotherapy is impossible to establish!'

—Ahmed Elzawawy and Wilfred Ngwa

Table 36.2. Contributions and benefits of PV, ICT, and RT companies.

	PV companies	ICT companies	RT companies
Common contribution	• Subject matter experience and existing references • Global market access through own offices, distributors, and partners • Contact with local governments, institutions, and regulators • Financing, education, and support programs • Sustainability and corporate responsibility experts and funds		
Special contribution	• Knowledge of electricity networks and energy policies, requirements, and opportunities • Regulatory requirements and grid-connection competence	• Experience in providing services to rural areas • Experience of PV-powered mobile network sites • Support through the ITU and other ICT organizations	• Knowledge of Healthcare and RT requirements in LMICs • Support from the IAEA and the UN in the fight against cancer • NGO and local community access • Global Health Catalyst pragmatism
Common benefits	• Positive marketing and impact on customers, partners, employees, shareholders, and stakeholders in general • New customers, new business, and partnership opportunities		
Special benefits	• New applications in the health-care and RT segments • New sales channels to rural areas • New contacts for utility PV projects	• New or optimized products for RT • Add-on sales • New locations for ICT equipment e.g. radio links and antennas	• Reliable electricity and communication services for RT practices

References and further reading

[1] The Global Goals 2020 The global goals https://globalgoals.org/

[2] Massat M B 2019 Applied Radiation Oncology. A world of difference: addressing the global need for radiation oncology systems https://appliedradiationoncology.com/articles/a-world-of-difference-addressing-the-global-need-for-radiation-oncology-systems

[3] Wirtz H, Müller-Polyzou R, Engbert A, Bücker R, Azangwe G, Kron T, Petrovic M, Hasan M and Okonkwo E 2020 Emerging technologies for improving access to radiation therapy. *The Modern Technology of Radiation Oncology: A Compendium for Medical Physicists and Radiation Oncologists* vol 4 ed J Van Dyk (Madison, WI: Medical Physics Publishing) pp 461–87

[4] Müller-Polyzou R, Reuter-Oppermann M, Engbert A and Wirtz H 2019 Digitalisierung in der Strahlentherapie 4.0: Chancen *u*nd Möglichkeiten der digitalen Strahlentherapie ed N Krämer and C Stoffers *Digitale Transformation im Krankenhaus: Thesen, Potenziale, Anwendungen, 1. Auflage.* (Kulmbach: Mediengruppe Oberfranken) pp 191–214

[5] Delaney M 2018 Solar power super charges cost savings and energy efficiency for hospitals. *Healthtech Magazine* https://healthtechmagazine.net/article/2018/05/solar-power-super-charges-cost-savings-and-energy-efficiency-hospitals

[6] Low Carbon Energy Company 2020 Solar panels for hospitals | Low Carbon Energy Company https://lowcarbonenergy.co/solar-panels/hospitals/

[7] Renewable Energy World 2019 World's largest hospital solar PV project online now in Amman, Jordan *Renewable Energy World* https://renewableenergyworld.com/2019/08/27/worlds-largest-hospital-solar-pv-project-online-now-in-aman-jordan/#gref

[8] Franco A, Shaker M, Kalubi D and Hostettler S 2017 A review of sustainable energy access and technologies for healthcare facilities in the Global South *Sustain. Energy Technol. Assess.* **22** 92–105

[9] SMA Solar Technology AG 2020 SMA energy systems » Business | SMA Solar (Accessed 28 August 2020) https://sma.de/en/business/sma-energy-system-business-overview.html

[10] IRENA 2020 International Renewable Energy Agency https://irena.org/

[11] IRENA 2020 Renewable Energy Capacity Statistics 2020: International Renewable Energy Agency (IRENA), Abu Dhabi www.irena.org

[12] Solargis 2020 Global Solar Atlas https://globalsolaratlas.info/map?c=–29.53523,–62.578125,2

[13] Maistrenko O 2020 Division for Human Health: DIRAC (DIrectory of RAdiotherapy Centres) https://dirac.iaea.org/Query/Map2?mapId=0

[14] PVsyst 2020 Photovoltaic Dimensioning Software https://pvsyst.com/

[15] Elekta 2012 German radiotherapy clinic harnesses sun to run systems, cuts dependence on power grid https://www.prnewswire.com/news-releases/german-radiotherapy-clinic-harnesses-sun-to-run-systems-cuts-dependence-on-power-grid-140123103.html (Accessed 26 August 2020)

[16] Giz 2020 Deutsche Gesellschaft für int. Zusammenarbeit https://giz.de/en/html/index.html

[17] Wikipedia 2020 Levelized cost of energy https://en.wikipedia.org/w/index.php?title=Levelized_cost_of_energy&oldid=975265415

[18] Global Health Catalysts 2020 https://globalhealthcatalyst.com/get-involved-copy

[19] Datta N R, Heuser M, Samiei M, Shah R, Lutters G and Bodis S 2015 Teleradiotherapy network: applications and feasibility for providing cost-effective comprehensive radiotherapy care in low- and middle-income group countries for cancer patients *Telemed. J. E. Health* **21** 523–32

[20] Balogun O, Rodin D, Ngwa W, Grover S and Longo J 2017 Challenges and prospects for providing radiation oncology services in Africa *Semin. Radiat. Oncol.* **27** 184–8
[21] Elekta 2020 Elekta Annual Report 2019/20 https://elekta.com/investors/reports/annual-reports/
[22] Ericsson 2016 Sustainable future https://ericsson.com/en/about-us/sustainability-and-corporate-responsibility/sustainable-development-goals
[23] Microsoft 2020 Sustainable development—Microsoft Corporate Social Responsibility https://microsoft.com/en-us/corporate-responsibility/un-sustainable-development-goals
[24] Radiating Hope 2020 Advancing Cancer Care Globally https://radiatinghope.org/
[25] Wikipedia, World PVOUT Solar-resource-map https://en.wikipedia.org/wiki/File:World_PVOUT_Solar-resource-map_GlobalSolarAtlas_World-Bank-Esmap-Solargis.png

Chapter 37

Helping African radiotherapy centers to overcome staff challenges: experience in Mozambique

Iracelma Neto, Sara Velha, André Lucas, Sara Navarro, Daniel Gonçalves, Catarina Souto and Francisco Alves

In this chapter, local colleagues in Mozambique and Mercurius Health (MH) present their experiences from a real-life project, identifying significant obstacles, contextual considerations, and unforeseen challenges as well as lessons learned, recommendations, and identified successes.

Purchasing equipment for radiation oncology is an issue, but the bigger issue is how to make a clinical oncology unit functional and how to sustainably run it at high quality levels. The shortage of local staff, i.e. radiation oncologists, medical physicists, technicians, radiation therapists, and nurses is a known problem. The second wing of the Win-Win initiative requires catalytic action and a search for solutions that can increase access to highly functional clinical oncology services in the underserved regions of the world. This also means: do not repeat, repeat, and repeat the telling of long tales about the problems, gaps, and tragic shortage of clinical oncology care for the majority of cancer patients in the world, which usually ends with some wishes or recommendations that are mostly repeated later on in other articles or declarations. Rather, the notion of the win-win movement implies a search for practical examples of solutions to different parts of the problem in the real world. In successive Global Health Catalyst Summit Win-Win Initiative sessions, Professor Francisco Alves has indicated in presentations and videos that Mercurius Health, SA, Portugal intervened by sending teams of radiation clinical oncologists, engineers, physicists, technicians, and radiotherapists to non-functioning, equipped radiotherapy services. Not only do they ensure the good functioning and running of radiotherapy departments, but they ensure that the local teams are trained. Their contract is usually for four years, but Francisco Alves stressed that he considers Mercurius Health would be more successful in their mission if they were to gradually

doi:10.1088/978-0-7503-3075-6ch37

retrieve their non-local staff before the end of the four-year period so that local colleagues could assume the complete running of the department. At the Summits, he gave examples of their achievements in Angola and Mozambique.

37.1 Background

Cancer, in any country in the world, remains an issue of the 21st century. It is recognized that radiotherapy is an important component of cancer control programs in about half of all cancer cases [1]. However, there is a global disparity in the access to this treatment modality [2]. More than 50% of patients requiring radiotherapy in low- and middle-income countries (LMICs) do not have access to treatment. The provision of adequate radiotherapy infrastructure and the availability of human resources are major hurdles to the provision of appropriate cancer care in Africa [3–6].

Mozambique is experiencing changes in its epidemiological profile due to the emergence of noninfectious diseases. According to the World Health Organization's (WHO's) Globocan 2018 report, Mozambique has an incidence of 25 631 new cases per year of patients with cancer, resulting in a mortality of 17 813 (69.5%) and is expected to reach 39 026 new cases in five years' time. The pathologies with the highest incidence are: Kaposi's sarcoma (24.7%), uterine cervix (16.7%), prostate cancer (6.4%) and breast cancer (5.3%) [7]. In the past, Mozambican patients requiring radiotherapy were transferred out of the country, but unfortunately, due to financial constraints, this option was not achievable for the vast majority of Mozambicans.

The Radiotherapy Service of Maputo Central Hospital (SRTHCM, in the original abbreviation), the first and only radiotherapy service installed in Mozambique, was recently opened. This project was only possible with investment support from the International Atomic Energy Agency (IAEA) and a partnership with Neopharma, a local private company that used the services of Mercurius Health as an on-site operational and 'know-how transfer' company for technical consultancy, commissioning, operation, and training of the local team. SRTHCM is equipped with high-precision technology and integrates a multidisciplinary team of local professionals and MH qualified professionals. This article describes the main challenges faced and the daily experience of an on-site team at the first radiotherapy center in Maputo, Mozambique.

37.2 Radiotherapy service implementation and operation

37.2.1 Technology installation and commissioning challenges

The SRTHCM was inaugurated on the 28th of March, 2019. The equipment installed at SRTHCM includes an Elekta Synergy® Platform (Elekta AB) digital linear accelerator (linac), with a maximum photon energy of 15 MV, an Elekta Flexitron® High Dose Rate (HDR) brachytherapy system, using a cobalt-60 afterloader and a Siemens SOMATOM® Perspective (Siemens Healthcare GmbH) computed tomography (CT) scanner, with a maximum tube voltage of 130 kVp. The external beam radiotherapy go live was initially planned for

September 2017; however, as delays are inevitable in a project as big as setting up the first radiotherapy facility in a country, treatments only started on the 28th of August, 2019.

Before clinical use and after the installation of the linac, the first work of a physicist is to perform a bunker survey and accept the linac [8]. These should usually not take much more than a week; however, due to a considerable number of drawbacks, a year and a half passed between initial mechanical acceptance tests and the signature of the CAT (Customer Acceptance Test). Most of the challenges faced were technical problems, customs clearance of equipment and parts, calibration of measuring equipment, remote connection, and coordinating the availability of the teams on site.

Part of the success of a project with this complexity is the involvement of different teams, with a variety of origins, jobs, plans, and deadlines to meet. This creates the need for good management of the expectations of all involved, which is only possible with a good chain of communication to facilitate the exchange of information between everyone working in the project, which is not always easy to accomplish.

Since the installation of the linac, the project has experienced three major issues, which highlighted the importance of a good plan for the infrastructure: overload of the UPS at the beginning of the acceptance tests; the bunker door fell onto the floor minutes before the end of the acceptance tests; and, as detected at the commissioning stage, during the wet season, the relative humidity of the facility was greater than the manufacturer limits, which caused recurrent failure of the linac and the CT scanner, with an huge impact on the commissioning schedule.

After a failure, it was often necessary to replace equipment parts, which are imported from Europe, and schedule corrective maintenance, which is performed by a manufacturer's specialized engineer. Siemens has representation in Mozambique, so they are nearby, but Elekta's representation is in South Africa. From our experience, order dispatch and customs clearance are bureaucratic and take a long time, increasing the breakdown time, which delays the resumption of treatment.

37.2.2 Specialized human resources training program

It has been shown that training programs for radiotherapy personnel in LMICs are few and inadequate. Sending trainees to other continents has not yielded the desired results of improving human resource self-sufficiency [9]. When returning to their own countries, the vast majority of local professionals is unable to apply the knowledge received from staff trained in well-equipped facilities, in their socio-economic and environmental realities [10–12]. With this in mind, the training that MH has been promoting demonstrates that it is possible to fulfill local needs by having a team of four professionals in Mozambique for two continuous years on a day-to-day basis in a radiotherapy department. The aim of this resident team is to ensure that the local multidisciplinary team of physicists, radiotherapists, nurses, and radio-oncologists is learning and acquiring confidence in each activity performed, keeping up with new knowledge and trends in the field through continuing education, and contributing to improving cancer care in Mozambique.

In order to monitor and improve the local team's knowledge and experience, a first analysis was carried out and a plan was designed for each professional within the radiotherapy department. The previous experience of the local teams in a radiotherapy department was outside the country, mostly in Brazil, for one year, in a radiotherapy center with linacs made by a different manufacturer.

37.2.3 Operational support provided to the radiotherapy center

Clinical protocols, work instructions, assessments, leaflets, and templates were created based on the reality and needs of SRTHCM. At the beginning, cultural and work methodology differences generated some difficulties, which were overcome with time. The daily tasks started to be distributed and aligned according to the common objective of delivering safe and compassionate care to cancer patients.

From 28th August 2019 to 22nd May 2020, 81 patients (21 male, 60 female; mean age 48.5 y; age range, 18–73 y) with different tumor stages were treated at SRTHCM using three-dimensional conformal radiotherapy (3D-CRT). An average of 16 patients was treated per day (60% with a curative intention). The main pathologies were uterine cervical cancer (37%), breast cancer (21%), bone metastasis (12%), and head and neck cancer (10%).

37.3 Conclusions

The SRTHCM implementation allowed radiotherapy treatments to be provided in Mozambique which, together with other medical specialties (surgery, oncology, pathology, clinical psychology, among others), will have a crucial role in cancer programs in this country.

This experience has shown that it is essential to create a multidisciplinary team of professionals, with continuous education and training of all involved in diagnosis, staging, and treatment, to optimize patient outcomes. Furthermore, all the work carried out and all the obstacles encountered will be taken into account when drawing up a more robust plan for implementing new services in challenging environments such as those in Africa. Problems related to the management of power generators or the extremely humid conditions encountered, which were not initially addressed, will certainly be included in a future plan.

The scarcity of radiation oncology resources is becoming more severe as cancer incidence increases in LMIC countries. This can be overcome with more investment in radiotherapy machines. A past study estimated that in the next two to three decades, approximately 12600 radiotherapy machines will be needed [13], and their geographic distribution in a given country will have to be considered, in order for them to be easily accessible to patients. In Mozambique, due to the lack of resources and qualified professionals, the SRTHCM can only perform a single work shift of 8 h per day and, since the service is centralized in Maputo, 46% of the patients already treated had to travel long distances and ask for social assistance and/or family support for accommodation in Maputo in order to receive radiotherapy treatments.

In SRTHCM, there will always be challenges to overcome, and the MH expert team is committed to supporting local teams to improve quality and promote the workflow efficiency of the activities performed. However, more national and international collaborations are needed to ensure that radiotherapy professionals on the front line in Africa are well trained in fighting this disease, thereby gradually extending access to this cancer treatment modality.

References and further reading

[1] Barton M B, Jacob S, Shafiq J, Wong K, Thompson S R and Hanna T P *et al* 2014 Estimating the demand for radiotherapy from the evidence: a review of changes from 2003 to 2012 *Radiother. Oncol.* **112** P140–4

[2] Yap M L, Hanna T P, Shafiq J, Ferlay J, Bray F and Delaney G P *et al* 2017 The benefits of providing external beam radiotherapy in low and middle-income countries *Clin. Oncol.* **29** P72–83

[3] Division for Human Health: DIRAC (Directory of Radiotherapy Centers) http://nucleus.iaea.org/HHW/DBStatistics/DIRAC/index.html

[4] Datta N R, Samiei M and Bodis S 2014 Radiation therapy infrastructure and human resources in low-and middle-income countries: present status and projections for 2020 *Int. J. Radiat. Oncol. Biol. Phys.* **89** 448–57

[5] Grover S *et al* 2015 A systematic review of radiotherapy capacity in low- and middle-income countries *Front. Oncol.* **4** 380

[6] Zubizarreta E H, Fidarova E, Healy B and Rosenblatt E 2015 Need for radiotherapy in low and middle income countries—the silent crisis continues *Clin. Oncol.* **27** 107–14

[7] International Agency for Research on Cancer homepage https://gco.iarc.fr/

[8] Podgorsak E B (ed) 2005 *Radiation Oncology Physics: A Handbook for Teachers and Students.* (Vienna: IAEA) https://www-pub.iaea.org/mtcd/publications/pdf/pub1196_web.pdf

[9] Ndlovu N, Woldermariam A and Tigeneh G *et al* 2013 Radiotherapy education in Africa: an IAEA survey *African Organization for Research and Training (AORTIC) International Conference Abstract Book* p 284

[10] Wroe L M, Ige T A and Asogwa O C *et al* 2019 Comparative Analysis of radiotherapy linear accelerator downtime and failure modes in the UK, Nigeria and Botswana *Clin. Onc.* **32** e111–8

[11] Atun R, Jaffray D A, Barton M B, Bray F, Baumann M and Vikram B *et al* 2015 Expanding global access to radiotherapy *Lancet Oncol.* **16** P1153–86

[12] Coleman C N, Pistenmaa D, Jaffray D, Gospodarowicz M, Vikram B and Myers S *et al* 2017 Effective global cancer care requires radiation therapy: defining a path from no radiotherapy to radiotherapy of high quality globally *J. Glob. Oncol.* **3** 16s

[13] Healy B J, van der Merwe D, Christaki K E and Meghzifene A 2017 Cobalt-60 machines and medical linear accelerators: competing technologies for external beam radiotherapy *Clin. Oncol.* **29** 110–5

[14] Ndlovu N 2019 Radiotherapy treatment in cancer control and its important role in Africa *ecancermedicalscience* **13** 942

Chapter 38

Rwanda Cancer Centre

Felix Sinzabakira and Pacifique Mugenzi

While the challenges and limitations of access to cancer care in low- and middle-income countries (LMICs) are well known and often cited. It is important to acknowledge and commend examples of advances in recent years, especially when those advances are initiated, supported, and valued by the national government, as has been seen in the case of Rwanda.

38.1 Introduction

Rwanda, officially the **Republic of Rwanda**, is a country where the African Great Lakes region and East Africa converge. It is one of the smallest countries on the African mainland; its capital city is Kigali. Rwanda has a population of over 12.6 million living on 26 338 km^2 (10 169 mi^2) of land, and is the most densely populated mainland African country. The population is young and predominantly rural.

38.2 Rwanda Military Hospital and Rwanda Cancer Centre

His Excellency President Paul Kagame, President of the Republic of Rwanda inaugurated the up-to-date Cancer Centre equipped with radiotherapy and chemotherapy services on the 4th of February, 2020. President Kagame spoke on the important role the new centre will play in the lives of patients living with cancer, and said that many more Rwandans will be able to get the care they need with their families close by.

The Government of Rwanda embarked on a journey to decrease the burden of disease through prevention, early detection, treatment, and care interventions. In 2016, the idea of a modern radiotherapy cancer centre, called the Rwanda Cancer Centre (RCC), was proposed at the Rwanda Military Hospital (RMH) in Kigali as the first step in ultimately providing a full-service cancer centre. At the time, the

doi:10.1088/978-0-7503-3075-6ch38

RMH already had advanced cancer services in place and the human resource skills required to run the radiotherapy and chemotherapy services.

Constructed by UNTEC (a French company) and funded by the Government of Rwanda, the Global Fund, and the Centers for Disease Prevention (CDC), the centre became operational in March 2019 and officially launched on 4 February, 2020, in observance of World Cancer Day.

Over the last ten years, Rwanda has made remarkable gains in health by placing the health and wellbeing of the Rwandan people at the forefront of the agenda. The health sector continues to strive for Universal Health Coverage (UHC), with the goal of ensuring preventable, curative, and supportive care for all. However, while the disease burden is increasingly becoming controlled, challenges remain, particularly those of noncommunicable diseases.

The cancer burden has particularly come to the forefront in LMICs, and Rwanda has worked to identify solutions to tackle the vast financial and human resource requirements of such diseases. Globally, cancer is among the leading causes of death, claiming over 70% of its victims in LMICs, where prevention and treatment remain limited. In 2018, estimates made by the International Agency for Research on Cancer (IARC) indicated that the incidence in Rwanda was 10 704 new cancer diagnoses, 4 520 registered cases among men and 6 184 registered cases among women, and an annual mortality rate of 7 662. In addition, 50% to 60% of all cancer patients require radiotherapy in the course of their treatment. The increasing cancer burden in Rwanda, and the limited access of the general population to treatment, required the Government of Rwanda to act. Four years ago, less than 10% of the population in need was able to access treatment and about one million USD was spent on international transfers for radiotherapy treatment. Patients were forced to seek radiotherapy care abroad by referral boards, using support provided by different funding entities including the Ministry of Health, the Ministry of Defense, and private insurance.

The newly completed radiotherapy unit is made up of two linear accelerators using volumetric modulated arc therapy (VMAT), which directly administers radiation to cancerous tumors, and one computed tomography (CT) scanner for treatment planning purposes. Thus far, 752 patients have been treated, and of the 752 treated patients, more than 57% have been covered by 'Mutelle de Sante' while others have been privately funded. Currently, the center is averaging 70 patients per day with the capability to treat up to 150 patients per day at full capacity. The facility will complement existing prevention, diagnosis, and treatment services, including a 20-bed chemotherapy unit already in operation. In addition, the center allows a full scale-up of screening and early detection for cancers such as cervical, breast, and those related to the hepatitis C virus.

Other hospitals that provide chemotherapy services includes the Butaro Cancer Center of Excellence, King Faisal Hospital, Centre Hospitalier Universitaire de Kigali (CHUK) and Centre Hospitalier de Butare (CHUB). They all refer patients who need radiotherapy to the Rwanda Cancer Centre that operates as part of Rwanda Military Hospital.

Future plans indicate that further diagnostic and inpatient services and nuclear medicine services will gradually be added in order to provide comprehensive cancer treatment and palliative care to those with late-state diagnoses. In addition, specialists are currently being trained in order to provide the necessary skill levels, and staff are currently undergoing training.

Chapter 39

The radiation oncology center in Kutaisi, Georgian Republic

Krystyna Kiel

In recent years, the Win-Win Initiative has proactively sought to engage collaborators in Eastern Europe and Asia, thus expanding global networks, services, and resources. This chapter shares experiences and gains made in Georgia through regular, repeated onsite visits in partnership with a responsive medical corporation.

The Republic of Georgia is a country isolated from Europe and Asia by the Black Sea and the Caucasus mountains. It has had very few years of independence and has been dominated by Russia or the Soviet Union. Its economy is based on tourism and wine exports. The success of the latter has been based on exports to ex-Soviet countries. The country has poor relations with Russia, which has significantly reduced foreign capital.

Georgia is small; it has approximately 3.7 million people and a unique language. It ranks 70th on the Human Development Index. In 2015, ~10% lived below the national poverty line and the average monthly household income was ~$426. A universal healthcare (UHC) program was established in 2013 [1]; a report by the World Bank in 2017 showed that access to good quality healthcare had improved, particularly for those less well off, but health budgets were consistently overspent [2]. Radiation therapy services are free to pensioners, veterans, and other subsets of the population, but for others, a 30% copayment is required. Similar coverage is available for diagnostic tests and chemotherapy (20%). There is some inequity between urban and rural populations. Although UHC coverage has improved in the past decade, 34% of the population had household health expenditures that exceeded 10%, and for 10% of the population, they were more than 25% of the household budget [3]. Funds for copayments are sometimes available from municipalities, on application.

There are both public and private medical schools; the former offer free tuition and have high admission standards. It is estimated that there are 18 000 medical students in Georgia, of whom 80% are foreigners [4]. After completing training at

doi:10.1088/978-0-7503-3075-6ch39

medical school, one can either work for little money in a primary care setting if one is available or obtain a residency. Graduates must pay for the residency for whatever length of time is required, based on state standards. The requirements for residency completion are based on specialty society recommendations. Examinations are computer based and are often available. References must be obtained to participate in examinations.

Most of the 270 hospitals in Georgia are privately operated. There are nine radiation oncology centers, seven with linear accelerators, two with brachytherapy capabilities, and seven within the capital of Tbilisi [5]. Patients can be self-referred but are often referred by other treating physicians (usually surgeons or medical oncologists). This may involve a small 'kickback fee'. There is little multidisciplinary discussion, which can result in inappropriate referrals and procedures, a lack of accountability, and inefficiencies for the patient, who may have to travel long distances for treatment. There is no requirement for continuing medical education for any physician. Electronic access to books and journals is individually obtained. English is not fluently spoken by many older physicians, nor by many younger physicians, which reduces their ability to attend international conferences or read journals. Some larger hospitals with international connections will host conferences in the country, which are translated. A group of Georgian expatriates host an annual conference in all medical specialties with invited foreign faculty. No credits are granted, but attendance is very good.

There is a residency fee, which costs £2450–3570 twice per year. There may be some salary, based on participation in procedures, at the discretion of the supervising physician. An oncology resident may have little practical exposure to medical oncology and instead provide surgical assistance in oncology procedures. The grant of a license requires a certification examination and a referral from the residency program. Competency examinations and answers are published on the internet and not always updated. There are three radiation oncology residencies in the Republic of Georgia and ten residents. Theoretically, an overall program curriculum is registered with the government, but no there is national oversight of performance and education. The residents are often assigned to paperwork, which is required for reimbursement by the government healthcare system.

In 2015, I was invited, along with a Chicago physicist, to help open a new radiation therapy department in Kutaisi. Evex Corporation renovated an old Soviet hospital. A Varian Trilogy® and a computed tomography (CT) simulator were purchased. It is unclear to me who advised the administrators.

Kutaisi is the third largest city in Georgia, 230 km from Tbilisi. It was a major industrial center before independence in 1991 and has not recovered. The average annual gross salary (pre 20% tax) is GEL 20 466 ($6 700). The national unemployment level was ~12% in 2018. The national pastimes for men are smoking, drinking wine, eating, and dancing.

Other than the issues encountered in any new department, several glaring issues were encountered. Qualified physicians were not in great supply. Some licensed physicians for radiation oncology only had experience with cobalt-60 machines, no experience in image guidance (including portal films), and no experience with modern technology. Physicists received their training on the job. Fortunately, there is a surplus of PhD nuclear physicists who can easily be retrained in medical physics. There are no formal radiation therapy training programs and therefore no radiation therapists. Nurses are undervalued and underpaid. Patients do not always know they have had cancer and families refuse to approach the subject.

The Evex Corporation paid for a four-month observational training period for two physicists, one resident physician, and one radiology technologist. The hospital corporation thought that one senior physician with cobalt-60 experience, a therapist, one resident, one radiologist for the CT simulator, and two physicists could run a department treating 40 patients. The group had a little hands-on experience while in Belarus, which had a very active radiation oncology program. The language of instruction was Russian and participants were not referred to medical literature. They then received the usual training from Varian at one of their European centers. A Varian teaching representative spent time in the department as is usual for a new machine. My physicist colleague helped with quality assurance and protocols, inspection issues, and the purchase of equipment. I helped two physicians (one with cobalt-60 experience and the other a resident sent to Belarus) to establish treatment and logistic protocols for treatment planning and treatment administration. We performed patient consultations together. We took each step of the treatment process and broke it down into instructions and protocols. We benefitted greatly from a radiation therapist who was brought in from Chicago. She developed protocols and trained the radiology technologist who was sent to Belarus and potential candidates for radiation therapy on the CT simulation and treatment machine. Over and over, they mimicked treatment setup and delivery. Radiation therapists were successfully recruited from medical school and from among dental school graduates, as salaries are higher than those earned by new primary care physicians.

Fortunately, Evex Corporation responded to our observations. They obtained quality assurance equipment and immobilization devices and increased the number of personnel, including physicians, nurses, therapists, and dosimetrists. Evex responded to our request that residents should receive a salary.

There is a surplus of medical and dental students in the country who cannot afford a residency. The salary for a radiation therapist is higher than that of a primary care physician assigned by the government to a remote station. We therefore could recruit very bright individuals to treat patients using the machine.

Access to cancer treatment is not only based on the distance to the place of treatment but also on affordability. There is a one-cost fee for any radiation therapy program in Kutaisi. Radiation treatment costs ~2800 dollars, whether you receive 1 fraction or 45 fractions and there is no difference in cost based on the complexity of treatment. Copayment for treatment ranges from 10%–30%. After consultation, the patient initially receives a referral paper with a recommendation for radiation therapy. The government health office then approves the treatment. The patient then returns to the hospital with the voucher and the money for the copayment in order to schedule a simulation. This is now handled electronically.

A patient may owe 280 dollars. The clerk in the hotel where I usually stay makes 75 dollars and a nurse makes $300 per month. A diagnostic CT scan is $50, but contrast is $150. Positron emission tomography (PET)/CT and new drugs are not paid for by the government. Herceptin was recently approved, but only for stage II and III breast cancer. We found that 30% of the consultations I initially saw did not return for treatment, due to the copayment.

My physics colleague from Chicago and I started a foundation to help with this copayment. In the last three years, we have supported nearly 200 patients.

Since we started, the department has grown. A TruBeam® was purchased with SRS and SBRT capabilities. Four-dimensional simulations and deep breath holding were added. Evex has been good in providing necessary QA equipment and immobilization equipment. The cost has not changed. They have also been responsive to our request for additional personnel. As is often the case, once an individual is well trained, they leave for a higher paying position elsewhere.

Unfortunately, the quality of formal training is very poor. Recently, the residency requirement was extended to four years. Since residents have to pay for residency, some residents have second jobs. Evex has agreed to grants that provide some salary and the residency fee. There are formal guidelines for residency training, but they are guidelines in name only. Physicists are trained on the job and in the department; our physicist provides formal training by Skype lectures.

Resident and continuing education can be a major issue. Many physicians speak very poor English. Access to textbooks and journals, either physical or electronic, is limited. There is no resident oversight or ongoing evaluation. Therefore, there is no incentive for self-education. There is no one to lecture locally. There is one examination at the end of residency. Most of the questions are published on the internet and no one has ever failed. There are no continuing education requirements in Georgia. As a result, only self-motivated physicians keep abreast of developments in their specialties. Non-English speakers do not benefit from international meetings. The quality of the medical care provided by some of the referring physicians is poor. Radiologists do not feel committed to their own quality assurance; therefore, imaging reports cannot always be trusted. Pathologists do not produce synoptic reports, as there is no request or other incentive for these. Many senior surgeons perform the same surgical procedures that they learned in the Soviet system. For instance, a 'radical mastectomy' includes partial mastectomies and level I axillary dissections.

Screening is free for breast cancer, prostate cancer, and colorectal cancer (Hemoccult testing). Because healthcare has a prohibitive cost, many do not seek help until their cancers are advanced. Because diagnostic testing cannot always be done appropriately (i.e. with contrast) or is unavailable (PET/CT scanning), making treatment decisions is often difficult, especially for young, inexperienced physicians.

My role in the department has evolved. Initially, I spent time on treatment protocols—how to simulate, how to mark the patients, how to make immobilization devices, how to document, what to contour, what to consider in treatment planning, what goals we should have in treatment plans. I brought multiple textbooks. The English-speaking resident and I created a list of cancers, what doses to prescribe, and organs at risk as a start. As news of the American doctor reached the public, we were inundated with consultations of all kinds. Each morning, I lectured to all the staff on the most common types of cancer. Each patient was a learning experience.

I receive an email for each patient, discussing the case. I review the contours and then the treatment plans. Suggestions are made and questions are answered. Often, I will ask the resident specific questions and ask them to report back on answers.

I now visit about 2–3 times per year, for 2–3 week periods. Each morning, we have patient discussions and/or lectures. I spend time with the physicists reviewing plans, since they have little physician input regarding concerns. I spent time with residents, particularly the new ones, contouring and providing teaching sessions. I perform consultations with all the physicians and concentrate on history taking and physical examination, a skill that is not well taught in the medical school. I find the poor English skills of some of the physicians very discouraging, as they do not read and do not acknowledge that they do not understand me. Occasionally, we make public service announcements promoting early screening, symptom recognition, and smoking cessation. By visiting the country regularly, I have learned about the issues and constraints that native physicians and patients face. For instance, PET/CT scanning is only available only in one institution, and any radioactive material must be imported from Turkey. The national insurance plan does not cover the exam, which is prohibitively expensive for Georgians. Many international guidelines for cancer care now include PET/CT scanning. Decisions must be made without such scans. This makes the experience of senior physicians invaluable.

The experience has been valuable for me and the Radiation Oncology Department. The quality of cancer care has improved. Treatment guidelines have been established. Managing international guidelines with fewer resources has been useful. I have convinced several physicians that an informed patient tolerates treatment better than otherwise and may have reasonable expectations. We are not limited by external insurance requirements and can choose radiation techniques in the best interests of the patient. Through the foundation, we have provided treatment to patients who would have skipped adjuvant treatment or foregone palliative care. I have two physicians of whom I am especially proud who will finish training soon, who want to improve the quality of care in their country. Evex has also recognized me by naming the cancer center after me, although I would challenge you to find my name!

I have come to love the people of Georgia, who have struggled and continue to do so politically and economically. I campaign regularly to reduce tobacco consumption and to urge screening.

I have visited other countries in other programs, but usually for one week. I would strongly recommend that an individual, or preferably a group of individuals, adopt a program. One would need to visit to develop a relationship. No one suffers from additional education. Textbook and electronic resources are important. Patient reviews and chart rounds on a regular basis are invaluable. Constant conversation with physicians and physicists helps.

I have provided opportunities for month-long visits to the United States. Observing patient–doctor interactions, the role of ancillary care, the importance of multidisciplinary interactions, and learning tricks for treatment planning and delivery has been invaluable. And there is nothing like an international conference. However, one must know English.

In summary, my own experience suggests that international involvement in the developing world should be based on an intimate involvement in the daily functioning of the department. Volunteer physicians need to learn about social issues and local limitations that impact the effective delivery of good medical care. The following are recommended:

(1) Regular visits by a core group of physicians and physicists
(2) Relationships developed between core individuals in the radiation oncology department and visitors.
(3) Regular interaction to discuss consultations, treatment plans, problems in treatment
(4) Bilateral discussion
(5) External review of treatment consultations and plans
(6) Availability for quick consultations
(7) Regular lectures, journal reviews, guideline reviews
(8) Increased access to medical lectures
(9) Visits to radiation oncology departments in developed countries
(10) Encouragement to learn sufficient English to read articles and attend international conferences

Note from the Editors:
To all readers: in order to consider the progress achieved in Kutaisi, Georgia in the field of radiation oncology, you are invited to compare it with the previous situation in Georgia, as documented in the report of our ICEDOC mission in Georgia, 22–29 July, 2000, annex 1, pages 13 and 14 available at: http://www.icedoc.org/Docs/Georgia-ICEDOC%20Report%20,%20recommendations,%20and%20annex%20I,%20II%20July2000..pdf

and

http://www.icedoc.net/Docs/Georgia-ICEDOC%20Report%20,%20recommendations,%20and%20annex%20I,%20II%20July2000..pdf.

Also, see: www.icedoc.org under 'ICEDOC's Experts'.

The great work of Professor Krystyna Kiel in Kutaisi is an excellent example of the type of support and meaningful interactions with local teams and populations that we encourage in the win-win movement. That is to say, we appreciate works, advice, and consultations that are translated into a tangible increase in clinical oncology services for patients by local colleagues and stakeholders anywhere in the world. This is of more value than hundreds of talks, declarations, conferences, plans, and publications. Please consider the ten recommendations of Professor Kiel. The provision of technical, scientific, and educational support to the doers, that is to say, local colleagues, is mandatory in order to make progress and record achievements in the forthcoming years. You are invited to help.

As we present 'a living book', the reader can access the video of Professor Krystyna Kiel at the GHC Summit at Harvard Medical School, May 24, 2021 by clicking on: https://youtu.be/XGYJ_GTgyfI [6].

—Ahmed Elzawawy
—Wilfred Ngwa

References

[1] Healthcare_in_Georgia https://en.wikipedia.org/wiki/Healthcare_in_Georgia_(country)#:~:text=In%20February%202013%2C%20the%20Government,health%20system%20reforms%20in%20Georgia

[2] Rukhadze T 2013 An overview of the health care system in Georgia: expert recommendations in the context of predictive, preventive and personalized medicine *EPMA J.* **4** 8

[3] 2017 Georgia Public Expenditure ReviewWorld Bank Group 2017 http://documents.worldbank.org/curated/en/630321497350151165/pdf/114062-PER-P156724-PUBLIC-PERFINAL.pdf

[4] Wera M Georgia's Medical Education Industry Needs Careful Monitoring https://www.timeshighereducation.com/opinion/giorgias-medical-education-industry-needs-carefulmonitoring

[5] Directory of Radiotherapy Centres https://dirac.iaea.org/Data/CountriesLight

[6] Krystyna K 2021 The Radiation Oncology in Kutaisi, Republic of Georgia, GHC Summit at Harvard Medical School May 24, 2021 https://youtu.be/XGYJ_GTgyfI

IOP Publishing

Approaching Global Oncology
The win-win model
Ahmed Elzawawy and Wilfred Ngwa

Chapter 40

Building capacity to control cervical cancer in Nigeria: a case study

Isaac F Adewole, T A O Oluwasola and I O Morhason-Bello

Cervical cancer control in Nigeria has evolved over the years amidst several multidimensional challenges, which often required a multipronged approach to manage. The Nigerian government has developed strategic pathways and frameworks that will ensure the availability, accessibility, and affordability of basic services for cervical cancer care. Experts, non-governmental organizations, professional organizations, and international donors are critical stakeholders that are needed in order to set a sustainable pathway for cervical cancer elimination.

40.1 Introduction

Cervical cancer remains a public health challenge in low- and middle-income countries, particularly in Africa, and it is ranked as the fourth most common cause of cancer incidence and mortality in women worldwide [1]. Cervical cancer is primarily caused by the persistence of a human papillomavirus (HPV) infection at the transformation zone of the cervix over an average period of ten years in a normal population.

According to GLOBOCAN estimates, the number of new cases of cervical cancer had increased worldwide from 471 000 in 2000 to 570 000 in 2018, giving an age-specific incidence ratio of 13.1/100 000 women-years [2]. Similarly, the mortality due to cervical cancer has increased to 311 000 annually, corresponding to 6.9/100 000. Almost 84% of all cervical cancers and 88% of all deaths caused by cervical cancer occurred in lower-resource countries [2].

In Africa, the highest burden of cervical cancer is in East Africa, followed by Southern and Western African countries [2, 3]. Nigeria has the highest burden of cervical cancer amongst the member countries in the Economic Community of West African States (ECOWAS). In 2018, 14 943 new cervical cancer cases and 10 403 related deaths occurred in Nigeria, accounting for 27.2% of the cervical cases and 20.0% of the cervical cancer deaths in West Africa [2].

doi:10.1088/978-0-7503-3075-6ch40

40.1.1 Synopsis of the key challenges associated with cervical cancer care in Nigeria

Cervical cancer is preventable by the administration of any of the three approved HPV vaccines in girls and boys before they reach the age at which sexual activity, sex education, or family life education programs take place and through screening for premalignant lesions of the cervix [4]. It is also curable with surgery and/or chemo-radiation in settings where early cervical cancer is diagnosed. Although the Nigerian government has approved HPV vaccines, they are yet to be incorporated into the national immunization program. The vaccine is only available to those that can afford to pay for it. In the same vein, there is no national program to screen premalignant lesions of the cervix. Again, screening is limited to occasional outreach programs funded by foundations or other stakeholders or is self-funded by privileged women. Evidence from Nigerian studies suggests that only a few women have a good knowledge of the risk factors, prevention strategies, and treatments for cervical cancer [5]. It is also worrisome that a large number of women have misconceptions of the etiological factors of the disease.

Another challenge is the late presentation of women with cervical cancer in Nigeria. The available data suggest that more than two-thirds of Nigerian women present with advanced cervical cancer at stage 2B or above, when definitive care is no longer feasible [6]. The delay in accessing specialized gynaecological oncology care in Nigeria might be due to poor understanding of the cause of the disease and the points of care, incorrect diagnosis and treatment by healthcare providers resulting in delayed referral, and financial constraints that prevent access to specialized care [6, 7]. Despite the fact that a National Health Insurance Scheme has been implemented for more than two decades in Nigeria, only about one in five of her citizens are covered. Currently, the insurance coverage does not cover all treatment modalities of cancer, including cervical cancer. There is also the growing fear of poor care outcomes. The fear is borne out of rumours, misconceptions, and a poor perception of cervical cancer characterized by progressive weight loss, foul-smelling vaginal discharge, urinary and fecal incontinence, as well as unbearable pain [6]. Apart from all these, women also nurse a fear of the possible loss of reproductive function and damage to contiguous structures from surgical or chemo-radiation treatments.

There is lack of prioritisation of investment in cervical cancer, compared to other competing health-related challenges among women [8]. The Federal Ministry of Health has a desk officer for the cervical cancer control program, the unit is poorly funded by the national health budget and many state governments in the country do not have a dedicated officer for cervical cancer control. The majority of the investment in cervical cancer control prevention in Nigeria has largely been funded by international donors, including the Clinton Health Access Initiative, USAID, JPEIGHO, and a host of other organizations. In 2018, The Federal Ministry of Health in collaboration with other stakeholders, including the Society of Obstetrics and Gynecology (SOGON) and the Gynecological Oncology Society of Nigeria (GOSON) produced the national algorithm for cervical cancer control; however, this program is yet to be supported by the Government for implementation.

The inadequacy of the human and infrastructural resources available to offer cutting-edge diagnostic and therapeutic services to women that present in different clinical stages of premalignant and malignant lesions in Nigeria remains a big challenge. For example, prior to 2015, there were only two radiotherapy machines functioning in the country that could offer brachytherapy and teletherapy. Chemotherapy is sometimes in short supply or prohibitively expensive for middle-class women with cervical cancer. The training of professionals—gynecological oncologists, colposcopists, oncological nurses, social health workers, and palliative care specialists is limited to 'ad hoc arrangements' between the scarce experienced specialists and a few interested mentees. The grossly inadequate number of available facilities in the country often leads to huge backlog of women with cervical cancer waiting for treatment. Nigeria has a peculiar seasonal disruption of its healthcare service due to health workers' strike action. Sometimes, public healthcare services are shut down for weeks and only rich individuals are able to afford private care facilities.

40.1.2 The effort to mitigate the challenges of cervical cancer care in Nigeria

Over the years, there have been notable local and international efforts to mitigate various teething challenges that detract from an optimal service for the control of cervical cancer. These efforts were targeted at one or multiple key issues that need to be fixed in order to improve the quality of service delivery.

40.1.2.1 Policy shift and priority setting

Although there have been some efforts by previous governments to prioritize cervical cancer control programs through promotion of yearly awareness programs in Nigeria, none has initiated a comprehensive strategic plan of action and implemented it. However, in 2015, the Federal Government of Nigeria through the Federal Ministry of Health included cancer prevention, treatment, and care as one of the four key programs of the administration. Other key deliverables were the reduction of maternal and neonatal mortality, the elimination of mother-to-child transmission of HIV, and public health emergencies.

In order to implement the health agenda for cancer control, the Federal government of Nigeria recently rose to the occasion and made significant contributions in this regard, in particular, with the launch of the National Cancer Control Plan for 2018–2022 [9]. This policy document was added to the roadmap for general control of cancer in Nigeria and itemized the importance of advocacy, developed the national framework for cancer prevention, and adopted international best practices for cancer care. The main mission of the National Cancer Control plan was to establish a framework that will ensure access to cancer screening and cancer care, leading to an improved quality of life for people affected by cancer [9]. The guiding principles for implementation hinged on seven points: (1) ownership and accountability by the government, which resulted in the decision to provide 75% of the required funds for implementation; (2) people-centered interventions and initiatives; (3) encompassing the entire cancer care continuum from primary prevention to tertiary care; (4) ensuring the involvement of the whole of society by understanding that multisectoral partnerships and community participation are essential to a successful implementation of the plan; (5) appropriate health system strengthening; (6) flexibility through a phased approach; and (7) continuous monitoring and evaluation of all processes [9]. For cervical cancer, the main objective was to attain 90% coverage for the HPV vaccine among the eligible population by 2022 and the main strategy is to extend the national immunization program to include HPV vaccination for children aged 9–13 years [9].

The government also provided budget to expand infrastructure, sought support from multinational companies such as SNEPCO, and collaborated with other African countries to partner with the American Cancer Society and other organizations to develop guidelines for cancer care on the continent. For example, SNEPCO paid for the purchase and installation of an Elekta linac radiotherapy machine at the National Hospital Abuja, Nigeria at a cost of one million US dollars, as part of the organization's corporate social responsibility. The arrangement also covered hands-on capacity building for the Nigerian radiation oncologists and physicists that are handling the machine. The Federal Government, through the Nigerian Sovereign Investment Authority (NSIA), funded the purchase and installation of a 3D 120 MLC Varian Vitalbeam linac radiotherapy machine, and this project was personally commissioned by President Muhammadu Buhari, Grand Commander of the Federal Republic (GCFR), during his first term in office (figure 40.1).

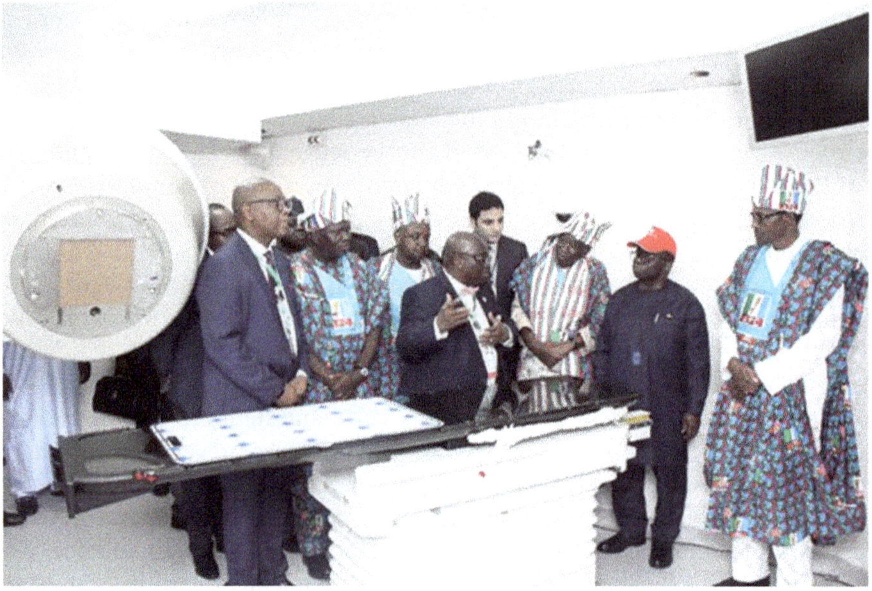

Figure 40.1. Photograph of the commissioning of the linac machine at Lagos University Teaching Hospital, Idi- Araba, 2018 by President Muhammadu Buhari, GCFR, speaking, and Hon. Professor Isaac Adewole, with red cap, Minister of Health, Federal Ministry of Health, Nigeria.

40.1.2.2 Expert projects

A couple of Nigerian experts have attracted grants from international donors and foundations to fund different aspects of the cervical cancer control program in Nigeria. Whilst some have focused on research or prevention programs such as screening and vaccination, a few others have engaged in a robust continuum of care approach from health promotion, prevention programs, capacity building training in the form of surgical exposure, to the purchase of key equipment for health facilities, in order to offer composite service delivery for cervical cancer patients [10, 11]. For example, the Operation Stop Cervical Cancer Program was implemented using a science grant provided by Mobil International (2006–2009). The grant was implemented by the University of Ibadan, Nigeria, and the MD Anderson Cancer Centre, USA in seven tertiary health facilities (teaching hospitals and federal medical centers) in Nigeria. The project offered intensive in-country training in screening protocols for cervical cancer, hands-on training in colposcopy, loop electrosurgical excision procedure (LEEP), radical surgery for early disease, and the setting up a cervical cancer screening unit. Biomedical engineers were also trained in the service and maintenance of equipment; nurses received training in sample collection for pap smears and visual inspection of the cervix with acetic acid or Lugol's iodine, including cryotherapy [12]. The cyto-screeners had refresher courses on the interpretation of slides using international guidelines.

After the intensive training, which was coordinated by a team of experts from the MD Anderson Cancer Centre and British Colombia University, each of the participating seven institutions in Nigeria was given equipment with which to set up a cervical cancer control unit. The equipment included: a colposcope, a LEEP machine, cryotherapy, and a host of other consumables. After the training, different institutions offered cervical cancer-related services, including an outreach program and step-down training [10]. Other funded programs have been implemented to provide better access to the cervical cancer program. Recently, the Clinton Health Access Initiative supported SOGON to implement pilot screening programs for premalignant lesions of the cervix in different regions of Nigeria.

40.1.2.3 Funding

The Nigerian government needs to make budgetary provision for cancer care, including the cervical cancer control program. It is important that government at all levels supports the HPV vaccination and screening program, procures the necessary equipment and provides scholarship for a short fellowship program for all cadres of health workers involved in cervical cancer care. Nigeria will need more investment in the procurement of radiotherapy machines to meet the IAEA requirement of a radiotherapy machine per one million people. Private organizations could also invest in cancer care as part of their corporate social responsibility. The role of non-governmental organizations (NGOs) has been well documented, and several NGOs across the country have continued to provide platforms for the screening and treatment of preinvasive cervical cancer lesions [13]. A particular NGO, the Pink Oak Cancer Trust, offers full payment for the care of indigent patients with early stage invasive cancer [14].

40.1.2.4 Training

In order to meet the rising demand for cervical cancer care, it is important to design training programs for health workers. Some countries in Africa have adopted modular training courses to quickly produce a critical mass of experts. For example, nurses and community health extension workers are trained in the use of visual inspection techniques for premalignant cervical lesion screening programs. Surgical sessions could also be regularly organized as a cheaper in-country alternative to overseas scholarships for individual training. Government will need to engage tertiary health institutions and professional bodies, such SOGON, GOSON, the National Postgraduate Medical College, the West African College of Surgeons, and medical schools to design and co-facilitate training with other renowned oncology centers.

40.1.2.5 Research and data gathering

Nigerian researchers will need to refocus on the critical aspects of epidemiology and the genomics of cervical cancer. It is important that local data on women with cervical cancer are collected at the population level in order to strengthen the quality of information in the cancer registry. The information should cover the presentation mode, the referral source, the histology, and the care outcome. It may be better that these data are centrally collected and transferrable between healthcare facilities without compromising data security and confidentiality. The role of traditional medicine practitioners and beliefs will need to be explored, considering their increasing patronage due to noncommunicable diseases in Nigeria.

40.1.2.6 Multidisciplinary sustainable collaboration

Nigerian health institutions will need to explore various angles of collaboration in order to tap knowledge and skills from each other and maximize the opportunity to offer optimal service. In addition, the promotion of large multicentre trials of different procedure and treatment protocols will help to generate generalizable evidence for national use [8].

40.2 Conclusions

There is a need to prioritize and invest in cervical cancer prevention and definitive care treatment. The provision of a policy environment that will support universal vaccination with the HPV vaccine to young girls and probably boys will assist in reducing the future burden of cervical cancer. It is imperative that a critical mass of enthusiasts are developed and promoted to offer quality care. A meticulous financing strategy that encapsulates all aspects of cervical cancer control, including infrastructural development and training, is germane to the successful implementation of this agenda. Nigeria has the potential to eliminate cervical cancer if this aim is given adequate priority and investment. It is possible and feasible, despite competing demands in the country.

References

[1] Arbyn M, Weiderpass E and Bruni L *et al* 2020 Estimates of incidence and mortality of cervical cancer in 2018: a worldwide analysis *Lancet Glob. Health* **8** e191–203

[2] Arrossi S *et al* 2017 Primary prevention of cervical cancer: american society of clinical oncology resource-stratified guideline *J. Glob. Oncol* **3** 611–34

[3] Bruni L, Albero G, Serrano B, Mena M, Gómez D, Muñoz J, Bosch F X and de Sanjosé S 2019 *Human papillomavirus and related diseases in the world* ICO/IARC Information Centre on HPV and Cancer (HPV Information Centre) 22 January 2019 https://hpvcentre.net/statistics/reports/XWX.pdf

[4] Buys T P *et al* 2012 Optical technologies and molecular imaging for cervical neoplasia: a program project update *Gend. Med* **9** S7–24

[5] Jedy-Agba E, Joko W Y and Liu B *et al* 2020 Trends in cervical cancer incidence in sub-Saharan Africa *Br. J. Cancer* **123** 148–54

[6] Morhason-Bello I O, Kareem Y O and Adewole I F 2020 Modeling for predictors of knowledge score on etiology and prevention strategies for cervical cancer among women of reproductive age in Ibadan *JCO Glob. Oncol* **6** 892–903

[7] Morhason-Bello I O, Odedina F, Rebbeck T R, Harford J, Dangou J M, Denny L and Adewole I F 2013 Challenges and opportunities in cancer control in Africa: a perspective from the African Organisation for Research and Training in Cancer *Lancet Oncol* **14** e142–51

[8] Nigeria National Cancer Control Plan 2018–2022 https://iccp-portal.org/system/files/plans/NCCP_Final[1].pdf

[9] Nwogu C E, Mahoney M, Okoye I, Ejiogu K, George S and Dy G *et al* 2016 Role of private enterprise in cancer control in low to middle income countries *J. Cancer Epidemiol.* **2016** 7121527

[10] Oladokun A, Morhason-Bello I O, Bello F A and Adewole I F 2010 The learning curve of radical hysterectomy for early cervical carcinoma *Afr. J. Med. Med. Sci.* **39** 329–32

[11] Oluwasola T A O and Oladewa A C 2018 Challenges of gynaecological cancer care in Nigeria—a review article *Afr. J. Med. Med. Sci.* **47** 227–37

[12] Operation Stop Cervical Cancer in Nigeria 2006 A Report on the Proceedings of a Site Representative Meeting and Training Session at the International Institute for Tropical Agriculture (IITA) in Ibadan, Nigeria, July 9–16, 2006 https://careersdocbox.com/Nursing/89158506-Operation-stop-cervical-cancer-in-nigeria.html

[13] Roblyer D, Richards-Kortum R, Park S Y, Adewole I and Follen M 2007 Objective screening for cervical cancer in developing nations: lessons from Nigeria *Gynecol Oncol* **107** S94–7

[14] Anorlu R I 2008 Cervical cancer: the sub-Saharan African perspective *Reprod. Health Matters* **16** 41–9

Chapter 41

Win-win collaborations initiative examples in Nigeria, Cameroon, and Pakistan

Wilfred Ngwa, Kingsley Ndoh, Francine Kouya, Dennis Palmer, Fiza Shaukat and Sumera Butt

In this chapter, current win-win collaboration initiatives catalyzed by the Global Health Catalyst Win-Win Initiative are highlighted, including collaborations that are leading to the establishment of cancer centers in low- and middle-income (LMIC) countries. We highlight specific initiatives in Nigeria, Cameroon, and Pakistan.

41.1 Ondo State Cancer Project

The Ondo State Cancer Control program is Nigeria's first innovative state government-initiated cancer control program to address the burden of cancer. The program hinges on awareness and education, early diagnosis, improved access to affordable cancer medicines, and the establishment of a state-of-the-art cancer treatment center that leverages the existing tertiary healthcare facilities in the state. The Ondo State Cancer Control Program was born from the passion of the first lady, Mrs Betty Akeredolu, to address cancer and other non-communicable diseases.

In October 1997, Betty Akeredolu, first lady of Ondo state was diagnosed with breast cancer. Unlike many wealthy Nigerians who would have opted to have their treatments outside the country, she received care in Nigeria. This choice exposed her to the reality of the inefficiencies and gaps in the management of cancer within the Nigerian healthcare system. She faced stigma from society. Though she was fortunate to have been diagnosed early, she realized that her case was the exception; most—if not all—women she saw at the oncology clinic had advanced breast cancer. After she had completed her treatment, undergone surveillance, and been declared cancer free, she founded the Breast Cancer Association of Nigeria (BRECAN), a non-profit advocacy organization aimed at creating awareness and galvanizing action and funding from the government, the private sector, and individuals against

doi:10.1088/978-0-7503-3075-6ch41

breast cancer. In 2017, shortly after her husband Rotimi Akeredolu became the governor of Ondo State, she decided to champion the cause of cancer control in Ondo state by leveraging the political will and support of the Ondo state government. Her mission is to make Ondo State a successful model for a government-initiated public–private partnership to create a high-quality and resource-appropriate comprehensive center for the prevention, diagnosis, and treatment of cancer in an LMIC setting. Its goals include:

- Increasing the rate of early diagnosis through awareness and education.
- Implementing sustainable programs to tackle vaccine-preventable cancers.
- Improving the clinical capacity available for cancer diagnosis and treatment.
- Expanding treatment capacity to include radiotherapy and brachytherapy.
- Improving affordable access to cancer medicines.

The state government developed a collaboration with the Global Health Catalyst Win-Win Initiative to catalyze the establishment of the cancer center, including collaboration for education and training, facilitating collaboration with radiotherapy manufacturers for win-win collaboration, research collaborations, and the establishment of a solar-powered cancer centre working with collaborators in Germany. Because of the COVID-19 pandemic, training was paused as travel around the world was disrupted. Construction was stalled because a significant portion of the government's health budget was being spent on COVID-19 control in the state.

The National Cancer Control Plan contains several initiatives and goals that are to be addressed by the plan. One of the goals is access to cancer medication and cancer care for most of Nigeria's population. In relation to this, two major organizations are working with the Nigeria Ministry of Health; one of them is the Clinton Health Access Initiative (CHAI) and the American Cancer Society and the other is BIO Ventures for Global Health, which works to improve access to innovative cancer medicine in Nigeria. There are also initiatives to improve radiotherapy care in Nigeria. A cancer center has been launched in Lagos; it is called the Lagos University Teaching Hospital National Sovereign Investment Authority Cancer Center (LUTH-NSIA). This represents an investment of 10 million dollars by the Nigerian Sovereign Fund at Lagos University Teaching Hospital. Radiotherapy machines have also been installed at the National Hospital, Abuja. Several activities are under way to improve cancer care in Nigeria. As everyone knows, Nigeria is the largest country in Africa in terms of population and in terms of GDP. Nigeria has the opportunity to be a leader in global oncology and to bridge the divide between wealthy countries and LMICs.

Ondo State is a unique state, as the wife of the governor who has participated at the GHC summit is a breast cancer survivor; she has been in the cancer advocacy space for over two decades after experiencing the gaps in healthcare in Nigeria when she was getting her cancer treatment. Thankfully, she is alive today and she is one of the shinning lights of cancer control in Nigeria. The government of Ondo State has gone to great lengths to bring many of the stakeholders together. In the whole of Nigeria, there are only about eight or nine radiotherapy centers. The World Health Organization recommends that there should be one radiotherapy machine per million people. Nigeria has 200 million people, so ideally there should be about 200 radiotherapy units in Nigeria, although right now there are only about nine. An op-ed in the Washington Post noted that dogs have better access to radiotherapy in the US than people in Nigeria. This sparked a lot of political debates and served as a wake-up call for leaders to act, so that in the future, when more people have access to treatment in Nigeria, such op-eds will not see the light of day.

Going forward, one thing that is often overlooked but needs to be addressed is the issue of human resources. We often think about equipment and other things, but we pay less attention to the people who are going to handle the equipment or carry out the treatments. So, one of the things Ondo State did recently is to sign a memorandum of understanding (MoU) with the GHC to collaborate on training, e.g. via the Global Oncology University initiative. A number of health workers have been identified, i.e. radiation oncologists and medical physicists who will start short-term (three- to six-month) fellowships. The purpose of these fellowships is not full training, as the selected candidates have had years of training. Rather, these will be continuous education opportunities to update their skills to be very conversant with the latest equipment, which is to be installed. When the COVID pandemic is under control, professional training will take place and the construction of the radiotherapy units will start. As the president of the Dana Farber Cancer Institute said during her welcome address at the GHC summit in 2019, cancer does not wait; no matter how many meetings we have, anyone who is diagnosed with cancer will still have cancer cells growing. So we need to act fast and the only way we can make meaningful progress is through collaboration and meetings as well as taking action with the win-win approach.

41.1.1 Pakistan

I am a radiation oncologist working at Shaukat Khanum memorial center hospital in Pakistan. I will be sharing how Shaukat Khanum is transforming cancer care in Pakistan. Pakistan is the fifth most populous country in the world. Despite its population of 220 million people, the GDP per capita and income per capita is very low. Pakistan ranks very low compared to other countries in terms of public health expenditure, which is less than 2%. This is the reason why most of the spending in Pakistan is from our own pockets; insurance and the government contribute very little to the health system. The annual cancer incidence in Pakistan is estimated to be 173 937 patients a year. This is an estimated amount, because we do not have a formal national cancer registry. There are only 30 hospitals with major oncology services. There are more than 50 general hospitals, but they have minor oncology facilities. Not only is the quantity lacking, but also the quality.

Shaukat Khanum became a model institute. The initiative was supported by the prime minister and his mother Shaukat Khanum, who is the inspiration behind the Shaukat Khanum cancer center. At Shaukat Khanum, cancer treatment is easily accessible to all citizens of Pakistan, irrespective of their background. The hospital is a model institute that alleviates the sufferings of cancer patients through state-of-the-art technology, irrespective of their ability to pay. Shaukat Khanum also promotes education and research. Our dream, as a hospital, has been fulfilled by the relentless efforts of the Shaukat Khanum team, which consists of Imran Khan who is chairman of the board of governors, Dr Faisal Sultan, the Chief executive officer, Dr Aasim Yuf who is the chief medical officer and Dr Asif Loya who is the medical director.

Shaukat Khanum hospital was founded in 1990 and completed in 1994 at a total cost of two million dollars. Our core values are that every patient should receive equal treatment. A private patient and a supported patient can be in the same room using the same hospital and clinical facilitates. Seventy-five percent of our patients are treated free of charge and 25% pay for their treatment. Shaukat Khanum currently employs 3 031 staff, which includes full-time consultants, visiting consultants, trainees, physicians, nursing staff, and allied medical and support staff. We also have clinical and support services staff. Our clinical services include medical oncology, pediatric oncology, clinical and radiation oncology, surgical oncology, anesthesia, internal medicine, pathology, radiology, nuclear medicine, and palliative care. For support services, we have nursing, pharmacy, finance, material management, human resources, quality assurance, a central sterile stores department, and management information systems.

In 2018, the clinical activity of the hospital had an exponential increase, in which there were almost 10 000 new patient registrations, around 13 000 admissions, 64 000 radiotherapy sessions, and 47 000 chemotherapy sessions. This is clear evidence that the hospital is busy. To continue meeting these demands, we need a larger workforce, more manpower, and more resources to keep the hospital running. The main income of the hospital comes from Zakat donations and hospital services (Zakat is a religious charity that helps to keep the hospital functioning). Hospital services make up 50% of the hospital's revenue. The three main sources of revenue keep increasing over time, which indicates how much trust people have for Shaukat Khanum, which is why they continue to donate.

So far, we have spent 430 million dollars on philanthropic treatment. This is one of the reasons why we get donations not only from Pakistan but from all over the world, for example, from the UK, the USA, Dubai International Humanitarian City (IHC), Canada, Australia, and Norway. Seventy percent of donations are domestic, 30% are overseas donations, and we benefit from charities across the world.

For research at Shaukat Khanum, we have defined research guidelines and research approval processes including scientific and ethical review boards. We have good clinical practice-compliant standard operating procedures, over 250 peer-reviewed publications, national and international collaborations, many phase-two and -three clinical trials running in the hospital, qualified research staff, and equipped basic science labs. Our research frame consists of three main domains: clinical research, cancer registry and clinical data management, and basic science labs. Recently, we have also introduced a tumor bank, which currently includes tumor banks for breast and colorectal cancer. It is also involved in molecular and genetic research. The clinical registry took the initiative to make its own registry, which is known as the Punjab cancer registry. It collects data on cancer incidence in the Punjab region. It is also involved in outcome research, which is collected locally in the hospital. Our clinical research office is involved with the institutional and scientific review board. We have clinical trials and international collaborations.

Shaukat Khanum not only provides clinical resources, but also faces brain drain, which is something the entire country is currently facing. To address this, Shaukat Khanum has started many postgraduate training programs. These training programs take place in all our facilities. We have programs for doctors, nursing staff, paramedics, and technicians. We have recently started a senior instructor program, in which we send our junior consultants for a two-year fellowship to a renowned cancer center either in the UK or the USA to receive training and return to work at Shaukat Khanum. This helps us to get professionals who are properly trained and to introduce new facilitates at Shaukat Khanum.

Shaukat Khanum is also playing a very important part in raising public awareness about cancers such as breast cancer, which is one of the commonest cancers. Every October, we run a breast cancer campaign in many schools and universities to educate students about its symptoms and how it is treated. We also include a tobacco campaign. Hospitals constantly invest in improving quality and in quality improvement projects such as ISO 9001. We have certification for hazard analysis and internal and external audits and are currently preparing for College of American Pathologists certifications from the college of American Pathologists. Shaukat Khanum is one of three hospitals in Pakistan that has been awarded quality approval by Joint Commission International (JCI, formerly JCAHO), which is the golden seal of quality the hospital has been providing for the last twenty years. Shaukat Khanum has also received many awards, such as the World Health Organization (WHO) Award in 2004, the Human Rights Society of Pakistan award 2008, and the Corporate Excellence Award in 2009, 2010, 2012, 2016, and 2018.

Due to the increasing demand created by more cancer patients, a new cancer hospital was built in Peshawar in December 2015. This has been very beneficial for the people of Pakistan and surrounding areas because they do not have to travel far for chemotherapy or radiological treatment. This hospital functions well and is in the third phase of surgical training; procedures will start in 2020. We successfully started radiation there this year.

The future of Shaukat Khanum is very bright, and the construction of a third Shaukat Khanum hospital has been started in Karachi. These three Shaukat Khanum hospitals bear testimony to the fact that quality cancer care can be provided in a third world country if you have dedicated and honest leadership and if resources are spent in the right way. However, I would like to say that this is just a model institute. There are many other hospitals in Pakistan that need to improve and need to follow the same model in order to improve the healthcare system in Pakistan.

The cancer center has established collaboration with the Global Health Catalyst Win-Win Initiative to support education and training, especially in stereotactic body radiotherapy. In 2019, lectures to provide this training were offered by Harvard radiation oncology professors, and there are plans to continue this.

41.2 Cameroon

My name is Dennis Palmer. I work at Mbingo Baptist Hospital. Mbingo is the most developed hospital in the Cameroon Baptist Convention health system in Cameroon. Mbingo originally started as a centre for leprosy in 1952. We still do leprosy work for the north-west region. More recently, the hospital has developed into a referral teaching hospital, especially in the last ten years, when we started our postgraduate training program. We currently have a surgical residency and an internal medicine residency. With the development of these training programs, we were pushed to improve the quality of the hospital. We now have much better laboratory services and imaging services. About six years ago, we were able to get a full-time pathologist, which enabled us to effectively diagnose the many patients who come to us with cancer. As a result of being able to diagnose these patients, we were able to develop pretreatment programs for them. We have a well-established surgical program, which is very helpful in managing patients. Within the last several years, we have advanced in our ability to treat these patients using chemotherapy. Two years ago, one of our internal medicine residency graduates, Dr Francin Kouya, came back after completing a fellowship in medical oncology and is now in charge of our oncology programs within the health ward.

Our oncology program in the Cameroon Baptist Convention Health Center started in 2003. It is divided into two big groups. The first group is pediatric oncology, which focuses on Burkitt lymphoma, which is the most common child cancer, making up about 50% of cases. We also treat Wilms tumor, which is the second most common, while the third most common is retinal blastoma. Children with leukemia are referred to Yaoundé at La Fondation Chantal Biya. For the adult program, we offer services to patients with breast and cervical cancer. After we treat patients with advanced stage two or three cancers, cases are referred to Yaoundé or Douala for radiotherapy. Another important program we have is the HIV program. We screen all our HIV-positive patients. They are also screened for cervical cancer. We screen approximately 200 patients every month.

The one major component of our oncology program that is not in place is radiation therapy. As in much of sub-Saharan Africa, there is almost no radiation therapy available for patients who would benefit from it. We had one very old cobalt machine in Douala, Cameroon but it has recently broken down, so we cannot currently offer anything to our patients. A project was proposed two years ago to install a radiation therapy unit in Mbingo, which would complete our treatment modality. The purpose of the project is to build a four-story building that will house all our cancer-related activities, and the radiation therapy bunkers will be nearby. We have a group of people that have been helping us to understand how to accomplish this. We are currently looking for funding that will allow a linear accelerator to be installed here in Mbingo. We know that the primary focus of the Global Health Catalyst Summit is the improvement of access to radiation therapy in sub-Saharan Africa and we think that our project will be one of the important ones that pursues this idea. The Global Health Catalyst is currently supporting the Mbingo Baptist Hospital to build the cancer center and supporting the training of our radiation oncology staff in Germany and South Africa. Construction of the bunker has begun, and the radiotherapy machine is secured and ready for shipment.

Chapter 42

Financing solutions for sustainable cancer control increase the availability of novel radiotherapy: a proposal from Uruguay, South America

Alvaro Luongo-Céspedes

42.1 Background

In Uruguay, there are 15 accelerators and two high-dose-rate brachytherapy devices; hence, the country averages five or more radiation therapy machines per million people. This is similar to the situation in other countries, such as the United States, Canada, most of Western Europe, Scandinavia, New Zealand, Japan, and Australia. In the remainder of South America, in the countries surrounding Uruguay, the number of radiotherapy machines per million people is less than one in a few countries and between three and five in the other countries.

We stress that counting the number of linear accelerators is not enough. A comprehensive approach, with a focus on technological aspects, should be considered. Examples of technological aspects are the year of equipment manufacture and the availability of different techniques, energies, and collimators. Additionally, quality management systems, quality controls, the number and technology type of simulators, the planning and execution of treatment, and the number of personnel available should be analyzed. In Uruguay, a secondary Metrology Laboratory was installed with the assistance of the International Atomic Energy Agency (IAEA).

Although international organizations carry out a considerable amount of technology transfer, much still remains to be done, as there is a huge lack of good-quality radiation oncology services in many parts of the world.

It is necessary to think in different ways about further innovations. As Albert Einstein said, 'If you always do what you always did, you will always get what you always got'.

doi:10.1088/978-0-7503-3075-6ch42

42.2 Things to ask ourselves and keep in mind

- What are the politics of technological updates?
- What technologies exist? In which countries do they exist, and how do they accompany the versions of radiotherapy?
- How do countries update the costs of radiotherapy treatment?
- How do they implement new technologies?

In thinking of additional innovations, it is important to think differently about early and timely diagnosis, about how one-third of cancers can be prevented, and about the use of technology transfer.

When deciding on radiotherapy equipment needs, an important consideration is the decision whether to purchase or rent. We also need to take into consideration that each country and each hospital has a unique situation and a different context. Although we might extrapolate conclusions, we need to make sure that these conclusions are thoroughly analyzed when considering whether to buy or to lease [1].

42.3 The experience of the National Cancer Institute of Uruguay

Five years ago, it was time for the National Cancer Institute of Uruguay to update its radiotherapy technology. As an organization, it was decided that the National Institute was going to lease and not buy new machines. Through international bidding, the latest technology was leased.

42.4 Why did we decide to lease and not to buy radiotherapy machines as a solution?

- We did not have enough available funds to purchase high-quality machines.
- We did not have guarantees that we would obtain financing for the purchase price.
- We needed to introduce updated, state-of-the-art technology for the benefit of our patients as soon possible.
- It is difficult and expensive for us to obtain proper preventive and corrective maintenance.
- It is extremely important that we reduce the number and length of machine downtime periods.
- We considered the issues associated with updating technologies along with the years of service obtained from equipment.

In the National Cancer Institute of Uruguay's hospital budget, only a small fraction was allocated to radiotherapy machines. Out of the total available funds, 42.64% was allocated to oncology drugs, 8.17% was allocated to medical–surgical materials, and only 8.057% was allocated to radiotherapy machines.

The National Cancer Institute of Uruguay has two linear accelerators (linacs) in its facility. The two linacs are used 49 273 times per year. On a monthly basis, 4 106 used are completed by the two linacs per month. This means 2053 uses per linac per month.

Every day, an average of 102 patients receive their radiotherapy treatment from the two linacs.

The cost of each linac application is $9 910, while the total cost per radiotherapy application is $30 940. Hence, the cost of the equipment can be calculated to be 32% of the application value.

From our five-year experience of leasing radiotherapy machines, we find the total costs of buying or leasing are approximately equal.

From this real experience, we summarize the benefits obtained as follows:

- No capital is needed
- Immediate introduction of new technology
- Service and spare parts are included in the lease contract
- Guaranteed reduction of service downtime for patients. In our case, downtime did not exceed 2% of the operational time
- The ten-year contract includes a commitment to an upgrade after five years.

Finally, we present our experience for the attention of interested stakeholders in the world, but we emphasize that every institution in each country needs to determine whether to buy or to lease based on what would be the best fit for its unique circumstances and what would result in increasing the availability of modern radiotherapy cancer care for its patients.

Reference

[1] Nisbet A and Ward A 2001 Radiotherapy equipment—purchase or lease? *Br. J. Radiol.* **74** 735–44

IOP Publishing

Approaching Global Oncology
The win-win model
Ahmed Elzawawy and Wilfred Ngwa

Chapter 43

Cancer control efforts: the Kenyan situation today

Nicholas A Othieno-Abinya

This chapter outlines the status of various aspects of comprehensive cancer care in Kenya, illustrating the shortfalls as well as the progress made in recent years, in part, through policy efforts and global partners.

43.1 Introduction

Kenya is situated in East Africa and borders Ethiopia to the north, south Sudan to the north-west, Uganda to the west, Tanzania to the south, and the Indian Ocean and Somalia to the east. It is divided into 47 counties, with Nairobi as the capital city. Mombasa and Kisumu are major metropolises, others are Nakuru, Eldoret, and Thika.

In Kenya, cancer is the third leading cause of death after infectious and cardiovascular diseases. In 2012, there were an estimated 37 000 new cancer cases, with 28 500 deaths out of a population of 46 000 000. Today, with a population estimated at 54 000 000, there are about 55 000 new cases annually. Given the improving cancer control infrastructure, the death rate is expected to decline, albeit slowly.

The top ten cancers in Kenya among men are:

1. Prostate
2. Oesophagus
3. Stomach
4. Colorectal
5. Mouth/Pharynx
6. Lymphoma
7. Leukaemia
8. Liver
9. Lung, trachea, bronchus
10. Brain and nervous system.

doi:10.1088/978-0-7503-3075-6ch43

The top ten cancers among women in Kenya are:

1. Breast
2. Cervix
3. Oesophagus
4. Colorectal
5. Stomach
6. Lymphoma
7. Ovarian
8. Mouth/Pharynx
9. Corpus uteri
10. Leukaemia.

Reference: Ann Korir (unpublished). KEMRI National Cancer Registry 2015–2016 cancerregistry@kemri.org.

Efforts to control cancer rely on **policy, investment in infrastructure, personnel development, programs, equipment, and supplies**. A well-planned research effort must support these efforts. The final pace-setter is financing and fiscal discipline.

Cancer control is about **prevention of the preventable, early detection, curative treatment, and palliation**.

Prevention, early detection, and treatment require reliable information on the cancer distribution in a population, and by extension, a cancer registry. Registries can be hospital-based or population-based.

43.1.1 Policy

The Cancer Bill (2011) paved the way for the country to roll out programs for cancer treatment and control strategies. The national cancer control strategy covered 2011–2016. On 2nd November 2011, the Kenyan parliament voted for cancer patients to be treated free of charge. That obviously fell short of appreciating the true cost of cancer treatment [2].

In 2016, health expenditure per capita in Kenya was US$ 169, and the total expenditure on health as a percentage of GDP was 5.7%.

The National Guidelines for Cancer Management were launched in 2013 [3]. In July 2019, the Kenya National Cancer Treatment protocols were launched by the Ministry of Health [4].

43.1.2 Infrastructure

Because of blind pride, each of the 47 counties in Kenya is striving to establish a comprehensive cancer centre, instead of giving way to the development of well-equipped, better-managed regional cancer centres. Despite this, the infrastructure in most of these counties cannot even address simple infections and infestations.

43.1.3 Personnel development

One of the eight major problems identified in the 2011 cancer bill was the lack of cancer specialists, which limits the achievement of the above goals. The country had a population approaching 46 million people and about 20 specialists, including six medical oncologists, involved in cancer treatment; all except one were based in Nairobi. Training facilities that had traditionally been accessed abroad were expensive and largely unavailable. There was clearly a need to train cancer specialists locally.

Cancer care personnel include oncologists, surgeons, nurses, palliative care physicians, radiotherapists, and other supportive care personnel.

A gynaecology oncology program was developed by the University of Toronto in 2014 in collaboration with Moi University, later taken over by the latter; so far, they have graduated seven gynaecology oncologists. In 2016, a medical oncology fellowship program was started at the University of Nairobi, spearheaded by Prof. N A Othieno-Abinya, and so far, six oncologists have graduated. In 2019, a gynaecology oncology fellowship program was initiated at the University of Nairobi, spearheaded by Prof. Omondi Ogutu and headed by Prof. S B O Ojwang, and in 2020, a master's program in radiation oncology was initiated at the University of Nairobi, spearheaded by Prof. N A Othieno-Abinya, though initially domiciled in the Department of Imaging and Radiation Medicine under Dr Gladys Mwango.

An oncology nursing program was started at the AgaKhan University Hospital in 2018, and in 2020, a similar program started at the Nairobi Hospital.

Today, the country has:

Medical oncologists	15
Radiation oncologists	7
Clinical oncologists	10
Gynaecology oncologists	10
Haematologists	5
Haematopathologists	45
Oncology nurses	40
Palliative care physicians	3
Radiophysicists	10
Therapy radiographers	27
Oncology clinical officers	34
Therapy radiographers	27
Oncology pharmacists	9
Nuclear medicine physicians	3
Nuclear medicine technologists	3
Palliative care nurses	328

At the International Cancer Institute based in western Kenya, there is a training program for lower-cadre healthcare personnel in aspects of cancer epidemiology and cancer management.

43.1.4 Programs

Cervical cancer screening has been integrated into the reproductive care system at the Ministry of Health, while breast cancer screening has mainly been carried out sporadically, aided by various nongovernmental organizations.

Nairobi's cancer registry has been located at the Kenya Medical Research Institute since 2001, following consultations between the United States National Cancer Institute, the International Agency for Research on Cancer (IARC), the Ministry of Health, and the Kenya Medical Research Institute. The registry is providing badly needed data and has now been extended to western and eastern parts of the country.

Planning for cancer prevention is guided by the Kenya Health Policy 2014–2030 and implemented through a strategic framework provided by the National Cancer Control Strategy (Ministry of Health: Kenya Cancer Policy 2019–2030).

Cancer organizations taking part in awareness campaigns include KENCASA and Women for Cancer. These are nonprofessional lobbyists with an interest in cancer awareness and screening.

The Kenya Society of Haematology and Oncology (KESHO) is a professional organization of physicians interested in cancer diagnosis and treatment, and has come a long way in helping with the regulation of cancer management in the country.

43.1.5 Facilities

Today, there are two public hospitals offering comprehensive cancer care. These are at the Kenyatta National Hospital and Kenyatta University Teaching, Referral, and Research Hospital, both in Nairobi County. The former has a linear accelerator and three cobalt-60 machines, and the latter has a linear accelerator.

The Moi Teaching and Referral Hospital in Eldoret has a cancer treatment centre without radiotherapy facilities. The same is true of the Jaramogi Oginga Odinga Teaching and Referral Hospital in Kisumu. Both are at advanced stages of realizing radiotherapy capability. The 'Win-Win International' movement of the Harvard Global Health Catalyst Summits has been instrumental in initiating efforts for the development of the Kisumu facility.

Other centres struggling to develop cancer treatment facilities are Kisii, Nakuru, Nyeri, Garissa, Meru, and the Coast Provincial General Hospital.

Private hospitals have taken a clear lead in the development of cancer treatment in the country. The Nairobi Hospital, the AgaKhan University Hospital, and the M.P. Shah Hospital, all in Nairobi, have two linear accelerators each. The Nairobi West Hospital and Texas Cancer Centre have a linear accelerator each.

A major point of deviation from the expected norm is unregulated medical tourism. More than 50% of the cancer patients who can afford treatment through insurance or from their own funds have tended to travel out of the country, in particular, to India, for treatment. This grossly undermines the efforts made to develop in-country facilities. Patients with Kaposi's sarcoma, for example, are encouraged to travel to India every week or every three weeks for the administration of paclitaxel.

43.2 Equipment and supplies

These are housed in the facilities that have made the effort to set up comprehensive programs for cancer control.

43.3 Partnerships

The World Health Organization (WHO), the US National Cancer Institute (NCI), the American Cancer Society (ACS), the International Agency for Research on Cancer (IARC), and the International Atomic Energy Agency (IAEA) are some of the organizations that have contributed in different ways to cancer care and capacity building in the country.

Takeda pharmaceutical, Takeda Foundation, and Merck Foundation are engaged in funding the medical oncology fellowship program and the master's program in radiation oncology at the University of Nairobi.

Global Health Catalyst Win-Win Initiative, has provided impetus for the development of cancer treatment centres. This has come about through the Harvard Global Health Catalyst Summits on cancer, spearheaded by Professors Wilfred Ngwa (Harvard Medical School, USA), Ahmed Elzawawy (Suez Canal University, Port Said, Egypt), Eduardo Cazap (Buenos Aires, Argentina), and David Kerr (Oxford University, UK).

Roche pharmaceuticals has also been instrumental in supporting awareness and screening activities. Other pharma, including AstraZeneca, have also supported programs, including the training of healthcare workers in breast cancer awareness, early diagnosis, and management principles through the Pambazuka program.

43.3.1 Research

Cancer research in Kenya, as in all sub-Saharan African countries, is still in its infancy (if not stillborn) and mainly based on small epidemiological surveys and hospital-based case series and case reports. Research efforts are mainly based at the Universities and to some extent the medical research institution. The National Cancer Institute is in place, but struggling for funding from the rather scarce resources.

Update of 31 January, 2022 by Professor N A Othieno-Abinya:

- In Kenya, we now have four metropolis with city status—Nairobi, Mombasa, Kisumu, Nakuru. Eldoret and Thika are other urban areas but without city status.
- We now have 17 gynecology oncologists and 15 clinical oncologists.
- There are now 5 public facilities with comprehensive cancer management capacity in Kenya:
  1. Kenyatta National Hospital, Nairobi;
  2. Kenyatta University Teaching, Referral and Research Hospital in Nairobi. It also has the second cyclotron and PET/CT facilities;
  3. Moi Teaching and Referral Hospital in Eldoret;
  4. Coast General Hospital in Mombasa;
  5. Nakuru Provincial General Hospital in Nakuru.
- The city of Kisumu and the Kisii county are still struggling to complete their radiotherapy capabilities.

Note from the Editors:
1. The original text was written by Professor Nicholas A Othieno-Abinya and revised by mid-2021. As Professor Abinya is one of the leaders of the GHC win-win movement, he is following the notions of its 'living book'. It is a breathing book with afterwards renewable data and innovations. We hope that it would be continuously an updated global forum receiving new progress and thoughts from all.
2. The goal of the first and the second wing of the Win-Win movement (www.icedoc.org/winwin.htm and www.globalhealthcatalysts.org) is to contribute in producing real increasing of access to cancer care in the real world. This hopefully could be achieved with the contribution of all stakeholders and not to just repeating the slogans that have lasted for decades and up to the present, like 'closing the gap', 'barriers and obstacles', 'inequity', 'universal cancer care', 'recognition and awareness of the problem'. However, the gap is widening between what is required and what is available for cancer care to millions of underserved cancer patients.

That is why, we welcome and highlight every real increase—like this recent update from Kenya—of functioning cancer facilities for our underserved patients everywhere in the world. This gives constructive hopes and optimism to all. This update is more meaningful than thousands of declarations, plans, agendas, conferences and publications if they are not resulting in really reducing the gap in cancer care services.

Ahmed Elzawawy and Wilfred Ngwa
February 5, 2022

References and further reading

[1] De Souza J A, Hunt B and Asirwa F C 2016 Global health equity: cancer outcome disparities in high-, middle-, and low-income countries *J. Glob. Oncol.* **34** 6–13

[2] 2017 Ministry of Health, Government of Kenya: National Cancer Control Strategy 2017–22 also 2011–16 https://www.iccp-portal.org/system/files/plans/KENYA%20NATIONAL%20CANCER%20CONTROL%20STRATEGY%202017-2022_1.pdf

[3] Othieno-Abinya N A, Odongo I and Ogaja E *et al* 2013 National Guidelines for Cancer Management. Ministry of Health, Kenya https://knh.or.ke/wp-content/uploads/2017/08/National-Cancer-Treatment-Guidelines2.pdf

[4] 2019 July 2019 Kenya National Cancer Treatment protocols were launched by the Ministry of Health https://www.health.go.ke/wp-content/uploads/2019/09/National-treatment-Protocols-2019.pdf

[5] Othieno-Abinya N A 2019 *Shadow in Perpetuity: The Hard Journey With Cancer* (Chişinău, Moldova: Lambert Academic Publishing)

Chapter 44

Global health catalyst summits

Lydia Asana, Noella Bih, Romy Mueller, Jana Wood, Ahmed Elzawawy and Wilfred Ngwa

The Global Health Catalyst summits are a flagship outreach component of the ecancerforall www.ecancerforall.com Win-Win Initiative described in previous chapters. These summits are a premier yearly event dedicated to catalyzing high-impact international collaborations and initiatives to eliminate global health disparities. The primary focus of each summit is the rising scourge of non-communicable diseases such as cancer, mental health issues, pain, and cardiovascular diseases, which are severely impacting global health and economic development. Since 2015, the yearly summits have led to numerous win-win collaborations in education, research, and outreach, benefitting both high-income and low-income countries. The success of the Global Health Catalyst summits has resulted in partnerships with faculty at globally recognized leading institutions, including the University of Pennsylvania, Oxford University (UK), the University of Heidelberg (Germany), and partners in low- and middle-income countries (LMICs). Each year, participants are encouraged and enabled to engage in win-win collaborations for global health and economic development.

44.1 Background

A well-known quote attributed to Martin Luther King Jr says, 'Of all the forms of inequality, injustice in health care is the most shocking and inhumane.' In 'Closing the Cancer Divide: An Equity Imperative', Knaul *et al* [1] discuss the shocking depth of the health inequality that exists in the availability and quality of cancer care in LMICs. The recent World Health Organization (WHO) Cancer Report [2, 3] describes the growing global burden of cancer and disparities as alarming, as over 60% of the global burden is in LMICs in Africa, Asia, and Central and South America, where 70% of cancer deaths occur. If the current trend continues, the burden of cancer is expected to increase to 22 million new cases annually by 2030; 81% of new cases and almost 88% of mortality will occur in LMICs. In African

doi:10.1088/978-0-7503-3075-6ch44

LMICs, where survival rates are amongst the lowest, the cancer burden is projected to reach an alarming 1.4 million new cases and 1 million deaths per year by 2030. In response to the growing global cancer burden and disparities, leaders in cancer research and policy from the United States and 14 economically diverse countries, meeting at the American National Cancer Institute, concluded that successful campaigns to control cancers and improve current strategies will increasingly depend on concerted international collaboration [4]. The major disparities in cancer deaths are, in part, a reflection of the major underlying disparities in radiation oncology [5–7]. Cancer research and education collaborations are crucial in driving innovation, policy, and cancer control efforts to address these disparities [8–10]. Significant barriers to initiating or supporting international collaborations in global oncology identified during recent global health catalyst cancer summits include: distance–time barriers, cultural barriers, and limited resources, including human capacity compounded by brain drain [11].

About the summits

The yearly Global Health Catalyst (GHC) cancer summits are designed to catalyze and strengthen new and existing high-impact international research and research education collaborations between high-income countries (HICs) such as the USA and LMICs. Institutions are challenged to address the growing global burden of cancer and cancer disparities [12]. To tackle distance–time barriers, GHC summits bring together leaders from LMIC institutions and their investigators to meet with global oncology leaders in HICs in order to develop a blueprint or roadmap for collaboration. The objective is to help initiate new collaborations, including co-mentored research collaborations that include investigators from both HIC and LMIC institutions. Furthermore, in today's hyperconnected world, information and communications technology (ICT) increasingly plays an integral role in healthcare and has great potential to bridge the distance–time barriers that limit collaboration [13, 14]. Here, ICT means tools that facilitate the capture, processing, storage, and exchange of information via electronic means. A GHC summit online platform has been designed to support and sustain collaborative activities beyond the face-to-face yearly summits. The online platform includes an app with features that provide access to summit content and a networking system with which interested individuals can easily find one another, form teams, share tools (including technologies), exchange ideas, access continuous research education, and explore relevant funding opportunities for co-mentored research that includes researchers from HICs and LMICs at all levels from student to faculty. The platform is used to continually engage a growing number of institutions each year from both HICs and LMICs, as well as community organizations such as diaspora groups, to support initiated collaborations.

Addressing cultural barriers to global oncology collaborations. Collaborative outreach that involves the diaspora would arguably help to reduce cultural barriers, given the lived experiences, and thus lead to better appreciation by diasporans of both HIC and originating LMIC cultures and strong connections to both. Diasporans constitute a significant part of minority populations in HICs such as the USA. The primary drivers of the disparities in incidence and deaths reflected in the World Health Organization reports for Africa also apply to disparities among African American populations in the USA.

Addressing limited resources/human capacity. The yearly GHC summits provide opportunities for HIC and LMIC researchers to collaborate in developing funding proposals for grants that can help to address resource limitations. Engaging the resource-laden diaspora also provides an opportunity to provide seed funding support for cancer projects involving HIC and LMIC institutions. For example, Africans in Diaspora (AiD) remits over $50 billion per year to Africa, which exceeds yearly global aid to the continent, while saving another $53 billion annually. Previous summits have highlighted the potential for resource support by the diaspora, leveraging some of these remittances and yearly budgeting from their organizations to support global health. This is exemplified by members of the Ethiopian-American Doctors' Group, who participated in previous summits and are building a cancer center with a radiation therapy facility in Ethiopia to significantly increase access for many East Africans. The AiD also constitutes one of the most educated diaspora groups in North America, and greater involvement in collaborations will undoubtedly continue to turn brain drain into brain circulation and global health gain. Their participation in research is also helping to advance understanding of the primary drivers of disparities in incidence and deaths prevalent among underrepresented minorities, such as African Americans in the USA.

Innovation

One innovation of the GHC summits is the unprecedented level of engagement of underrepresented minorities (URMs) in global health and the African diaspora in American–African collaborations which have the potential to turn brain drain into brain circulation and global health gain. The integration of URMs into healthcare efforts is in consonance with the mission of the National Cancer Institute. Another innovative advantage is the complementary nature of combining the face-to-face meetings with the development of an ICT-powered GHC meeting platform that continues to catalyze collaborations and mutually beneficial global oncology interactions across distance–time barriers after the summit. In addition, the summits catalyze support from diaspora organizations and industry to provide seed funding beginning at 5000 USD for co-mentored research collaborations that include investigators from cancer institutions in the USA and Africa. This allows, for example, a US investigator to partner in research with an investigator in Tanzania, where relatively modest funds could allow the generation of preliminary data for publication that could be used to secure further funding to sustain the research.

Significance

The GHC summits are designed to catalyze mutually beneficial collaborations between cancer research and education investigators from HICs and LMICs. The commitment to catalyzing new collaborations each year and strengthening others is very significant. Catalyzing these collaborations means bringing together oncology health professionals from LMICs and HICs each year to share knowledge at the summit and present a joint proposal which could receive seed funding or be jointly submitted for funding support by industry, diaspora organizations, foundations, or other external funding agencies, including other NIH funding mechanisms. The GHC summit online platform serves as a valuable resource that facilitates ongoing collaboration beyond the face-to-face meetings at GHC summits. The app provides a systematic avenue for investigators to easily: find each other and form teams, share tools and technologies, receive advanced research education/training, and obtain funding for co-mentored research that can lead to joint publications, as highlighted in recent publications following the GHC summit. Co-advising/supervising research trainees in LMIC institutions could help to build more local capacity and enable further innovation in research areas focused on addressing the growing burden of cancer and disparity. As highlighted below, GHC summit participants are also drawn from industry. This is significant, as it facilitates the transfer of new knowledge, the translation of innovations into practical healthcare solutions, economic growth, and sustainable development.

44.2 Summary evaluation of previous GHC summits

The GHC summits have received funding support from University of Pennsylvania Center for Global Health, the Radcliffe Institute for Advanced Studies at Harvard University, the Joint Center for Radiation Therapy foundation, the Biomedical Research Institute of the Brigham and Women's Hospital, and the University of Heidelberg has provided a guest professorship for Wil Ngwa to start a program in Germany. Some outcomes and lessons resulting from summits in the USA, Europe, and Africa include:

1. *Knowledge generated and joint publications involving both USA and African partners.* The summits have provided a platform for knowledge sharing, resulting in numerous publications involving both American and African oncology health professionals. For example, publications have identified key barriers to American–African collaborations and potential solutions, such as collaborations that use advanced ICT to further global radiation oncology research, education, and care. Barriers to collaboration include distance– time barriers, limited resources, limited human capacity, and cultural barriers, which will be addressed by this project.
2. *Engagement of over* 100 *URM diaspora organizations to participate in and support global oncology.* This has led to the formation of different AiD groups united against cancer and the initiation of tumor boards by diaspora oncology health professionals using ICT such as Zoom to remotely support cancer centers in Africa and collaborate in research. Some of these outcomes are highlighted in support letters from a sample of these URM and AiD group leaders.
3. *Engagement of young people in the USA and Africa.* In an effort to introduce young people to the world of global health, raise awareness of global disparities, and inspire early engagement in global cancer efforts, particularly in radiation oncology, young people including high-school and college students as well as recent graduates and others have participated in

general summit sessions as well as interactive youth sessions onsite and remotely, giving young people a voice with which to contribute ideas, solutions, and strategies for engaging other young people. By serving as volunteers, young people have also had unique opportunities to interact with accomplished professionals. Many of these young people have reported being educated, inspired, and challenged to contribute to addressing global health disparities in innovative ways.

4. *Needs assessment for multi-center clinical trials collaborations.* The summits have resulted in collaborative efforts to establish a multicentre clinical trials network also supported by an NIH-funded ICT-powered platform, namely the Quality Assurance and Review Center platform.
5. *African Journal of Medical Physics.* For the first time, this journal provides a platform for the publication and dissemination of research results and innovation that includes a significant number of editorial board members from Africa and the USA. The platform will also be used for the dissemination of outcomes from collaborative projects.
6. *Lancet Oncology Commission for sub-Saharan Africa.* The 2019 summit resulted in the launch of a landmark *Lancet Oncology* commission for Sub-Saharan Africa, led by the principal investigators and with the significant involvement of commissioners from both American and African institutions; it is expected to help drive cancer policy related to Africa for years to come.
7. *Development of recommendations on global health for the American government.* Past summits have also led to the development of recommendations on global health for the American government, with a focus on cancer. This has involved the participation of the Chair of the USA House Subcommittee On Africa, Global Health, Global Human Rights, and International Organizations.
8. *Global Oncology University Education platform*: This platform, is dedicated to education efforts complementing face-to-face workshops to build capacity for oncology in Africa and greater participation by the USA. For example, this has allowed oncology health professionals from different American institutions to pool their time and collaborate in giving online lectures benefitting both African and American trainees in areas such as how to write research papers, the development of funding proposals, responsible conduct in research, etc. This innovation has received an award for Education Innovation from the American Association of Physicists in Medicine, and has also contributed to the launch of an online education and training platform by the African Organization for Research and Training in Cancer (AORTIC).
9. Many partnerships and collaborations, including some between diaspora organizations and industry.
10. New initiatives, organizations, and projects that complement the work of the summits and extend to other related areas have been reported.

These initial outcomes and others provide momentum which will be built upon for years to come. A key consensus emerging from previous summits is the need for more effective approaches to catalyze collaborations, especially in oncology, including leveraging ICT and the diaspora to catalyze and advance global oncology collaborations.

Plans: Future summits will scale and be organized in more regions of the world to continue to catalyze high-impact international collaborations. Abstract submissions will be accepted from participants from institutions with a main focus on oncology and related cross-disciplinary collaborations with a potential for high impact, as identified in summits of previous years. Previous GHC summits have had an approximately equal participation of women and men in all aspects of the summit, or possible more women. At least a third of all participants are minorities, including African Americans, who have traditionally been underrepresented in science. The involvement of minorities is a major strength of the summit. The conference facilities are also highly accessible to people with disabilities. Going forward, the organizing committee is committed to ensuring that this level of participation is maintained and further encouraged when selecting conference abstracts and inviting keynote speakers and panellists. When registering, conference participants will be offered the opportunity to indicate their childcare or other family care needs. Based on the information provided during registration, the organizing committee will ensure that adequate care services are available at the conference site to allow individuals with family care responsibilities to attend. The availability of care services will be included when publicizing the conference.

The conference will continue to be publicized through placements in journals, magazines, newspapers, radio, television, and social media, the conference website, advertisements at other conferences in HICs and LMICs, and distribution via the growing GHC summit participant lists. The proceedings of the summit will be published in the Journal of Global Oncology and the 'Red Journal'.

Throughout the summit, participant feedback opportunities are provided, including an evaluation questionnaire to be completed by participants, which evaluates the content, speakers, and outcomes. Following each summit, the core organizing committee convenes regular follow-up conference calls with session chairs/moderators and sample participants to evaluate the summit, and works together in putting together the proceedings of the summit. The yearly summit evaluation and oversight committee will continuously evaluate outcomes and work to ensure success and growth.

References and further reading

[1] Gerhard D 2013 Closing the cancer divide: an equity imperative *Yale J. Biol. Med.* **86** 282–3

[2] 2017 *Highlights from the WHO Global Conference on NCDs: Enhancing policy coherence to prevent and control noncommunicable diseases, 18–20 October 2017, Montevideo, Uruguay. Meeting Report* WHO https://www.who.int/conferences/global-ncd-conference/montevideo-report.pdf

[3] Stewart B W and Wild C P 2014 *World Cancer Report 2014* WHO IARC 1–2 https://publications.iarc.fr/Non-Series-Publications/World-Cancer-Reports/World-Cancer-Report-2014

[4] Atun R *et al* 2015 Expanding global access to radiotherapy *Lancet Oncol.* **16** 1153–86

[5] Samiei M 2013 Challenges of making radiotherapy accessible in developing countries *Cancer Control* **2013** 85–94 http://www.cancercontrol.info/cc2013/challenges-of-making-radiotherapy-accessible-in-developing-countries/

[6] Abdel-Wahab M, Bourque J M, Pynda Y, Izewska J, Van der Merwe D, Zubizarreta E and Rosenblatt E 2013 Status of radiotherapy resources in Africa: an Int. Atomic Energy Agency analysis *Lancet Oncol* **14** e168–75

[7] Ngwa W and Ngoma T 2016 *Emerging Models for Global Health in Radiation Oncology.* (Bristol, UK; Philadelphia, PA: IOP Publishing)

[8] Ngwa W *et al* 2016 Closing the cancer divide through ubuntu: information and communication technology-powered models for global radiation oncology *Int. J. Radiat. Oncol. Biol. Phys.* **94** 440–9

[9] Ngwa W *et al* 2015 Potential for information and communication technologies to catalyze global collaborations in radiation oncology *Int. J. Radiat. Oncol. Biol. Phys.* **91** 444–7

[10] Varmus H and Kumar H S 2013 Addressing the Growing International Challenge of Cancer: A Multinational Perspective *Sci. Transl. Med.* **5** 175cm2

[11] Zietman A 2014 Bringing radiation therapy to underserved nations: an increasingly global responsibility in an ever-shrinking world *Int. J. Radiat. Oncol. Biol. Phys.* **89** 440–2

[12] Dad L, Shah M M, Mutter R, Olsen J, Dominello M, Miller S M, Fisher B, Lee N and Komaki R 2014 Why target the globe?: 4-year report (2009–2013) of the Association of Residents in Radiation Oncology Global Health Initiative *Int. J. Radiat. Oncol. Biol. Phys.* **89** 485–91

[13] Coleman C N and Many O 2014 Bringing cancer care to the underserved globally: a challenging problem for which radiation oncology can pioneer novel solutions *Int. J. Radiat. Oncol. Biol. Phys.* **89** 443–5

[14] Mayr N A *et al* 2014 International Outreach: What Is the Responsibility of ASTRO and the Major International Radiation Oncology Societies? *Int. J. Radiat. Oncol. Biol. Phys.* **89** 481–4

Part VII

Future directions

IOP Publishing

Approaching Global Oncology
The win-win model
Ahmed Elzawawy and Wilfred Ngwa

Chapter 45

Final notes and future directions

Ahmed Elzawawy and Wilfred Ngwa

We have come to the 'see you soon' note. It is *au revoir* and not *adieu*! In this chapter, we highlight final notes on the win-win approach to global oncology and possible future directions. This is in addition to those highlighted in previous chapters.

45.1 Affordability with respect and dignity. We mean here financial, physical, and social dignity

When all is said, indeed, the goal of the Win-Win Movement and the unifying purpose that compelled such a geographically and professionally diverse set of stakeholders to earnestly collaborate is the belief that cancer should not automatically mean a death sentence for anyone in the world. Whether a cancer patient has a chance to beat cancer should not depend on their zip code, latitude, or nationality.

As Robin Williams said in the film Patch Adams 'You treat a disease, you win, you lose. You treat a person, I guarantee you, you'll win, no matter what the outcome'. In the face of a disease such as cancer, after doing all that is needed through scientific and evidence-based medical care, we may conquer the disease or we may not, but every effort should be made to provide care for all cancer patients through:

(a) Better-value medical cancer care
(b) Affordable care for all patients
(c) Consideration and respect for dignity

As has been repeatedly mentioned in this work, disparities in the availability of cancer care are widespread. Not only is there a need to increase the number of opportunities for cancer care, such care must be of better value than is currently available in many parts of the world in terms of affordability, accessibility, and value-based and patient-centered care.

doi:10.1088/978-0-7503-3075-6ch45

Affordability is a significant barrier to healthcare and individual patient capabilities need to be considered by national health ministries. The contributions in this work have raised awareness about the limitations imposed by cost, but also presented innovative and context-specific recommendations for reducing costs, which ultimately benefits all patients.

While the value of medical care and affordability are significant factors that often involve multi-layered interactions and collaborations, treating patients with respect and dignity boils down to interactions between patients and caregivers. By considering physical, psychological, social, and financial factors that may affect a patient's response to treatment opportunities, caregivers can communicate to each patient that they are worth caring for.

With all our efforts, many patients may live. Despite all our efforts, we may lose some. However, in either situation every patient should be treated with dignity. This is an area in which every individual involved in patient care can, and should contribute. There are also rooms for health systems to incorporate broad policies and practices that encourage and reward treating patients with dignity.

45.2 Who are the patients?

It is worth stating the obvious: nobody is immune to cancer. Despite even the best efforts to live active healthy lives, there are factors, such as genetics, that we have little control over. Patients could be our family members, friends, or anyone in our lives. Today's care providers could one day be patients. It could be you. It could be me. This reality is not meant to foster a defeatist mentality—there are certainly lifestyle efforts that can reduce the risk of cancer and practices such as regular screenings that can lead to early detection or warning signs—but overall, anyone could find themselves affected by cancer, either directly or indirectly.

45.3 Not just a traditional book, but a stimulus for effective global change

This book is a call to action or a renewal of effort for all who are involved in cancer treatment and care: all stakeholders, all communities, all scientific cancer societies; all organizations: international, national, governmental, and non-governmental; to all health industries; to all investors: public, private, and public–private partnerships; and to all who may provide scientific creativeness, inventions, ideas; and approaches: let us come together to accomplish more! To do so, we advocate 'Three Cs and One P' (3Cs1P): coordination, cooperation, collaboration, and partnership. We have repeatedly expressed that our desire is to spark and promote a large-scale forum—for all—focused on making tangible strides in the affordability of better-value cancer care for millions of underserved or unserved patients in the world. This book is directed to all cancer care stakeholders in the world. It is an effort to inform, inspire, and appreciate the diverse efforts already underway. It is to the 'doers' that credit is due. This book is simply a tool and the win-win movement simply a vehicle. The Global Health Catalyst Win-Win Movement is an opportunity for coordinated collaboration intended to serve as a complement to existing efforts. The benefits of our collaborations can be enjoyed and celebrated by all.

45.4 Beyond good intentions

As has been repeatedly highlighted in this book, and despite precious efforts that include numerous organizations, plans, reports, and excellent agendas, the limitations of access to cancer treatment are enormous and ever increasing. As such, the realization of the global win-win forum is a matter of urgency.

The win-win movement recognizes that remarkable change for the better can only be achieved by:

(a) Scientific methods, innovation, and creativity
(b) Considering the interests and incentives of all stakeholders in the real world; win-win
(c) Advocating a global win-win campaign and forum, open to all parties, but with full recognition of, and respect for, the independence and distinct inner workings of all parties involved
(d) Newer strategies for the mobilization of resources, promotion, and marketing to increase cancer treatment services around the world. One of these strategies is proposed in this book: 'The win-win modified blue ocean strategy'. The proposed approaches will be under continuous development by all, e.g. in publications, in virtual meetings, and at Global Health Catalyst summits.

45.5 Flexibility of thoughts

The notion of the 'the Fourth Way', that was coined by Ahmed Elzawawy in 2013 [1] suggests the adoption of more free streaming of ideas and flexibility of thoughts that continuously evolve and lead to impactful improvements for all stakeholders. Such approaches consider the legitimate incentives of all parties and the mobilization of all potential resources.

Applying the notions of the 'Fourth Way' smartly in the field of oncology [2, 3] could support the realization of economically-sustainable and accessible cancer care, the promotion of cancer care, and more innovation for triple-value-based diagnostic and treatment technologies in the real world. As explained by Sir Muir Gray *et al* [4], 'triple value' denotes the improved impact of value for patients, populations and communities, and technology

45.6 Unleash your thoughts and ideas

The thoughts and books of Todd Henry point out that it is a huge loss that graves are full of plenty of ideas that were buried and never expressed. The theory of accidental creativity suggests that if some of these thoughts had been developed, they may have resulted in much progress and many benefits for our planet [5, 6].

In the field of cancer treatment and care, many may have accidental ideas or thoughts that may be dismissed as crazy or immature. Such thoughts sometimes result in forgotten or suppressed ideas that remain hidden for many years.

Whatever you think about your idea or thought, release it. Some of these ideas or suggestions could be crystallized into creative scientific contributions that serve to effectively increase access to cancer care in the world.

45.7 The need for 'a living book' as the model for publications in the 3rd decade of the 21st century

In recent years, the publication of classic hard copy and electronic books has faced challenges. After journeying through the processes from conception to publication, and after being accessed by readers for a variable length of time, some of the published material may become outdated. Moreover, e-journals, Youtube videos, web information, interactive media, e-learning, and virtual conferences have become readily available sources of information.

There is a great need for innovative approaches to making resources readily available around the globe.

One of the new terms that Ahmed Elzawawy coined in this book is 'a living book' that comprises:

(a) Hard and/or electronic book copies

(b) Links to websites, videos, Youtube content for some keynotes that accompany the text of some chapters and in the references, in addition to traditional references.

(c) Web-based opportunities for readers to send their feedback, suggestions, and ideas relevant to the topics of the book and its objectives. For example, in this book, there are two links that can be used to send e-mails with feedback: http://icedoc.net/feedback.html and http://icedoc.org/feedback.html.

(d) Relevant feedback received will be shared with the book contributors and willing experts. It is open for all experts and key players to join.

(e) Summaries of relevant feedback, in addition to short updates of the previously published chapters of this book, will appear on our different websites, including Global Health Catalyst Win-Win Initiative, ecancerforall http://www.icedoc.org/Books.htm and http://www.icedoc.net/Books.htm. Some of the feedback in Spanish and English will appear in the new win-win section of the website of the Latin American and Caribbean Medical Oncology Society (SLACOM) led by Prof. Eduardo Cazap in partnership with the Network of Latin American Cancer Institutes (RINC).

With the above five points, a published book will be a living book grows with the reader, and will provide interactive opportunities. According to Elzawawy's proposals for living books, there is an optional sixth point, which is relevant to this work, due to its wide reach and long-term goals. Additional content and summaries of filtered feedback from readers will constitute special parts in the next editions or books, resulting in a series of living books in this decade.

Among many lessons, the COVID-19 pandemic has served as a reminder that anything can happen, resulting in a renewed awareness of the need for succession planning.

Should the original editors of this work not be available for future additions to the living books series, the work will continue and other leaders in the field can continue to keep the series alive. Together with all the involved experts and contributors, we provide a foundation that could continue and grow with all interested parties in the coming years. All readers have the opportunity to contribute and even to lead.

45.8 Virtual meetings and GHC summits

To boost further progress and development, the topics of this book and reader feedback will be the subjects of virtual meetings and future Global Health Catalyst Summits. The Global Health Catalyst summits at Harvard, in Europe, and in Africa have become an epitome of the win-win collaboration that needs to happen to eliminate global health disparities in oncology. Recent funding from the National Institutes of Health to support these yearly events recognizes their value and has elevated this to a cross-institutional and global forum for all. Everyone is invited.

45.9 The need for a 'win-win think tank'

One of ideas that we intend to develop progressively in the upcoming virtual meetings and summit is the formation of a think tank. The idea of a think tank helped President Franklin D Roosevelt during the period of recession in the 1930s [7]. The term 'think tank' was also used as military jargon during World War II to describe a safe place where plans and strategies could be discussed, but its meaning began to change during the 1960s, when it came to be used in the United States to describe private and nonprofit policy research organizations.

We define precisely that the objective of **the virtual, web-based 'win-win think tank'** would be **focused on** how to realize—in this decade—an enormous increase in the affordability of better-value cancer care in the world using win-win scenarios and scientific approaches.

This could be realized using contributions from concerned experts and in partnership with other interested groups.

45.10 The Global Oncology University, GO-U (www.ghcuniversity.org)

GO-U will receive more attention and a higher priority for its development in the coming year. Human capacity building is the backbone of the progress we hope for.

45.11 The need for volunteers and young colleagues from different parts of the world

From the abovementioned points and this book in general, it can be seen that much remains to be done. The involvement of enthusiastic volunteers from different parts of the world will help in the upcoming years. Among these volunteers, there is a particular desire to engage young volunteers from around the globe. A corps of young Global Health Catalyst win-win advocates is part of the global team of win-win team members, alongside professional experts and consultants. As noted in two chapters of this book, we are keen for the young catalyst win-win collaborators to be more involved in assisting with the arrangement of most activities. We count on them for the future continuation of the win-win movement.

45.12 Final words

Behind the win-win initiative and this book, there is a message of sympathy and love for all in the world, but we emphasize that our work, strategies, and methods are completely based on explorations of scientific approaches and pragmatic ways to achieve measurable objectives in this decade in the real world.

To all readers: This book and the Global Health Catalyst Win-Win Movement are yours as well! Let us go forward together for the sake of the global oncology win-win model to serve millions of underserved human beings with cancer in the world in this decade. No one should lose. It is a win-win!

On behalf of all contributors in this book and the Ambassadors, leaders and faculty of the global health catalyst win-win movement.

—Ahmed Elzawawy and Wilfred Ngwa

References

[1] Elzawawy A 2013 The Fourth Way. http://icedoc.org/anticancer5.htmhttp://icedoc.net/anticancer5.htm

[2] Elzawawy A 2015 The shortage of essential cancer drugs and generics in the United States of America: global brain storming directions for the world *Int. J. Cancer Clin. Res.* **2** 016

[3] Elzawawy A and Kerr D 2013 Variation in the availability of cancer drug generics in the United States of America *Ann. Oncol.* **24** 17–22

[4] The Oxford Centre for Triple Value Healthcare https://3vh.org/

[5] Henry T 2013 *Die Empty: Unleash Your Best Work Every Day* (New York: Penguin)

[6] Henry T 2015 *Die Empty: Unleash Your Best Work Every Day* (audiobook excerpt). https://youtu.be/ZBGsZ0EmBOw

[7] Hernando M G, Pautz H and Stone D 2018 Think tanks in 'hard times'—the Global Financial Crisis and economic advice *Policy Soc.* **37** 125–39